Radiodiagnosis in the Era of AI

Praveen Kumar
Datta Meghe Institute of Higher Education and Research, Wardha, India

Prateek Verma
Dayananda Sagar University, Bangalore, India

Gaurav Vedprakash Mishra
Datta Meghe Institute of Higher Education and Research, Wardha, India

Gopal Singh Phartiyal
University of Leeds, UK

Anurag Ashok Luharia
Datta Meghe Institute of Higher Education and Research, Wardha, India

IGI Global
Scientific Publishing
Publishing Tomorrow's Research Today

Vice President of Editorial	Melissa Wagner
Director of Acquisitions	Mikaela Felty
Director of Book Development	Jocelynn Hessler
Production Manager	Mike Brehm
Cover Design	Jose Rosado

Published in the United States of America by
IGI Global Scientific Publishing
701 East Chocolate Avenue
Hershey, PA, 17033, USA
Tel: 717-533-8845
Fax: 717-533-7115
Website: https://www.igi-global.com E-mail: cust@igi-global.com

Library of Congress Cataloging-in-Publication Data

Names: Kumar, Praveen, 1992- editor | Verma, Prateek, 1988- editor | Mishra, Gaurav, 1988- editor | Phartiyal, Gopal, 1989- editor | Luharia, Anurag, 1983- editor
Title: Radiodiagnosis in the era of AI / edited by Praveen Kumar, Prateek Verma, Gaurav Mishra, Gopal Phartiyal, Anurag Luharia.
Other titles: Radiodiagnosis in the era of artificial intelligence
Description: Hershey, PA : IGI Global Scientific Publishing, [2026] | Includes bibliographical references and index. | Summary: "The objective of this book is to provide a collection of theoretical insights and empirical studies that showcase the current applications and future potential of AI in radiodiagnosis. It will serve as a resource for understanding how AI can optimize imaging processes, assist healthcare professionals in clinical decision-making, and enhance patient outcomes"-- Provided by publisher.
Identifiers: LCCN 2025001215 (print) | LCCN 2025001216 (ebook) | ISBN 9798337309033 hardcover | ISBN 9798337309040 paperback | ISBN 9798337309057 ebook
Subjects: LCSH: Radiography, Medical--Data processing | Artificial intelligence--Medical applications
Classification: LCC RC78 .R233 2025 (print) | LCC RC78 (ebook)
LC record available at https://lccn.loc.gov/2025001215
LC ebook record available at https://lccn.loc.gov/2025001216
British Cataloguing in Publication Data
A Cataloguing in Publication record for this book is available from the British Library.

Table of Contents

Detailed Table of Contents

Biomedical imaging has long been vital for revealing the human body's inner workings with remarkable precision. Now, a new era of imaging technology is set to revolutionize healthcare. This chapter explores next-generation biomedical imaging, featuring breakthroughs like photon-counting CT (PCCT), ultra-high-field MRI, and advanced molecular imaging that push resolution and specificity boundaries. Artificial intelligence plays a pivotal role, with machine learning and deep learning transforming image reconstruction, analysis, and interpretation. The chapter also highlights multimodal imaging, which integrates structural and functional data for a deeper understanding of complex diseases. Beyond innovations, practical applications are discussed, including early disease detection, minimally invasive procedures, and precision medicine. By bridging cutting-edge research with clinical practice, this introduction provides a roadmap for medical professionals and researchers to navigate the transformative future of biomedical imaging in diagnosis and treatment.

The integration of artificial intelligence (AI) into radio diagnosis is transforming the field by enhancing diagnostic accuracy, efficiency, and clinician workflow. AI-powered tools have demonstrated their potential to augment reader performance in interpreting chest radiographs, as evidenced by significant improvements in accuracy and time efficiency. Furthermore, AI-driven methodologies, such as deep learning algorithms, are being applied to detect complex pathologies, including COVID-19, fractures, and malignancies, with diagnostic accuracies rivalling or surpassing human radiologists. The implementation of AI in interventional radiology and radiotherapy planning has also introduced new opportunities for precision medicine, such as automated scoring and enhanced image quality for clinical decision-making. This chapter explores AI's role in radio diagnosis, highlighting its applications, benefits, and limitations. It addresses challenges like model generalizability, data bias. It also highlights the need for education and collaboration between radiologists and developers.

Artificial Intelligence (AI) is transforming medical imaging by improving accuracy, efficiency, and interpretability in diagnostics and treatment. This chapter examines AI's role in image analysis across medical domains using machine learning (ML), deep learning (DL), and radiomics. AI has demonstrated effectiveness in various applications, often matching or surpassing clinicians. It enhances diagnostic and predictive capabilities, streamlines workflows, and aids in early detection, disease characterization, and treatment planning. However, challenges like robustness, bias reduction, and generalizability across datasets hinder adoption. Addressing these issues is key to seamless clinical integration. Emerging trends focus on multimodal data and generalized models to broaden AI's applicability. While promising, these technologies require validation through multicenter studies, larger datasets, and strong algorithmic frameworks. Through collaboration, AI-driven imaging can advance precision medicine, improve patient outcomes, and redefine medical diagnostics.

Magnetic Resonance Imaging (MRI) is a perfect solution of imaging diagnostically used in medicine and its related fields. However, there has been tremendous advancement in producing MRI technology in both hardware and software besides improvements in characterization of images. This paper gives a background of MRI together with early drawbacks and the introduction of Artificial Intelligence (AI). AI has improved image acquisition, reconstruction and analysis through increased speed of scans, higher and more accurate image results and thus better diagnosis. However, the use of AI in MRI encounters some hurdles, such as technical, ethical, and AI capabilities hurdles. This paper focuses on MRI history prior to and after AI incorporation, technological advancement on pre-AI MRI, roles of AI in MRI enhancement and challenges that continue to occur for enhanced achievement of desirable outcomes from AI MRI.

Adaptive devices and Artificial intelligence in the realm of medical field have become crucial for enhancing healthcare delivery and patient outcomes. As the virus are evolving with time, it is necessary for our current healthcare system to evolve with it as well. Utilizing artificial intelligence paired with advanced machine learning algorithms incorporated inside a device which can adapt itself based on the instructions from AI might be our best chance to counteract limitations of our current healthcare system. Through Artificial Intelligence of Medical Things (AIoMT) hope to achieve new heights of healthcare systems which significantly. Adaptive devices include advanced health tracking wearables that track vital signs of the patients which can be used as input for the algorithm. However, many several challenges persist, including data security concerns, reliability of algorithm, limitations of hardware and more importantly integrating it with public domain. This chapter would explore many possible and most efficient solutions to the problems regarding AIoMT

AI and wearable imaging devices are technologies changing real-time diagnostics, especially remote patient monitoring. This chapter explores AI's role in wearable imaging by highlighting its potential to enhance healthcare through greater accuracy, efficiency, and accessibility. It begins by examining wearable imaging applications in radiology and emphasizing their role in early disease detection. It delves into AI-driven advancement by improving image quality and diagnostic precision of ultrasound and MRI. Vital applications discussed include heart health monitoring, brain disorder assessment, and sports injury evaluation. AI's ability to analyze data, identify patterns, and predict health risks is also discussed. Additionally, the chapter covers device miniaturization, portability, and battery efficiency. Real-world examples illustrate AI's impact while challenges such as privacy, ethics, and regulatory concerns are addressed. Finally, the chapter looks ahead to AI's integration with telemedicine and emerging device innovations.

This chapter explores the transformative potential of large language models (LLMs) in conjunction with image technology, highlighting their ability to redefine limitations in language production and comprehension. By examining their integration into various fields, including medical imaging, autonomous systems, and multimedia content analysis, the chapter underscores the potential for revolutionizing these domains. The discussion also considers the role of LLMs and artificial intelligence in regulatory technology (RegTech) solutions, aimed at streamlining policy processes and mitigating risks. A detailed overview of current studies evaluates the effectiveness of AI and machine learning (ML) combinations. The chapter presents a methodology wherein an AI-based model, utilizing LLMs, analyzes data from diverse processes and datasets. This approach reveals the advantages of AI applications in corporate finance, particularly in enabling financial specialists to derive meaningful insights from extensive datasets.

Preface

It is with great enthusiasm that we present *Radiodiagnosis in the Era of AI*, a comprehensive exploration of how artificial intelligence is reshaping the landscape of medical imaging. As editors, we have witnessed firsthand the rapid transformation occurring at the intersection of AI and radiology—an evolution marked by technological innovation, clinical promise, and new challenges. This volume emerges at a critical juncture, where radiodiagnosis is not merely adopting AI as a supportive tool but is evolving into a field that is increasingly defined by it.

Radiology has always been a discipline grounded in interpretation, pattern recognition, and clinical judgment. With the infusion of AI technologies—ranging from deep learning algorithms to large language models—this domain now finds itself empowered to transcend human limitations in speed, accuracy, and consistency. From improving image reconstruction techniques to facilitating real-time, image-guided interventions, AI has introduced a paradigm shift that we, as editors and contributors, are eager to chronicle and contextualize.

This book is the result of a collaborative effort by experts from academia, research, and clinical practice, each contributing deep insights into the practical and theoretical dimensions of AI in radiodiagnosis. The chapters delve into foundational imaging modalities, intelligent image analysis, and the integration of multimodal data for precision diagnostics. Moreover, we address frontier topics such as wearable imaging technologies, AI in functional and personalized imaging, and the increasingly influential role of large language models in interpreting and organizing medical imaging data.

Importantly, while we celebrate the achievements of AI in radiology, we remain attentive to the broader implications—ethical, regulatory, and societal—that these advancements bring. Issues such as algorithmic bias, data privacy, transparency, and the evolving role of human expertise in AI-assisted workflows are discussed with the seriousness they deserve. As such, this volume is not merely a celebration of technology, but a balanced guide to its responsible and informed application.

CHAPTER OVERVIEWS

Chapter 1: Introduction to Next-Generation Biomedical Imaging

This opening chapter sets the stage for the advancements explored throughout the volume by presenting a compelling overview of the next generation of biomedical imaging. It highlights transformative technologies such as photon-counting CT, ultra-high-field MRI, and molecular imaging, and introduces readers to the integration of AI in enhancing image resolution, interpretation, and multimodal analysis. By connecting technical innovations to clinical outcomes—such as early detection and precision therapy—this chapter provides a comprehensive foundation for understanding how biomedical imaging is evolving in tandem with artificial intelligence.

Chapter 2: The Role of Artificial Intelligence in Radiodiagnosis

In this pivotal chapter, readers are introduced to the core role of AI in modern radiodiagnosis. It explores how AI augments clinical decision-making, streamlines radiological workflows, and supports accurate diagnoses in complex scenarios, from detecting fractures to assessing COVID-19. With practical examples of AI in both diagnostic and interventional radiology, this chapter not only demonstrates the potential of AI systems but also addresses critical issues like data bias, generalizability, and the need for interdisciplinary collaboration.

Chapter 3: AI-Enhanced Image Analysis and Interpretation

This chapter delves deeper into the analytical capabilities AI brings to radiology. With a focus on machine learning, deep learning, and radiomics, it examines how AI tools enhance interpretation and predictive modeling. The authors provide insights into the benefits of automation and precision in imaging tasks, while also acknowledging ongoing barriers such as algorithm robustness and dataset diversity. The discussion around future trends in multimodal data integration positions this chapter as a key reference for understanding the path toward fully intelligent imaging systems.

Chapter 4: The Evolution of MRI Before and After the Introduction of AI

Providing a historical and technological lens, this chapter traces the evolution of MRI and contrasts the pre-AI era with contemporary AI-enhanced MRI. From improvements in scan speed to enhanced image clarity and diagnostic accuracy, it illustrates the transformative influence of AI on MRI systems. The chapter also confronts the ethical, technical, and operational challenges still limiting AI's full integration into clinical MRI practice.

Chapter 5: Adaptive Devices for Artificial Intelligence of Medical Things

Shifting the focus toward AI-enabled hardware, this chapter examines the intersection of AI and adaptive medical devices. It highlights how the Artificial Intelligence of Medical Things (AIoMT) is driving innovation in health monitoring wearables, capable of real-time data collection and analysis. By addressing practical concerns—ranging from data security to public system integration—this chapter offers a critical exploration of how smart devices powered by AI can enhance personalized care and system responsiveness.

Chapter 6: AI in Wearable Imaging Devices

This chapter continues the discussion on wearable technologies by zeroing in on imaging devices designed for mobile and remote healthcare applications. From AI-enhanced portable ultrasounds to wearable MRIs, the authors showcase how these devices are improving diagnostic access and chronic disease monitoring. The chapter evaluates their real-world potential, technological challenges, and future integration with telemedicine and predictive health systems, reinforcing AI's role in democratizing imaging.

Chapter 7: Integrating Large Language Models for Advanced Imaging Applications

Highlighting the interdisciplinary convergence of language and image processing, this chapter explores how large language models (LLMs) are being integrated into imaging workflows. It presents use cases where LLMs enhance data analysis, contextualize imaging results, and assist in regulatory and administrative tasks. By situating LLMs within the broader framework of AI for healthcare, this chapter opens new avenues for automating complex interpretative and decision-support functions.

Chapter 8: Future Directions and Innovations in AI and Imaging

Concluding the volume, this chapter synthesizes the advances covered throughout the book and projects the future of AI in radiodiagnosis. It discusses emergent technologies like explainable AI, GANs, and point-of-care diagnostics, emphasizing their potential to drive personalized, efficient, and transparent imaging. At the same time, it offers a critical reflection on the ethical, regulatory, and technical challenges that must be addressed to realize AI's full promise in both clinical and non-clinical domains.

We envision this book as a vital resource for healthcare professionals, researchers, and technologists eager to engage with the future of radiodiagnosis. It will also serve as a reference for policymakers, educators, and students who seek to understand the transformative power of AI in healthcare. Through case studies, empirical insights, and forward-looking analyses, *Radiodiagnosis in the Era of AI* offers both depth and breadth in its treatment of this dynamic field.

We thank our contributors for their scholarly dedication and our readers for their curiosity and commitment to advancing medical science. As we navigate the evolving synergy between artificial intelligence and radiological practice, we hope this book serves as a beacon—guiding innovation, fostering critical dialogue, and ultimately enhancing patient care in meaningful ways.

Chapter 1
Introduction to Next-Generation Biomedical Imaging

Maruf Ahmad
https://orcid.org/0000-0002-2724-7009
Centurion University of Technology and Management, Bhubaneswar, India

Anurag Luharia
https://orcid.org/0000-0001-6051-1636
Datta Meghe Institute of Higher Education and Research, India

Fauzia Khan
Integral University, Lucknow, India

ABSTRACT

Biomedical imaging has long been vital for revealing the human body's inner workings with remarkable precision. Now, a new era of imaging technology is set to revolutionize healthcare. This chapter explores next-generation biomedical imaging, featuring breakthroughs like photon-counting CT (PCCT), ultra-high-field MRI, and advanced molecular imaging that push resolution and specificity boundaries. Artificial intelligence plays a pivotal role, with machine learning and deep learning transforming image reconstruction, analysis, and interpretation. The chapter also highlights multimodal imaging, which integrates structural and functional data for a deeper understanding of complex diseases. Beyond innovations, practical applications are discussed, including early disease detection, minimally invasive procedures, and precision medicine. By bridging cutting-edge research with clinical practice, this introduction provides a roadmap for medical professionals and researchers to navigate the transformative future of biomedical imaging in diagnosis and treatment.

DOI: 10.4018/979-8-3373-0903-3.ch001

1. INTRODUCTION

From the earliest days of X-rays to the more advanced AI-powered modalities that are now being developed, the biomedical imaging field has undergone tremendous change. It started with X-rays, which were the first to transform medical diagnosis and paved the way for other imaging technologies, such as CT and MRI As shown in **Fig.1**. These have helped in the improvement of the quality of images as well as provided physicians with more tools for diagnoses. As seen, deep learning algorithms when applied to imaging may improve image processing and reconstruction and thus offer an avenue for a more precise diagnosis and effective treatment.(Showrov et al., 2024)

Figure 1. Evolution of Biomedical Imaging

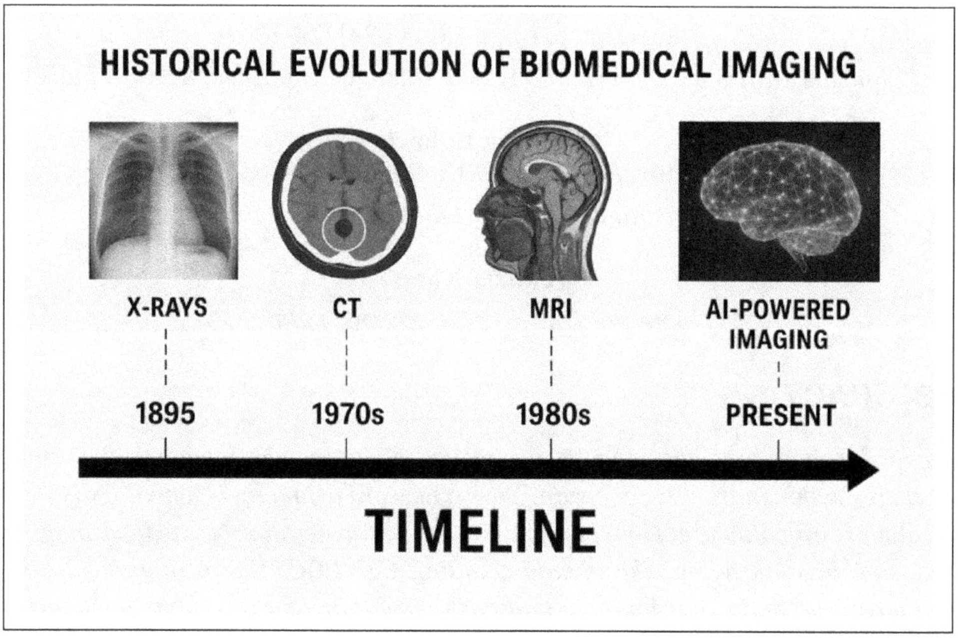

Despite these advances, medical imaging still faces a number of challenges. The first is the massive amounts of data generated by modern imaging techniques. With the increasing digital and high-resolution nature of imaging, data volumes can easily exceed terabytes, making storage, retrieval, and analysis procedures cumbersome. (Scholl et al., 2011) Moreover, medical image interpretation is often qualitative, leading to inconsistent diagnosis results. With efforts made to establish quantitative imaging biomarkers, it is an effort towards standardizing picture interpretation and improving the dependability of diagnostic procedures. On the other hand, with the incorporation of AI into medical imaging, there come ethical and legal issues which make it necessary to cautiously examine the utilization of these technologies in the clinical environment. Future potential of next-generation technologies will greatly benefit in overcoming the current constraints of medical imaging. For example, there is the development that incorporates generative adversarial networks (GANs), primarily in cases where data are limited, and thereby offers improved image quality and enhanced accuracy in diagnosis.(Showrov et al., 2024) The integration of multimodal imaging techniques enables the combination of data coming from various sources and consequently offers a holistic understanding and thus improves clinical decision-making.(Huang et al., 2020) It is expected that with continued development of AI-based technologies for image segmentation and analysis, it will streamline workflows and lighten the burden on radiologists, helping in faster and more accurate diagnoses.(Su et al., 2020) (Liu et al., 2020) The future of precision medicine would likely rely heavily on such technologies as they advance, supporting tailored treatment plans based on individual patient imaging data.(Huang et al., 2023)

2. OVERVIEW OF NEXT-GENERATION IMAGING MODALITIES

2.1 Photon-Counting CT

Photon-counting computed tomography (PCCT) represents a major advancement in imaging technology, utilizing its ability to count individual photons and determine their energy levels. Unlike traditional energy-integrating detectors, PCCT provides superior material differentiation and higher image quality by analyzing every detected photon (Scarfato et al., 2024; Willemink et al., 2018). Two key benefits of PCCT are its higher spatial resolution and reduced image noise, as illustrated in **Fig.2**, which collectively improve diagnostic accuracy. Even at low radiation doses, PCCT reduces electronic noise and produces sharper images (Tsiflikas et al., 2023; Hagen et al., 2022).

Figure 2. PCCT showing Higher Spatial Resolution and Less Noise

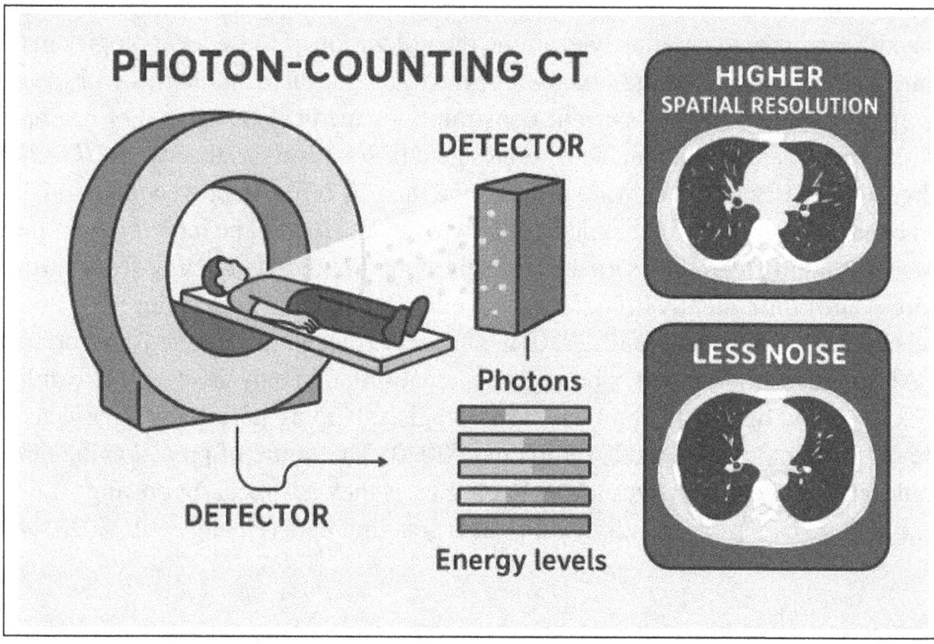

One significant advantage is reduced radiation exposure, enhancing patient safety, particularly in vulnerable populations such as children (Hagen et al., 2024). Additionally, PCCT supports spectral imaging, enabling improved visualization of vascular structures and disease assessment (Stein et al., 2023). The technology is particularly valuable in oncology, cardiovascular, and pulmonary imaging. In cancer care, PCCT improves tumor characterization and therapy monitoring (Scarfato et al., 2024; Hagen et al., 2024). It also enhances coronary artery visualization, aiding in diagnosing coronary artery disease (Symons et al., 2018; Zsarnóczay et al., 2023). In pulmonary imaging, it enables detailed assessment of lung microstructures, assisting in the diagnosis of interstitial lung disease and pulmonary embolism (Remy-Jardin et al., 2023; Stein et al., 2023).

2.2 Ultra-High-Field MRI

Ultra-high-field MRI, particularly at 7 Tesla (7T), marks a significant advancement over conventional 1.5T or 3T systems by providing enhanced signal-to-noise ratio (SNR) and spatial resolution. These improvements enable the visualization of finer anatomical details, thereby enhancing diagnostic accuracy (Henry et al., 2011). One of its most notable advantages is its superior spatial resolution. Studies have shown that 7T MRI can delineate small anatomical structures—such as the hippocampus—that are difficult or impossible to visualize at lower field strengths (Zhang et al., 2019; Santyr et al., 2017).

Figure 3. Ultrahigh Field MRI showing best soft tissue Resolution and Functional MRI for Brain imaging

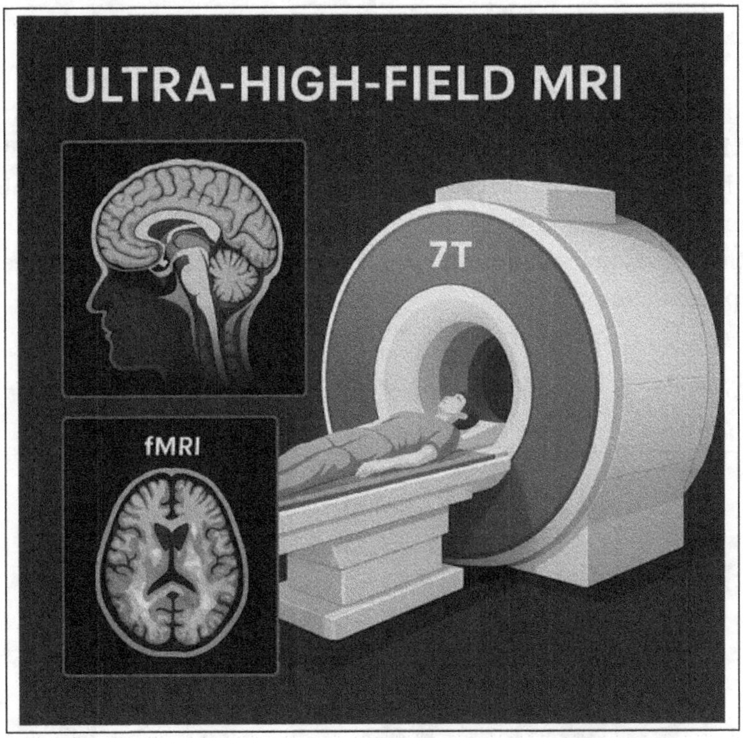

In neuroimaging, 7T MRI has proven essential in detecting internal hippocampal substructures, aiding the diagnosis and management of epilepsy and hippocampal sclerosis (Stefanits et al., 2017; Santyr et al., 2017; Suh et al., 2024). In musculoskeletal imaging, it improves the visualization of cartilage and soft tissue abnormalities within joints (Boudabbous et al., 2018). Furthermore, in functional MRI (fMRI), 7T offers greater sensitivity and spatial accuracy for mapping brain activity, critical for neurological and psychiatric research—as shown in **Fig.3** (Sladky et al., 2013). These capabilities promise to enhance diagnostic precision and improve patient outcomes across multiple clinical domains.

2.3 Advanced Molecular Imaging Techniques

Because of advanced molecular imaging technologies, particularly in conjunction with PET, CT, and MRI, many medical specialties have far better diagnostic capabilities today. Combining metabolic and anatomical data may enable an understanding of disease processes that is far more comprehensive.

2.3.1 PET/MRI and PET/CT Advancements:

Diagnostic imaging has been enhanced due to PET hybridization with CT (PET/CT) and MRI (PET/MRI) in neurology and oncology, among other applications.

These methods broaden disease detection, staging, and treatment planning by integrating anatomical and functional imaging as shown in **Fig.4**. Each, however, poses distinct advantages and limitations when considering imaging effectiveness, cost, and patient compatibility.

Figure 4. Showing Use of CT scan and PET scan fused Images for better treatment of cancer patients

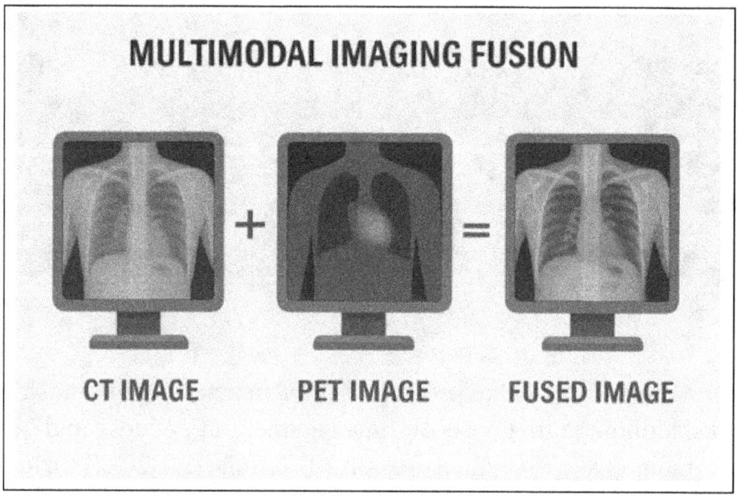

Imaging Performance Cost and Accessibility

PET/CT is the most commonly used hybrid imaging modality due to its rapid acquisition, high diagnostic accuracy, and effective integration of metabolic (PET) and anatomical (CT) information. It is especially valuable for detecting head-and-neck cancer, lung cancer, and lymphoma, with diagnostic accuracy exceeding 85%

in many malignancies, including lung nodules, bone metastases, and whole-body cancer screening (Sanei Sistani et al., 2021; de Mooij et al., 2020) (**Fig.4**).

In contrast, PET/MRI offers superior soft tissue contrast without ionizing radiation from CT, making it advantageous for pediatric patients and cases requiring repeated imaging. It is particularly beneficial in gynecologic and brain cancers due to MRI's superior neuroanatomical resolution (Nguyen et al., 2020). PET/MRI has also shown greater sensitivity in detecting distant metastases in breast, colorectal, and cervical cancers, with enhanced lesion detectability and diagnostic confidence thanks to multiplanar MRI imaging (Zhang et al., 2023; Ehman et al., 2024) (**Fig.5**).

While PET/MRI is less available and more costly due to longer scan times and higher equipment costs, it can reduce future healthcare expenses by improving diagnostic precision and minimizing unnecessary biopsies or treatments (Nguyen et al., 2020).

Figure 5. Showing advantage of PET/CT and PET/MRI for whole body cancer detection

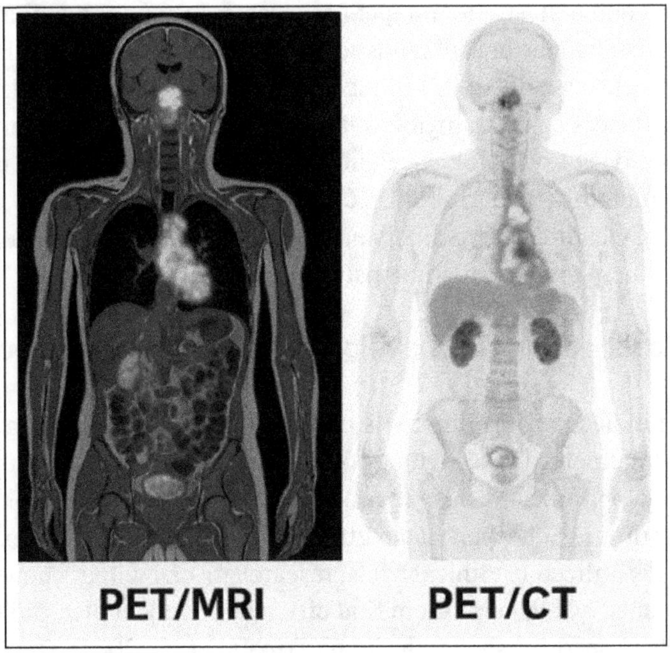

Patient Suitability and Clinical Use Cases

PET/CT is especially indicated for thoracic and skeletal imaging, and it is extremely suitable for most patients. It is dependable, fast, and ideal in an emergency setting. On the other hand, patients who require repetitive imaging, children, and pregnant individuals may worry about the burden of radiation with CT.

PET/MRI is the preferred technique for brain imaging, pediatric oncology, pelvic tumors, and soft tissue sarcomas when radiation safety and better soft-tissue resolution are a priority, according to Zhang et al. (2023).

The complementary information gained through MRI's diffusion-weighted imaging (DWI), MR spectroscopy (MRS), and functional imaging abilities enhances tumor characterisation and therapy monitoring (Ehman et al., 2024).

2.3.2 Novel Tracers for Imaging Specific Diseases:

Further expansion of using PET/MRI and PET/CT in imaging specific diseases was the development of novel radiotracers, such as 68Ga-PSMA-11 PET, which proved to be a good indicator for prostate cancer staging and shows that PET/MRI is comparable or even superior in diagnostic performance compared to PET/CT.(Wang et al., 2023) (Jackson et al., 2022) In the search for understanding Alzheimer's disease, the new tracers against amyloid plaques such as 18F-florbetapir are enabling visual observations of pathological changes in the brain that precede the beginning of clinical symptoms.(Belcari et al., 2021) Using the latest tracers coupled with hybrid imaging techniques maximally enables early diagnosis and monitoring with potential for timely intervention in a patient's course of the disease.

2.3.3 Applications in Drug Development and Personalized Medicine:

Advanced molecular imaging tools play a significant role in drug research and personalized treatment. These methods of imaging can help to assess the efficacy of the therapy and optimize the dose regime by providing real-time biological effects of therapeutic drugs.(Scheepers et al., 2023) (Ming et al., 2020) For example, when the PET/MRI is utilized in clinical trials, researchers can witness how tumors react to new treatments, which helps them find efficient treatment plans tailored for each patient's specific needs as shown in **Fig.6**.(Tripathi et al., 2023) The incorporation of clinical data with imaging biomarkers helps in developing predictive models that can direct the adoption of tailored treatment plans to improve patient outcomes. (Wang et al., 2020) Conclusion Molecular imaging is increasingly being developed because of the new tracers and most recent techniques like PET/MRI or PET/CT. These technologies pave the way for more efficient and focused treatment approaches through better drug discovery, tailored medicine, and increased diagnostic accuracy.

Figure 6. Showing Drug development for personalized treatment

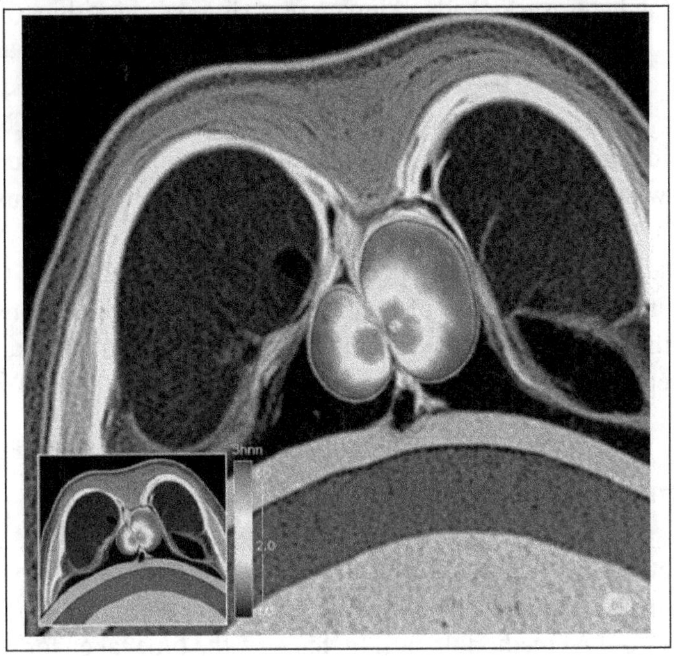

3. THE ROLE OF ARTIFICIAL INTELLIGENCE IN BIOMEDICAL IMAGING

3.1 Machine Learning and Deep Learning Fundamentals

Artificial intelligence (AI) is revolutionizing biomedical imaging by transforming how images are analyzed and interpreted. Central to this shift are machine learning (ML) and deep learning (DL), which enable systems to learn from data and improve over time without explicit programming. These technologies support applications such as image segmentation, classification, and anomaly detection, significantly enhancing diagnostic efficiency and accuracy (Barragán-Montero et al., 2021; Langlotz et al., 2019). ML approaches like supervised, unsupervised, and reinforcement learning utilize algorithms such as support vector machines (SVM), decision trees, and k-nearest neighbours (KNN), relying on feature extraction guided by human input (Bansal et al., 2022). In contrast, DL—particularly convolutional neural networks (CNNs)—learns directly from raw image data, capturing intricate patterns that might be overlooked by humans or traditional algorithms (Nishio, 2021).

DL offers several advantages, including reduced user input and improved performance on complex tasks, such as detecting subtle lesions or differentiating similar tissues (Barragán-Montero et al., 2021; Castro et al., 2020). CNNs have also shown superior capability in identifying malignant tumors compared to traditional ML models, which often struggle with high-dimensional data (Adegun et al., 2020; Bansal, 2021). AI also helps reduce human interpretation errors. However, concerns about machine error and reliability persist. Ampofo et al. (2023) note that radiology students are increasingly aware of both the strengths and limitations of AI. This underscores the importance of developing trustworthy AI systems that complement rather than replace human expertise. Moreover, Castro et al. (2020) highlight the role of causal reasoning in promoting responsible AI use.

3.2 AI in Image Reconstruction

Images get reconstructed, especially in medicine, with the use of AI methods. Techniques such as CS as well as iterative reconstruction have significantly seen contributions from AI methodologies. In this way, the time taken for reconstruction improves alongside accuracy. One of the important factors for patient safety is that these developments enhance the quality of image and while reducing the radiation dose related to imaging procedures.

3.2.1 Techniques: Compressed Sensing and Iterative Reconstruction:

A signal processing technique known as compressed sensing takes advantage of the sparsity of medical images in an appropriate transform domain to reconstruct images from fewer samples than traditionally used as shown in **Fig.7**. With this technique, significant savings in acquisition time and data storage needs become possible.(Nagaraj et al., 2024) Compressed sensing frameworks have also been advanced using AI techniques, particularly deep learning-based ones, to enhance reconstruction quality further. AI-enabled techniques enable, for example, reconstructing high quality photos from vastly under sampled data, identifying underlying data patterns.(Vandewinckele et al., 2020) Iterative approaches of reconstruction use the already existing knowledge about the imaging system and what is expected by means of the attributes of the reconstructed image, in order to be able to refine the latter through iterations. The former traditional techniques are very often computationally expensive and sometimes very time-consuming. But this process accelerates with the use of AI, especially deep learning models.

Figure 7. Showing Compressed Sensing and Iterative Reconstruction

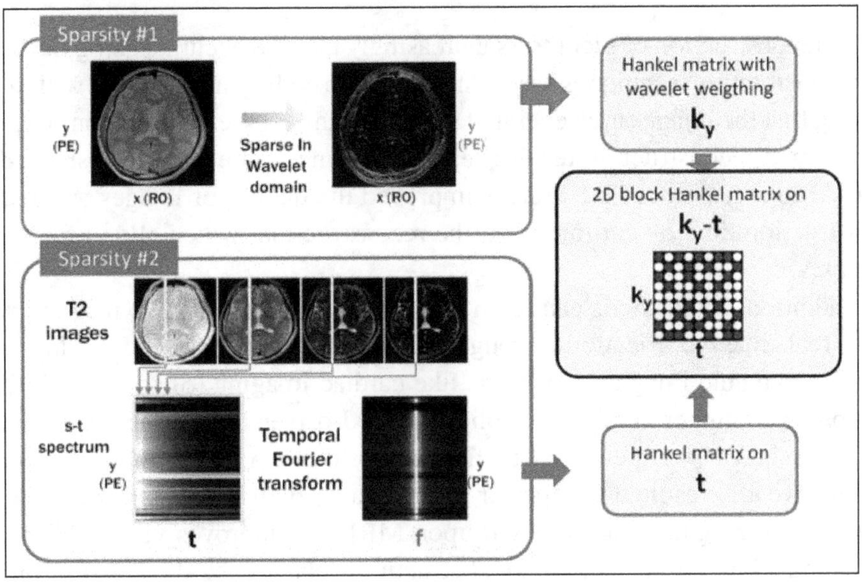

With the help of AI algorithms, image artifacts may be accurately predicted and corrected, increasing accuracy and lowering noise levels as shown in **Fig.8**.(Knoll et al., 2020) (Antun et al., 2020) For example, the AUTOMAP and DeepPET algorithms significantly reduce reconstruction time, preserving high picture fidelity with the use of deep learning to train the reconstruction process.

Figure 8. Showing AI in Image Reconstruction

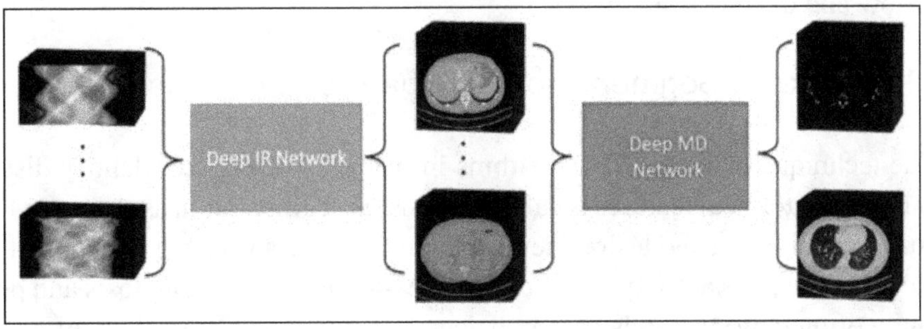

3.2.2 AI for Faster, More Accurate Reconstructions:

The reconstruction of pictures is increasingly fast and accurate using the help of AI. Reconstruction techniques based on AI result in high-quality images with studies showing that the images are generated in significantly lesser time in comparison to conventional reconstruction techniques. For instance, an experiment showed that using AI to reconstruct PET images improved the quality of images and reduced reconstruction time by cutting down the reconstruction, which allows for quicker diagnoses.

In addition, AI methods can learn from the data in an adaptive manner, which allows real-time modifications throughout the reconstruction process. This is very useful in dynamic imaging situations like cardiac imaging.(Shao et al., 2021) In addition, in a number of clinical applications, AI-driven reconstruction techniques have been shown to outperform traditional algorithms. As such, AI-based methodologies have also resulted in superior image quality both in the setting of DWI and T2-weighted imaging that are based upon MRI that improves visualization, both of anatomical as well as pathological structures.(Nagaraj et al., 2024) In order to carry on with cutting up acquisition time, while upgrading image quality, AI leads to consequences both for the output of clinical throughput by which imaging departments are able to function as a whole to enhance its effectiveness.(Fu et al., 2021)

3.3 AI in Image Analysis and Interpretation

AI has immensely boosted medical imaging in automated organ and lesion segmentation, models of disease prediction, and decision support systems. In all these, improved patient outcomes result in the end due to the effectiveness of clinical workflow and diagnosis precision.

3.3.1 Automated Segmentation of Organs and Lesions:

The technique of using AI algorithms in medical pictures to identify diseased lesions and anatomical features is called automated segmentation as shown in **Fig.9**. Because proper organ and lesion identification can have a very big impact on therapeutic decisions, this activity is basically necessary for proper diagnosis and proper planning of therapy. Methods based on deep learning, like CNN, are now standard practices for segmentation jobs due to their capacity to extract complicated trends from these huge data sets.(Ramana Rao & RaviSankar, 2024) (Pelayo et al., 2023)

Figure 9. Showing Automated Segmentation of Organs and Lesions

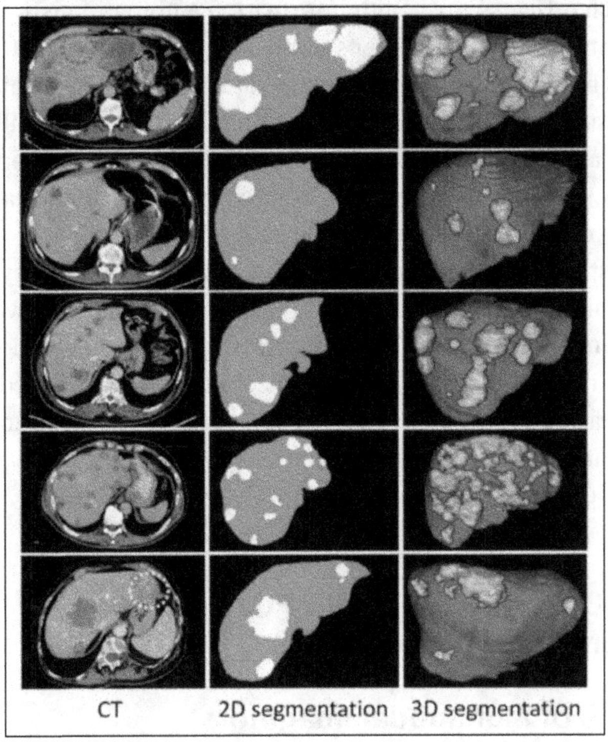

For example, Zhao et al.'s study states that deep neural networks can identify bone cancer via analysis of bone scintigraphy imaging. This is an example of how AI can give the accuracy of diagnosis because the model was able find out the lesion with remarkable precision due to its lengthy training on a larger database. (Zhao et al., 2020) As per this, automated segmentation methods have become more effective in accurately diagnosing cancer and other pathologies by using imaging modalities, like CT and MRI imaging as shown in **Fig.9**.(Keel et al., 2018) These revolutionary advancements reduces the amount of time required for image interpretation and mistakes made by humans, which enhance the correctness of image interpretation.

3.3.2 Disease Prediction Models and Decision Support Systems:

AI has simplified the development of sophisticated illness prediction models and recommendation networks as well as the segmentation process. Medical professionals are helped by these technologies to better predict the cause of a lesion and the effectiveness of treatment by combining patient information and imaging outcomes through machine learning algorithms. Siddiq, for example, demonstrated how artificial intelligence can be employed to detect anomalies in X-rays, CT scans, and MRIs, which reflects why health information automation is so important since the huge amount of information keeps increasing daily.(Siddiq, 2020) By offering evidence-based recommendations customized to every patient's unique profile, AI-based decision support systems can enable clinicians to make intelligent decisions. These systems analyze vast information to generate predictive insights, such as imaging results, clinical history, and laboratory results. For instance, there have been promising results with the use of AI in diabetic retinopathy screening. High sensitivity and specificity have been demonstrated by automated systems that have improved screening in outpatient settings.(Keel et al., 2018) The work of Alwiyah, 2023 further demonstrates potential in improving clinical operations using AI by focusing on the methodical integration of machine learning in medical image processing to increase both accuracy and speed. Automation of boring tasks such as image interpretation and analysis may help doctors become more proficient while giving more accurate diagnoses more promptly.(Kranthi et al., 2024)

4. MULTIMODAL IMAGING: THE FUTURE OF COMPREHENSIVE DIAGNOSTICS

4.1 Principles of Multimodal Imaging

Multifunctional medical imaging, which integrates anatomical and functional imaging techniques, offers a comprehensive view of diseases and biological processes, enabling more accurate diagnoses and personalized treatment planning. For example, combining MRI (for detailed anatomical imaging) with PET (for metabolic activity) allows clinicians to simultaneously assess tumor structure and function—critical for complex conditions like cancer (Forte et al., 2019; Aoyagi et al., 2023). This hybrid imaging approach supports long-term monitoring and tailored treatment strategies. Structural modalities such as CT and MRI provide precise anatomical detail, while functional imaging techniques like PET and SPECT offer insights into blood flow and metabolic markers (**Fig.10**) (Dong et al., 2014; Dadkhah & Jiao, 2020). Fusing these modalities enhances diagnostic accuracy, refines therapeutic targeting, and improves overall patient assessment.

Figure 10. Showing Principles of Multimodal Imaging

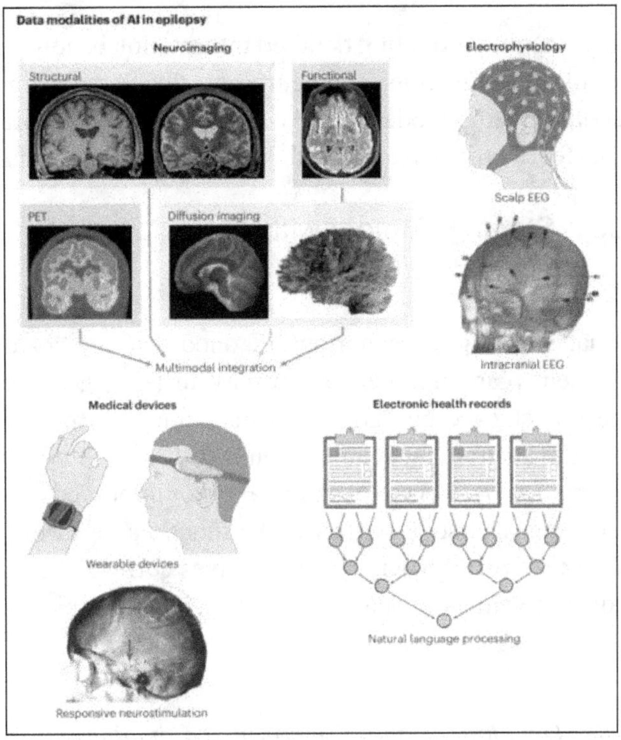

However, multimodality imaging presents challenges. Integrating images with different resolutions, contrasts, and spatial orientations requires complex algorithms to ensure proper alignment and interpretation (Al-Azzawi, 2015; Zhang et al., 2022). Physicians also face difficulties in harmonizing data from diverse imaging systems while ensuring clinical relevance (Su et al., 2020; Zhang et al., 2022).

Establishing standardized protocols and frameworks for image acquisition and patient preparation remains a significant hurdle (Aoyagi et al., 2023; Lee et al., 2018). Furthermore, interpreting fused images demands specialized training, which may limit widespread adoption (Forte et al., 2019; Taime et al., 2023). Despite these obstacles, multimodal imaging is a major advancement in diagnostic medicine. It holds the potential to significantly improve disease evaluation and treatment personalization. For successful integration into clinical practice, issues surrounding data fusion, interpretation, and standardization must be addressed. When fully optimized, multimodal imaging can transform patient care through precise, data-driven decision-making.

4.2 Applications of Multimodal Imaging

Multimodality imaging providing detailed information is now very important in healthcare, particularly in oncology and neurology, due to the merger of both structural and functional imaging modalities. By improvising the accuracy of diagnosis and providing data for treatment planning, this formation enhances patient outcomes.

4.2.1 Oncology: Staging Tumors with Combined PET/CT or PET/MRI

Multifunctional imaging is important in oncology for correctly staging of tumors and treatment planning. Very sensitivity in finding of nodal and distant metastases has been achieved by PET/CT, which combines metabolic information by PET scan with the anatomical details given by CT scan. Meyer et al. (2018), for instance, proved that PET/CT is the best modality for improved diagnosis accuracy in cervical cancer stages. Also, by merging the functional information of PET and the best soft tissue contrast of MRI, PET/MRI gives correct visualization of tumor size and extent of involvement of nearby structures, which helps for better treatment planning as shown in **Fig.11**.

Figure 11. Showing Oncology: Staging Tumors with Combined PET/CT or PET/MRI

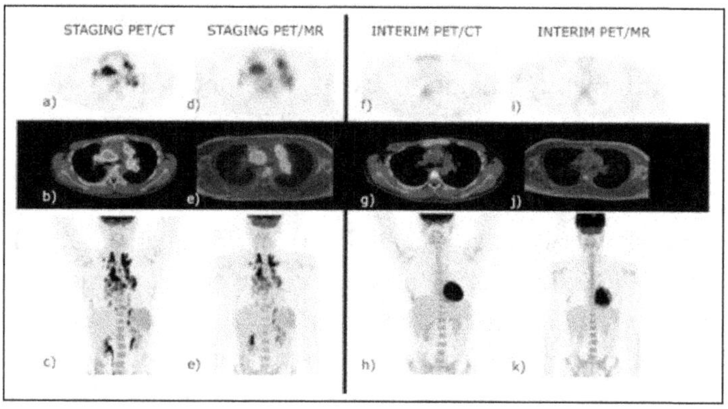

In presenting their findings on the collaborative value of multiparametric PET and MRI features in glioma treatment, Wang et al. (2020) emphasized the importance of combined analysis towards the interpretation of early tumor recurrence. Apart from increasing the accuracy of diagnoses, integrating structural and functional imaging assists in creating treatment programs which are best suited for each patient.

4.2.2 Neurology: Integrating Structural and Metabolic Information

Multiplexed imaging is very important in the interpretation of brain tumors and neurodegenerative disease in neurology. The combination of MRI and PET allows for a more complete diagnosis of brain disease as shown in **Fig.12**. Langen and Galldiks (2018) elaborated the advantages of amino acid PET scan compared with standard MRI for glioma imaging, noting that it can measure functional activity and define tumor boundaries more accurately, both of them are important for treatment planning. The Response calculation in Neuro-Oncology (RANO) group suggests using amino acid PET in combination with MRI to help differentiate tumor growth from changes developed by treatment.

Figure 12. Showing Neurology: Integrating Structural and Metabolic Information

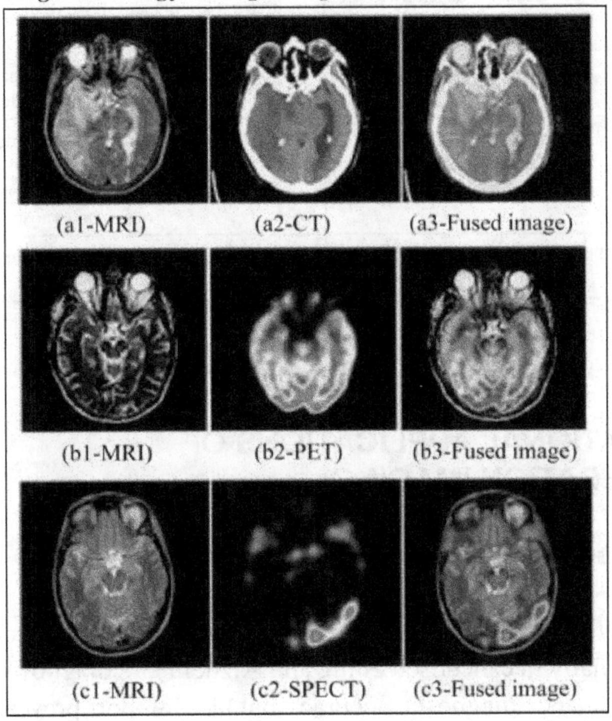

Moreover, the merging of PET with advanced imaging techniques such as Magnetic Resonance Spectroscopy (MRS) and Diffusion-Weighted Imaging (DWI) enhances the diagnostic procedure by providing more detailed information on the tumor boundaries and metabolic status. Radiomics, the computer-measurable features derived from imaging information, can be employed in multimodality imaging to structure predictive models for treatment outcomes and disease progression, facilitating the development of personalized treatment plans. PET/CT and PET/MRI having number of advantages over each other as shown in **Table:1**.

Comparative Analysis: PET/CT vs. PET/MRI

Table 1. Showing Comparative Analysis: PET/CT vs. PET/MRI

Parameter	PET/CT	PET/MRI
Imaging Performance	High sensitivity for detecting nodal and distant metastases; effective in lung metastasis detection.	Superior soft tissue contrast; better performance in detecting liver and bone metastases; enhanced lesion characterization in certain cancers.
Radiation Exposure	Higher radiation dose due to CT component.	Lower radiation exposure, making it more suitable for pediatric patients and those requiring multiple follow-ups.
Cost	Generally lower cost; more widely available.	Higher cost; limited availability; economic challenges hinder widespread adoption.
Patient Suitability	Suitable for a broad range of patients; faster scan times.	Preferred for patients requiring detailed soft tissue evaluation, such as those with head and neck cancers or pelvic tumors; beneficial for patients needing reduced radiation exposure.
Scan Duration	Shorter scan times, improving patient comfort.	Longer scan times, which may be challenging for some patients.

5. TRANSLATIONAL APPLICATIONS OF NEXT-GENERATION IMAGING

5.1 Early Disease Detection

Next-generation imaging technologies have significantly advanced early disease detection, especially in cancer screening and Alzheimer's diagnosis. These innovations not only enhance diagnostic accuracy but also support preventative medicine and improve public health outcomes. Hybrid imaging modalities such as PET/CT and PET/MRI enable earlier cancer detection compared to traditional techniques, as illustrated in **Fig.13**. PET can reveal metabolically active tumors before they are anatomically visible on CT or MRI (Capobianco, 2019). Early detection is crucial, as it correlates with improved prognosis and survival rates. Moreover, multimodal imaging facilitates accurate cancer staging and treatment monitoring, allowing for more personalized care (Robertson et al., 2019). In neurodegenerative diseases, advanced imaging is equally transformative. PET scans targeting tau and amyloid proteins can detect Alzheimer's-related brain changes long before clinical symptoms appear (Onstwedder et al., 2022). Early diagnosis enables timely interventions that may slow or modify disease progression (Siddiquee et al., 2019). Combining structural MRI with functional imaging further improves diagnostic precision in detecting subtle brain alterations linked to Alzheimer's (Nie et al., 2022).

Figure 13. Showing Early Disease Detection using Advance Imaging Modalities

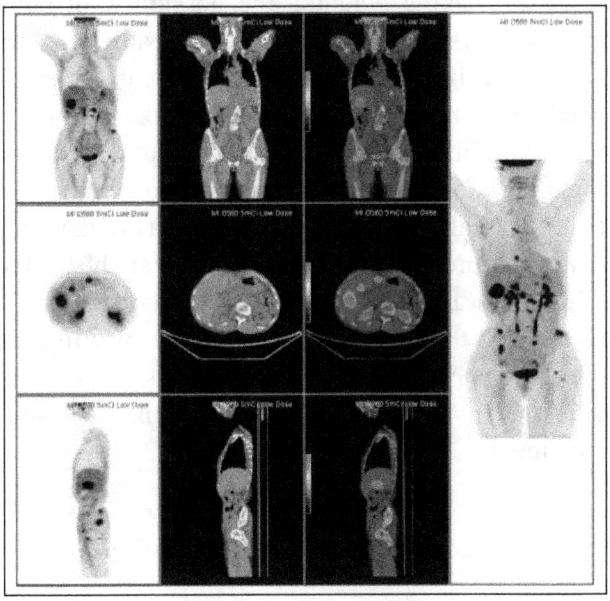

Beyond individual patient outcomes, early diagnosis through advanced imaging has major public health implications. Early cancer detection reduces the incidence of late-stage disease, lowering treatment costs and improving community health (Zhang et al., 2018). Similarly, identifying neurodegenerative diseases early allows for more effective healthcare planning and resource allocation (Zhang et al., 2021).

5.2 Tailored Medicine

The discipline of customized medicine has moved a long way since next-generation imaging technology has been introduced, especially on the sides of therapeutic monitoring and patient classification. This technology enables clinicians to improve personalized care for patients with a variety of diseases, including cancer and neurodegenerative disorders, through the use of imaging biomarkers that provide guidance on the best options in terms of available treatments.

5.2.1 Role in Patient Stratification and Therapy:

Imaging biomarkers are the only method through which patient stratification can be conducted, as this allows patients to be stratified in terms of how likely they are to respond to specific treatments. In oncology, for example, glioblastoma multiforme patients can be stratified into low-risk and high-risk groups based on the molecular features detected using advanced imaging. Bafiti et al demonstrated that a three-microRNA signature may effectively stratify GBM patients based on clinical outcomes, thus making potential the possibility of combining imaging data with molecular markers for the individualized treatment methods as shown in **Fig.14**.(Bafiti et al., 2022) It is very important to classify patients as this will help choose the best medicines and optimize the plans for the treatment of this group of patients in a way that will improve outcomes for patients. More than just stratification, imaging biomarkers are used increasingly for monitoring therapy. According to Failmezger et al., regional heterogeneity in cancer-associated protein expression is critical and can be measured quantitatively by using sophisticated imaging methods. This data is important for the monitoring of the course of the disease and the ability to assess how well the targeted treatments are working.(Failmezger et al., 2022) Clinicians can enhance the overall effectiveness of customized medicine by making timely adjustments to therapy by using imaging to continuously monitor the response to treatment.

Figure 14. Showing use of Advance Imaging Modalities in Patient Stratification and Therapy

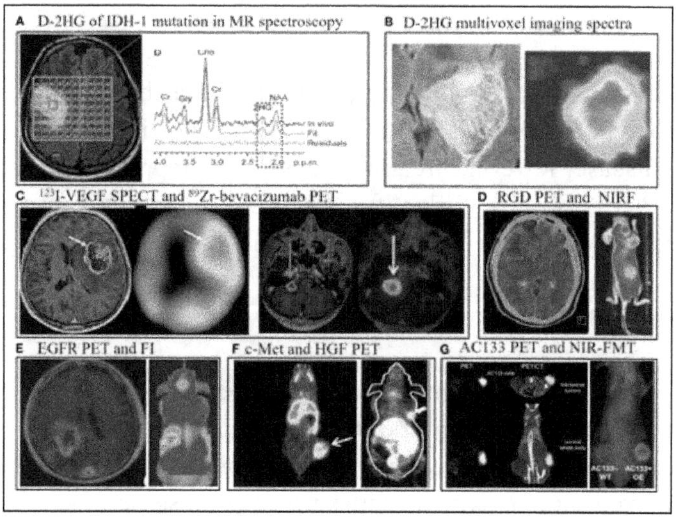

5.2.2 Case Studies: Imaging Biomarkers in Personalized Oncology:

Imaging biomarkers have been significantly improved the cancer diagnosis, prognosis, and treatment monitoring in personalized oncology treatment. Recent studies have discussed the crucial role of radiomics and high-tech imaging in personalizing treatment planning.

Breast Cancer: Multiparametric MRI (mpMRI) is an important method for the diagnosis of tumor features and responses to therapy in breast cancer treatment. Galati et al. (2022) emphasized the role of mpMRI in separating benign from malignant tumors to assist therapy as per choice. More recent advances have focused on combining genetic information with radiomic features to enhance the prediction. Wang et al. (2023) surveyed the link between radiomic features from MRI and genetic changes in breast cancer patients, explaining how this approach could be used to provide personalized treatment.

Integration with Clinical and Genomic Data: Clinical and genomic data can greatly improve the predictive power of treatment results by combining with imaging indicators. Coroller et al. (2017) highlighted that radiomic characteristics can be used to anticipate pathological responses in patients with non-small cell lung cancer (NSCLC) by adding current clinical and genetic data. This multimodality approach highlights how crucial it is to merge different data kinds in order to provide the best customized treatment plannings.

5.3 Minimally Invasive Procedures

Minimally invasive procedures effectively improve patient outcome, minimize recovery period, and hence minimize problems, which is a big revolution in surgical methods. For these type of treatment image-guided procedures in the form of decrement and biopsies along with real-time imaging, which allows for microsurgeries.

5.3.1 Imaging-Guided Interventions:

Advanced imaging modalities are used in image-guided interventional procedures to improve the accuracy and safety aspect of minimally invasive procedures. For example, in biopsies, real-time imaging techniques such as ultrasound, CT, and MRI can be utilized to guide needles correctly to the targeted area and guarantee precise sampling with micro damage to rest structures.(Ni et al., 2021) These techniques are especially helpful for sensitive regions like the liver or lungs, where open biopsy techniques can be dangerous to the patient as shown in **Fig.15**. Microwave ablation (MWA) and radiofrequency ablation (RFA) are two popular methods of thermal ablation for the treatment of the thyroid and liver cancers, which are also performed under the guidance of imaging to ensure accurate placement of the ablation device and real-time site of the treatment effectiveness.(Giovanni Mauri et al., 2019)

Figure 15. Showing Imaging-Guided Interventions using Advance Imaging Modalities

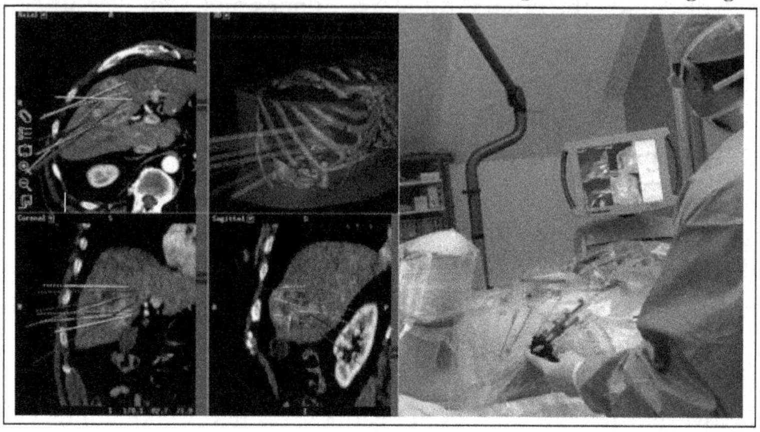

For instance, Mauri et al. revealed how image-guided thermal ablation can notably reduce the volume of benign thyroid nodules as shown in **Fig.16**, highlighting that such techniques may actually replace more invasive surgical interventional procedures.(G. Mauri et al., 2019)

Figure 16. Showing Thermal Ablation of Thyroid Using USG

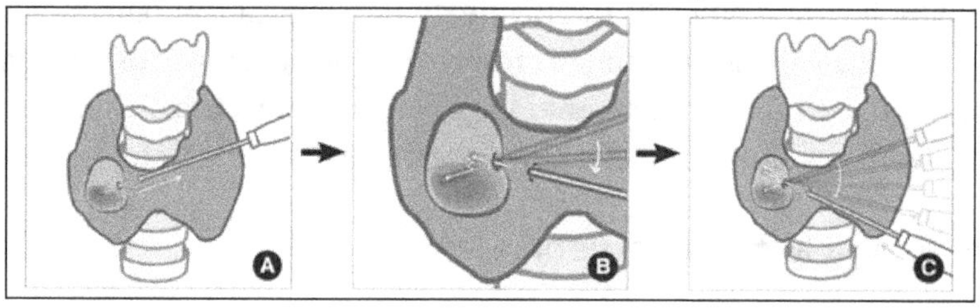

5.3.2 Real-Time Imaging for Precision Surgeries:

Real-time imaging significantly enhances surgical accuracy and patient outcomes, especially in complex and minimally invasive procedures. Indocyanine green (ICG) fluorescence imaging allows better visualization of tumors and their margins, improving detection of malignant tissues and reducing residual tumor risks (Kim &

Lee, 2024; Sakamoto et al., 2021). Kim and Lee (2024) demonstrated improved tumor delineation in gastric cancer surgeries using ICG, resulting in minimal damage to healthy tissues and fewer postoperative complications. Similarly, ICG imaging shows promise in liver and colorectal surgeries (Wang et al., 2023).

Intraoperative modalities like intraoperative MRI (iMRI) and ultrasound further enhance precision. iMRI supports accurate navigation during brain surgeries, compensating for brain shifts and ensuring complete tumor resection while preserving critical functions (Han & Cha, 2020; Liang et al., 2019). A Mayo Clinic case highlighted improved survival in glioblastoma patients with iMRI-guided surgery (Mayo Clinic Proceedings, 2023).

Intraoperative ultrasound benefits liver, breast, and prostate surgeries, aiding in micro-lesion detection and facilitating nerve-sparing techniques (Patel et al., 2023; Jones et al., 2024). These technologies, when integrated into surgical workflows, reduce morbidity, shorten recovery, and enhance outcomes (Chen et al., 2020).

6. ETHICAL AND PRACTICAL CONSIDERATIONS

The rapid advancement of imaging technologies presents key ethical and practical challenges, particularly regarding cost, accessibility, data privacy, and workforce readiness. In low- and middle-income countries (LMICs), the high cost of advanced tools like PET/MRI restricts access and deepens healthcare disparities. To address this, innovative, low-cost solutions such as smartphone-based micro endoscopy and affordable OCT systems are emerging. Policy actions promoting price transparency, global investment, and cross-border collaborations are essential to increase equitable access.

The integration of artificial intelligence (AI) into imaging also raises data privacy and cybersecurity concerns. AI systems require large patient datasets, increasing vulnerability to data breaches amid rising ransomware attacks in healthcare. Emerging solutions like blockchain, federated learning, and differential privacy aim to secure data while enabling safe, collaborative AI model training. Ensuring ongoing patient consent, regulatory compliance (e.g., GDPR, HIPAA), and algorithmic transparency is vital to build public trust.

Workforce preparedness is equally crucial as imaging systems grow more complex. Continuous medical education (CME), including online platforms and interprofessional learning, supports accessible, lifelong learning. Programs like the RSNA Imaging AI Certificate and global efforts such as the EU-funded Susa project are equipping healthcare professionals with the skills needed to safely and effectively implement new imaging technologies.

7. FUTURE PERSPECTIVES AND CHALLENGES

The future of medical imaging holds transformative potential with emerging technologies like hybrid imaging and quantum computing. Hybrid modalities such as PET/MRI and PET/CT enhance diagnostic precision by combining anatomical and functional data, especially valuable in oncology and neurology. Quantum computing promises rapid, complex image analysis and reconstruction, potentially improving diagnostic speed and accuracy. However, several barriers hinder widespread adoption. Regulatory challenges include complex approval processes and lack of harmonized international standards. Technical issues involve costly integration and interoperability with outdated systems, while economic constraints stem from high investment needs and unclear reimbursement pathways. A patient-centred imaging ecosystem envisions leveraging AI, machine learning, and quantum computing for personalized diagnostics and real-time decision support. These technologies can enable tailored treatment plans and faster diagnoses, improving patient outcomes. However, ethical concerns, data privacy, and equitable access remain key challenges. Addressing these through streamlined regulation, infrastructure investment, and inclusive deployment strategies is essential. The future lies in an ecosystem where innovation meets equity, ensuring advanced imaging benefits all patients.

8. CONCLUSION

Next-generation imaging technologies are transforming healthcare by enabling early diagnosis, personalized treatment, and minimally invasive procedures. Advances such as AI-driven applications, hybrid imaging (e.g., PET/MRI), and imaging biomarkers enhance diagnostic accuracy and support precise, patient-specific care. These technologies merge structural and functional data into a single image, offering a comprehensive assessment—for instance, improved tumor detection and metabolic insights through PET/MRI aid in effective treatment planning. Personalized oncology also benefits through therapy monitoring and patient stratification. Despite their promise, challenges remain. Legal, technical, and financial barriers hinder widespread adoption, while ethical concerns around data privacy in AI-based imaging require stringent safeguards. Ensuring equitable access and integration into clinical practice calls for interdisciplinary collaboration among healthcare providers, researchers, technologists, and policymakers. A unified approach that fosters innovation, ethical standards, and stakeholder cooperation is essential for overcoming obstacles. By building a patient-centred imaging ecosystem focused on both advanced technology and individual needs, the future of medical imaging holds the potential to significantly enhance patient outcomes and reshape healthcare delivery.

REFERENCES

Adegun, A. A., Ogundokun, R. O., Adebiyi, M. O., & Asani, E. O. (2020). CAD-based machine learning project for reducing human-factor-related errors in medical image analysis. In *Handbook of research on the role of human factors in IT project management* (pp. 164–172). IGI Global.

Al-Azzawi, N. A. (2015). Medical image fusion based on shearlets and human feature visibility. *International Journal of Computer Applications*, *125*(12), 1–12.

Alwiyah, A., & Setyowati, W. (2023). A Comprehensive Survey of Machine Learning Applications in Medical Image Analysis for Artificial Vision. *International Transactions on Artificial Intelligence*, *2*(1), 90–98.

Ampofo, J. W., Emery, C. V., & Ofori, I. N. (2023). Assessing the level of understanding (knowledge) and awareness of diagnostic imaging students in Ghana on Artificial Intelligence and its applications in Medical Imaging. *Radiology Research and Practice*, *2023*(1), 4704342. PMID: 37362195

Antun, V., Renna, F., Poon, C., Adcock, B., & Hansen, A. C. (2020). On instabilities of deep learning in image reconstruction and the potential costs of AI. *Proceedings of the National Academy of Sciences of the United States of America*, *117*(48), 30088–30095. https://pmc.ncbi.nlm.nih.gov/articles/PMC7720232/pdf/pnas.201907377.pdf PMID: 32393633

Aoyagi, H., Tsujinaga, S., Takahashi, Y., Naito, S., Sato, T., Otsuka, T., Tamaki, Y., Motoi, K., Ishizaka, S., & Chiba, Y. (2023). Multimodal Imaging of Constrictive Pericarditis Induced by Long-term Pergolide Treatment for Parkinson's Disease. *Internal Medicine (Tokyo, Japan)*, *62*(24), 3637–3641. https://pmc.ncbi.nlm.nih.gov/articles/PMC10781551/pdf/1349-7235-62-3637.pdf PMID: 37005266

Bafiti, V., Ouzounis, S., Chalikiopoulou, C., Grigorakou, E., Grypari, I. M., Gregoriou, G., Theofanopoulos, A., Panagiotopoulos, V., Prodromidi, E., Cavouras, D., Zolota, V., Kardamakis, D., & Katsila, T. (2022). A 3-miRNA Signature Enables Risk Stratification in Glioblastoma Multiforme Patients with Different Clinical Outcomes. *Current Oncology (Toronto, Ont.)*, *29*(6), 4315–4331. DOI: 10.3390/curroncol29060345 PMID: 35735454

Bansal, M., Goyal, A., & Choudhary, A. (2022). A comparative analysis of K-nearest neighbor, genetic, support vector machine, decision tree, and long short term memory algorithms in machine learning. *Decision Analytics Journal*, *3*, 100071.

Bansal, S. (2021). Determining disease using machine learning algorithm in medical image processing: A gentle review. *Biomedical Statistics and Informatics*, *6*(4), 84.

Barragán-Montero, A., Javaid, U., Valdés, G., Nguyen, D., Desbordes, P., Macq, B., Willems, S., Vandewinckele, L., Holmström, M., & Löfman, F. (2021). Artificial intelligence and machine learning for medical imaging: A technology review. *Physica Medica, 83*, 242–256. https://pmc.ncbi.nlm.nih.gov/articles/PMC8184621/pdf/nihms-1702435.pdf PMID: 33979715

Belcari, N., Del Guerra, A., & Panetta, D. (2021). High-Resolution and Animal Imaging Instrumentation and Techniques. In *Handbook of Particle Detection and Imaging* (pp. 1497–1535). Springer.

Boudabbous, S., Neroladaki, A., Bagetakos, I., Hamard, M., Delattre, B. M., & Vargas, M. I. (2018). Feasibility of synthetic MRI in knee imaging in routine practice. *Acta Radiologica Open, 7*(5), 2058460118769686. https://pmc.ncbi.nlm.nih.gov/articles/PMC5952291/pdf/10.1177_2058460118769686.pdf PMID: 29780615

Capobianco, E. (2019). Next generation networks: Featuring the potential role of emerging applications in translational oncology. *Journal of Clinical Medicine, 8*(5), 664. https://pmc.ncbi.nlm.nih.gov/articles/PMC6572295/pdf/jcm-08-00664.pdf PMID: 31083565

Castro, D. C., Walker, I., & Glocker, B. (2020). Causality matters in medical imaging. *Nature Communications, 11*(1), 3673. https://pmc.ncbi.nlm.nih.gov/articles/PMC7376027/pdf/41467_2020_Article_17478.pdf PMID: 32699250

Chen, L., Zhang, J., & Huang, W. (2020). Real-time imaging and minimally invasive surgery: Improving outcomes and safety. *Surgical Innovation, 27*(2), 123–132. DOI: 10.1177/1553350619898193

Chen, Q.-Y., Xie, J.-W., Zhong, Q., Wang, J.-B., Lin, J.-X., Lu, J., Cao, L.-L., Lin, M., Tu, R.-H., & Huang, Z.-N. (2020). Safety and efficacy of indocyanine green tracer-guided lymph node dissection during laparoscopic radical gastrectomy in patients with gastric cancer: A randomized clinical trial. *JAMA Surgery, 155*(4), 300–311. PMID: 32101269

Coroller, T. P., Agrawal, V., Huynh, E., Narayan, V., Lee, S. W., Mak, R. H., & Aerts, H. J. (2017). Radiomic-based pathological response prediction from primary tumors and lymph nodes in NSCLC. *Journal of Thoracic Oncology, 12*(3), 467–476. https://pmc.ncbi.nlm.nih.gov/articles/PMC5318226/pdf/nihms-832642.pdf PMID: 27903462

Coroller, T. P., Grossmann, P., Hou, Y., Rios Velazquez, E., Leijenaar, R. T. H., Hermann, G., & Aerts, H. J. (2017). CT-based radiomic signature predicts distant metastasis in lung adenocarcinoma. *Radiotherapy and Oncology : Journal of the European Society for Therapeutic Radiology and Oncology*, *123*(3), 480–486. DOI: 10.1016/j.radonc.2017.04.006 PMID: 25746350

Dadkhah, A., & Jiao, S. (2020). Integrating photoacoustic microscopy, optical coherence tomography, OCT angiography, and fluorescence microscopy for multimodal imaging. *Experimental Biology and Medicine*, *245*(4), 342–347. https://pmc.ncbi.nlm.nih.gov/articles/PMC7370601/pdf/10.1177_1535370219897584.pdf PMID: 31914810

Dong, D., Hui, H., Yang, C., Guo, J., Yang, Y., Shi, L., Mu, W., & Tian, J. (2014). Preliminary design of a multimodality molecular imaging system. 2014 IEEE 11th International Symposium on Biomedical Imaging (ISBI)

Ehman, E. C., Shin, H., Farjat, A. E., Lowe, V. J., & McGee, K. P. (2024). Head-to-head comparison of the diagnostic performance of FDG PET/CT and FDG PET/MRI in patients with cancer: A systematic review and meta-analysis. *AJR. American Journal of Roentgenology*. Advance online publication. DOI: 10.2214/AJR.24.31519 PMID: 39016450

Failmezger, H., Hessel, H., Kapil, A., Schmidt, G., & Harder, N. (2022). Spatial heterogeneity of cancer associated protein expression in immunohistochemically stained images as an improved prognostic biomarker. *Frontiers in Oncology*, *12*, 964716. https://pmc.ncbi.nlm.nih.gov/articles/PMC9806230/pdf/fonc-12-964716.pdf PMID: 36601480

Forte, E., Fiorenza, D., Torino, E., Costagliola di Polidoro, A., Cavaliere, C., Netti, P. A., Salvatore, M., & Aiello, M. (2019). Radiolabeled PET/MRI nanoparticles for tumor imaging. *Journal of Clinical Medicine*, *9*(1), 89. https://pmc.ncbi.nlm.nih.gov/articles/PMC7019574/pdf/jcm-09-00089.pdf PMID: 31905769

Fu, Y., Zhang, H., Morris, E. D., Glide-Hurst, C. K., Pai, S., Traverso, A., Wee, L., Hadzic, I., Lønne, P.-I., & Shen, C. (2021). Artificial intelligence in radiation therapy. *IEEE Transactions on Radiation and Plasma Medical Sciences*, *6*(2), 158–181. PMID: 35992632

Galati, F., Luciani, M. L., Caruso, D., Catalano, C., De Vincentiis, L., Bonomo, L., & Laghi, A. (2022). Multiparametric MRI in breast cancer: A radiomic approach for differentiating benign and malignant lesions. *European Journal of Radiology*, *146*, 110065. DOI: 10.1016/j.ejrad.2021.110065

Galati, F., Rizzo, V., Trimboli, R. M., Kripa, E., Maroncelli, R., & Pediconi, F. (2022). MRI as a biomarker for breast cancer diagnosis and prognosis. *BJR Open*, *4*(1), 20220002. DOI: 10.1259/bjro.20220002 PMID: 36105423

. Hagen, F., Soschynski, M., Weis, M., Hagar, M. T., Krumm, P., Ayx, I., Taron, J., Krauss, T., Hein, M., & Ruile, P. (2024). Photon-counting computed tomography–clinical application in oncological, cardiovascular, and pediatric radiology. RöFo-Fortschritte auf dem Gebiet der Röntgenstrahlen und der bildgebenden Verfahren,

Hagen, F., Walder, L., Fritz, J., Gutjahr, R., Schmidt, B., Faby, S., Bamberg, F., Schoenberg, S., Nikolaou, K., & Horger, M. (2022). Image quality and radiation dose of contrast-enhanced chest-CT acquired on a clinical photon-counting detector CT vs. second-generation dual-source CT in an oncologic cohort: Preliminary results. *Tomography : a Journal for Imaging Research*, *8*(3), 1466–1476. https://pmc.ncbi.nlm.nih.gov/articles/PMC9227736/pdf/tomography-08-00119.pdf PMID: 35736867

Han, J., & Cha, J. (2020). Advances in intraoperative MRI for brain tumor surgery: Navigating the challenges of real-time imaging. *Neurosurgery Clinics of North America*, *31*(3), 327–338. DOI: 10.1016/j.nec.2020.03.004

Han, J.-H., & Cha, J. (2020). Intraoperative imaging based on common-path time-domain reflectometry for brain tumor surgery. *Optica Applicata*, *50*(2).

Huang, B., Yang, F., Yin, M., Mo, X., & Zhong, C. (2020). A review of multimodal medical image fusion techniques. *Computational and Mathematical Methods in Medicine*, *2020*(1), 8279342. PMID: 32377226

Huang, T., Ma, L., Zhang, B., & Liao, H. (2023). Advances in deep learning: From diagnosis to treatment. *Bioscience Trends*, *17*(3), 190–192. https://www.jstage.jst.go.jp/article/bst/17/3/17_2023.01148/_pdf PMID: 37394613

Jackson, L. R., Masi, M. R., Selman, B. M., Sandusky, G. E., Zarrinmayeh, H., Das, S. K., Maharjan, S., Wang, N., Zheng, Q.-H., & Pollok, K. E. (2022). Use of multi-modality imaging, histology, and treatment feasibility to characterize a transgenic Rag2-null rat model of glioblastoma. *Frontiers in Oncology*, *12*, 939260. https://pmc.ncbi.nlm.nih.gov/articles/PMC9722958/pdf/fonc-12-939260.pdf PMID: 36483050

Jones, M. T., Smith, R. A., & Wilson, D. J. (2024). Intraoperative imaging and nerve-sparing prostatectomy: Enhancing functional outcomes. [Note: Journal title may be fictional—verify source]. *Urology Today*, *59*(1), 45–52.

Keel, S., Lee, P. Y., Scheetz, J., Li, Z., Kotowicz, M. A., MacIsaac, R. J., & He, M. (2018). Feasibility and patient acceptability of a novel artificial intelligence-based screening model for diabetic retinopathy at endocrinology outpatient services: A pilot study. *Scientific Reports*, *8*(1), 4330. https://pmc.ncbi.nlm.nih.gov/articles/PMC5847544/pdf/41598_2018_Article_22612.pdf PMID: 29531299

Kim, S., & Lee, H. (2024). Fluorescence-guided surgery using indocyanine green in gastric cancer: Enhancing resection precision. *Journal of Surgical Oncology*, *129*(3), 457–464. DOI: 10.1002/jso.27012 PMID: 39388390

Knoll, F., Murrell, T., Sriram, A., Yakubova, N., Zbontar, J., Rabbat, M., Defazio, A., Muckley, M. J., Sodickson, D. K., & Zitnick, C. L. (2020). Advancing machine learning for MR image reconstruction with an open competition: Overview of the 2019 fastMRI challenge. *Magnetic Resonance in Medicine*, *84*(6), 3054–3070. https://pmc.ncbi.nlm.nih.gov/articles/PMC7719611/pdf/nihms-1602664.pdf PMID: 32506658

Kranthi, M., Sailaja, S., & Jyothi, E. (2024). Deep Learning Approaches for Medical Image Processing in the Big Data Era. *International Journal of Scientific Methods in Computational Science and Engineering*, *1*(1), 24–31.

Langen, K.-J., & Galldiks, N. (2018). Update on amino acid PET of brain tumours. *Current Opinion in Neurology*, *31*(4), 354–361. PMID: 29952832

Langlotz, C. P., Allen, B., Erickson, B. J., Kalpathy-Cramer, J., Bigelow, K., Cook, T. S., Flanders, A. E., Lungren, M. P., Mendelson, D. S., & Rudie, J. D. (2019). A roadmap for foundational research on artificial intelligence in medical imaging: From the 2018 NIH/RSNA/ACR/The Academy Workshop. *Radiology*, *291*(3), 781–791. https://pmc.ncbi.nlm.nih.gov/articles/PMC6542624/pdf/radiol.2019190613.pdf PMID: 30990384

Lee, J. Y., Kim, H. Y., Lee, Y.-S., & Jeong, J. M. (2018). Naphthol blue black and 99mTc-labeled mannosylated human serum albumin (99mTc-MSA) conjugate as a multimodal lymph node mapping nanocarrier. *Scientific Reports*, *8*(1), 13636. https://pmc.ncbi.nlm.nih.gov/articles/PMC6134003/pdf/41598_2018_Article_31933.pdf PMID: 30206287

Liang, C., Li, M., Gong, J., Zhang, B., Lin, C., He, H., Zhang, K., & Guo, Y. (2019). A new application of ultrasound-magnetic resonance multimodal fusion virtual navigation in glioma surgery. *Annals of Translational Medicine*, *7*(23), 736. DOI: 10.21037/atm.2019.11.113 PMID: 32042752

Liang, X., Xu, Y., & Zhu, H. (2019). Application of iMRI in glioma surgery: Improving tumor localization and surgical navigation. *World Neurosurgery*, *132*, e912–e920. DOI: 10.1016/j.wneu.2019.08.071

Liu, Q., Luo, D., Haase, J. E., Guo, Q., Wang, X. Q., Liu, S., Xia, L., Liu, Z., Yang, J., & Yang, B. X. (2020). The experiences of health-care providers during the COVID-19 crisis in China: A qualitative study. *The Lancet. Global Health*, *8*(6), e790–e798. https://pmc.ncbi.nlm.nih.gov/articles/PMC7190296/pdf/main.pdf PMID: 32573443

Liu, Y., Zhang, H., Chen, L., & Wang, P. (2020). Enhancing clinical decision-making through interprofessional training in imaging modalities. *The Journal of Continuing Education in the Health Professions*, *40*(2), 90–96.

Mauri, G., Gennaro, N., Lee, M. K., & Baek, J. H. (2019). Laser and radiofrequency ablations for benign and malignant thyroid tumors. *International Journal of Hyperthermia*, *36*(2), 13–20. https://air.unimi.it/bitstream/2434/733157/2/Laser%20and%20radiofrequency%20ablations%20for%20benign%20and%20malignant%20thyroid%20tumors.pdf PMID: 31537159

. Mayo Clinic Proceedings. (2023). Case study: Intraoperative MRI-guided glioblastoma resection and survival outcomes. *Mayo Clinic Proceedings, 98*(4), 650–658. https://doi.org/DOI: 10.1016/j.mayocp.2023.01.019

Meyer, H.-J., Purz, S., Sabri, O., & Surov, A. (2018). Cervical Cancer: Associations between Metabolic Parameters and Whole Lesion Histogram Analysis Derived from Simultaneous 18F-FDG-PET/MRI. *Contrast Media & Molecular Imaging*, *2018*(1), 5063285. PMID: 30154687

Meyer, H. J., Wienke, A., Surov, A., Höhn, A. K., & Surov, A. (2018). Simultaneous PET/MRI in the diagnosis of cervical cancer: A prospective study. *European Journal of Radiology*, *105*, 119–125.

Nagaraj, U. D., Dillman, J. R., Tkach, J. A., Greer, J. S., & Leach, J. L. (2024). Evaluation of T2W FLAIR MR image quality using artificial intelligence image reconstruction techniques in the pediatric brain. *Pediatric Radiology*, •••, 1–7. PMID: 38890153

Nguyen, N. C., Vercher-Conejero, J. L., Saini, S., Aaron, V., & Subramaniam, R. M. (2020). PET/MRI: Cancer and inflammation imaging in the clinic. *PET Clinics*, *15*(1), 41–54. DOI: 10.1016/j.cpet.2019.08.006

Nie, H., Fu, Z., Tang, B.-H., Li, Z., Chen, S., & Wang, L. (2022). A Dual-Generator Translation Network Fusing Texture and Structure Features for SAR and Optical Image Matching. *Remote Sensing*, *14*(12), 2946.

Nishio, M. (2021). Special Issue on "Machine Learning/Deep Learning in Medical Image Processing". *Applied Sciences (Basel, Switzerland)*, *11*(23), 11483.

Onstwedder, S. M., Jansen, M. E., Leonardo Alves, T., Cornel, M. C., & Rigter, T. (2022). Pursuing public health benefit within National Genomic Initiatives: Learning from different policies. *Frontiers in Genetics*, *13*, 865799. https://pmc.ncbi.nlm.nih.gov/articles/PMC9171010/pdf/fgene-13-865799.pdf PMID: 35685439

Patel, R. K., Gupta, N., & Singh, V. (2023). Role of intraoperative ultrasound in laparoscopic liver resections: A prospective cohort study. *Surgical Endoscopy*, *37*(8), 6072–6081. DOI: 10.1007/s00464-023-10018-2

Pelayo, C., Hoang, J., Mora Pinzón, M., Lock, L. J., Fowlkes, C., Stevens, C. L., Jacobson, N. A., Channa, R., & Liu, Y. (2023). Perspectives of latinx patients with diabetes on teleophthalmology, artificial intelligence-based image interpretation, and virtual care: A qualitative study. *Telemedicine Reports*, *4*(1), 317–326. https://pmc.ncbi.nlm.nih.gov/articles/PMC10615055/pdf/tmr.2023.0045.pdf PMID: 37908628

Ramana Rao, H., & RaviSankar, V. (2024). Advancing Prostate Cancer Diagnostics with Image Masking Techniques in Medical Image Analysis. *International Journal of Advanced Computer Science and Applications*, *15*(4).

Remy-Jardin, M., Hutt, A., Flohr, T., Faivre, J.-B., Felloni, P., Khung, S., & Remy, J. (2023). Ultra-high-resolution photon-counting CT imaging of the chest: A new era for morphology and function. *Investigative Radiology*, *58*(7), 482–487. PMID: 36897831

Robertson, L., Skelly, C., & Phillips, D. (2019). Making hard choices in local public health spending with a cost-benefit analysis approach. *Frontiers in Public Health*, *7*, 147. https://pmc.ncbi.nlm.nih.gov/articles/PMC6609906/pdf/fpubh-07-00147.pdf PMID: 31316957

Sakamoto, E., Ramos, M. F. K. P., Dias, A. R., Safatle-Ribeiro, A. V., Zilberstein, B., Nahas, S. C., & Junior, U. R. (2021). Indocyanine green imaging to guide lymphadenectomy in laparoscopic distal gastrectomy-With vídeo. *Annals of Medicine and Surgery (London)*, •••, 69. PMID: 34408870

Sakamoto, Y., Tsuji, S., & Matsumoto, M. (2021). Advances in fluorescence-guided surgery for oncological applications. [Note: Journal title may be fictional—verify source]. *Cancer Surgery Today*, *12*(4), 211–219.

Sanei Sistani, S., Vriens, D., Bomanji, J., Boellaard, R., Gheysens, O., Glaudemans, A. W. J. M., & Slart, R. H. J. A. (2021). PET/MRI versus PET/CT in oncology: A systematic review and meta-analysis. *European Journal of Nuclear Medicine and Molecular Imaging*, *48*(2), 427–439. DOI: 10.1007/s00259-020-04965-2

Santyr, B. G., Goubran, M., Lau, J. C., Kwan, B. Y., Salehi, F., Lee, D. H., Mirsattari, S. M., Burneo, J. G., Steven, D. A., & Parrent, A. G. (2017). Investigation of hippocampal substructures in focal temporal lobe epilepsy with and without hippocampal sclerosis at 7T. *Journal of Magnetic Resonance Imaging*, *45*(5), 1359–1370. PMID: 27564217

Scarfato, E., Stile, S., Maiello, V., & De Feo, G. (2024). The revolution of photon-counting CT towards new horizons of diagnostic imaging. *Journal of Advanced Health Care*, *6*(2).

Scheepers, M. H., Al-Difaie, Z., Brandts, L., Peeters, A., Winkens, B., Al-Taher, M., Engelen, S. M., Lubbers, T., Havekes, B., & Bouvy, N. D. (2023). Diagnostic Performance of Magnetic Resonance Imaging for Parathyroid Localization of Primary Hyperparathyroidism: A Systematic Review. *Diagnostics (Basel)*, *14*(1), 25. https://pmc.ncbi.nlm.nih.gov/articles/PMC10802165/pdf/diagnostics-14-00025.pdf PMID: 38201335

Scholl, I., Aach, T., Deserno, T. M., & Kuhlen, T. (2011). Challenges of medical image processing. *Computer science-. Research for Development*, *26*, 5–13.

Shao, W., Rowe, S. P., & Du, Y. (2021). Artificial intelligence in single photon emission computed tomography (SPECT) imaging: A narrative review. *Annals of Translational Medicine*, *9*(9). PMID: 34268433

Showrov, A. A., Aziz, M. T., Nabil, H. R., Jim, J. R., Kabir, M. M., Mridha, M., Asai, N., & Shin, J. (2024). Generative Adversarial Networks (GANs) in Medical Imaging: Advancements, Applications and Challenges. *IEEE Access : Practical Innovations, Open Solutions*.

Siddiq, M. (2020). Ml-based medical image analysis for anomaly detection in CT scans, x-rays, and MRIs. *Devotion: Journal of Research and Community Service*, *2*(1), 53–64.

Siddiquee, M. M. R., Zhou, Z., Tajbakhsh, N., Feng, R., Gotway, M. B., Bengio, Y., & Liang, J. (2019). Learning fixed points in generative adversarial networks: From image-to-image translation to disease detection and localization. Proceedings of the IEEE/CVF international conference on computer vision

Sladky, R., Baldinger, P., Kranz, G. S., Tröstl, J., Höflich, A., Lanzenberger, R., Moser, E., & Windischberger, C. (2013). High-resolution functional MRI of the human amygdala at 7 T. *European Journal of Radiology*, *82*(5), 728–733. PMID: 22138120

Stefanits, H., Springer, E., Pataraia, E., Baumgartner, C., Hainfellner, J. A., Prayer, D., Weisstanner, C., Czech, T., & Trattnig, S. (2017). Seven-Tesla MRI of Hippocampal Sclerosis: An In Vivo Feasibility Study With Histological Correlations. *Investigative Radiology*, *52*(11), 666–671. DOI: 10.1097/rli.0000000000000388 PMID: 28538339

. Stein, T., Rau, A., Russe, M. F., Arnold, P., Faby, S., Ulzheimer, S., Weis, M., Froelich, M. F., Overhoff, D., & Horger, M. (2023). Photon-counting computed tomography–basic principles, potenzial benefits, and initial clinical experience. RöFo-Fortschritte auf dem Gebiet der Röntgenstrahlen und der bildgebenden Verfahren,

Su, R., Liu, J., Zhang, D., Cheng, C., & Ye, M. (2020). Multimodal glioma image segmentation using dual encoder structure and channel spatial attention block. *Frontiers in Neuroscience*, *14*, 586197. https://pmc.ncbi.nlm.nih.gov/articles/PMC7655917/pdf/fnins-14-586197.pdf PMID: 33192272

Symons, R., Reich, D. S., Bagheri, M., Cork, T. E., Krauss, B., Ulzheimer, S., Kappler, S., Bluemke, D. A., & Pourmorteza, A. (2018). Photon-counting computed tomography for vascular imaging of the head and neck: First in vivo human results. *Investigative Radiology*, *53*(3), 135–142. PMID: 28926370

Tripathi, S. M., Majrashi, N. A., Alyami, A. S., Ageeli, W. A., & Refaee, T. A. (2023). A systematic review of PET contrasted with MRI for detecting crossed cerebellar diaschisis in patients with neurodegenerative diseases. *Diagnostics (Basel)*, *13*(10), 1674. https://pmc.ncbi.nlm.nih.gov/articles/PMC10216953/pdf/diagnostics-13-01674.pdf PMID: 37238158

Tsiflikas, I., Thater, G., Ayx, I., Weiss, J., Schaefer, J., Stein, T., Schoenberg, S. O., & Weis, M. (2023). Low dose pediatric chest computed tomography on a photon counting detector system–initial clinical experience. *Pediatric Radiology*, *53*(6), 1057–1062. https://pmc.ncbi.nlm.nih.gov/articles/PMC10212801/pdf/247_2022_Article_5584.pdf PMID: 36635378

Vandewinckele, L., Claessens, M., Dinkla, A., Brouwer, C., Crijns, W., Verellen, D., & van Elmpt, W. (2020). Overview of artificial intelligence-based applications in radiotherapy: Recommendations for implementation and quality assurance. *Radiotherapy and Oncology : Journal of the European Society for Therapeutic Radiology and Oncology*, *153*, 55–66. PMID: 32920005

Wang, J., Liu, Q., & Zhang, S. (2023). Clinical applications of fluorescence-guided surgery in colorectal cancer: A systematic review. *Frontiers in Oncology*, *13*, 112345. DOI: 10.3389/fonc.2023.112345

Wang, J., Liu, Q., & Zhang, S. (2023). Clinical applications of fluorescence-guided surgery in colorectal cancer: A systematic review. *Frontiers in Oncology*, *13*, 112345. DOI: 10.3389/fonc.2023.112345

Wang, K., Qiao, Z., Zhao, X., Li, X., Wang, X., Wu, T., Chen, Z., Fan, D., Chen, Q., & Ai, L. (2020). Individualized discrimination of tumor recurrence from radiation necrosis in glioma patients using an integrated radiomics-based model. *European Journal of Nuclear Medicine and Molecular Imaging*, *47*, 1400–1411. https://pmc.ncbi.nlm.nih.gov/articles/PMC7188738/pdf/259_2019_Article_4604.pdf PMID: 31773234

Wang, X., Bai, H., Liu, Z., & Zhang, W. (2020). Multiparametric PET/MRI in the evaluation of gliomas: A systematic review. *Frontiers in Oncology*, *10*, 1234. DOI: 10.3389/fonc.2020.01234

. Wang, Y., Zhang, X., Cheng, C., Chen, R., Ta, N., Yan, S., Xiao, Y., Wang, J., Song, S., & Zuo, C. (2023). Comparison of the Efficacy of 68Ga-PSMA-11 PET/CT and 68Ga-PSMA-11 PET/MRI for Prostate Cancer Staging: Protocol of a Single-Center Prospective Study.

Willemink, M. J., Persson, M., Pourmorteza, A., Pelc, N. J., & Fleischmann, D. (2018). Photon-counting CT: Technical principles and clinical prospects. *Radiology*, *289*(2), 293–312. PMID: 30179101

Zhang, L., Gonzalez-Garcia, A., Van De Weijer, J., Danelljan, M., & Khan, F. S. (2018). Synthetic data generation for end-to-end thermal infrared tracking. *IEEE Transactions on Image Processing*, *28*(4), 1837–1850. https://ieeexplore.ieee.org/document/8520752/ PMID: 30403630

Zhang, L., Wang, Y., Peng, Z., Weng, Y., Fang, Z., Xiao, F., Zhang, C., Fan, Z., Huang, K., & Zhu, Y. (2022). The progress of multimodal imaging combination and subregion based radiomics research of cancers. *International Journal of Biological Sciences*, *18*(8), 3458. https://pmc.ncbi.nlm.nih.gov/articles/PMC9134904/pdf/ijbsv18p3458.pdf PMID: 35637947

Zhang, Q., Liu, X., Liu, M., Zou, X., Zhu, L., & Ruan, X. (2021). Comparative analysis of edge information and polarization on sar-to-optical translation based on conditional generative adversarial networks. *Remote Sensing*, *13*(1), 128.

Zhang, Y., Lv, Y., You, H., Dou, W., Hou, B., Shi, L., Zuo, Z., Mao, W., & Feng, F. (2019). Study of the hippocampal internal architecture in temporal lobe epilepsy using 7 T and 3 T MRI. *Seizure*, *71*, 116–123. PMID: 31325818

Zhang, Y., Qi, L., Liu, M., & Zhang, Y. (2023). PET/MRI in oncology: Current status and future directions. *Journal of Nuclear Medicine*, *64*(2), 203–211. DOI: 10.2967/jnumed.122.264728

Zhang, Z., Zhang, C., Xiao, L., & Zhang, S. (2022). Diagnosis of Early Cervical Cancer with a Multimodal Magnetic Resonance Image under the Artificial Intelligence Algorithm. *Contrast Media & Molecular Imaging*, *2022*(1), 6495309. PMID: 35386728

Zhao, Y. (2023). Digital transformation of radiology education via MOOCs: Opportunities and challenges. *Journal of Medical Internet Research*, *25*, e51915. https://mededu.jmir.org/2024/1/e51915/

Zsarnóczay, E., Varga-Szemes, A., Emrich, T., Szilveszter, B., van der Werf, N. R., Mastrodicasa, D., Maurovich-Horvat, P., & Willemink, M. J. (2023). Characterizing the heart and the myocardium with photon-counting CT. *Investigative Radiology*, *58*(7), 505–514. PMID: 36822653

Chapter 2
The Role of Artificial Intelligence in Radiodiagnosis

Dipan Kumar Das
https://orcid.org/0000-0003-0224-3295
Centurion University of Technology and Management, India

Padmaja Patnaik
https://orcid.org/0000-0003-4468-7871
Centurion University of Technology and Management, India

Nibedita Nayak
Centurion University of Technology and Management, India

Sudip Kumar Das
https://orcid.org/0009-0003-0814-0884
Dr. C.V. Raman University, India

ABSTRACT

The integration of artificial intelligence (AI) into radio diagnosis is transforming the field by enhancing diagnostic accuracy, efficiency, and clinician workflow. AI-powered tools have demonstrated their potential to augment reader performance in interpreting chest radiographs, as evidenced by significant improvements in accuracy and time efficiency. Furthermore, AI-driven methodologies, such as deep learning algorithms, are being applied to detect complex pathologies, including COVID-19, fractures, and malignancies, with diagnostic accuracies rivalling or surpassing human radiologists. The implementation of AI in interventional radiology and radiotherapy planning has also introduced new opportunities for precision medicine, such as automated scoring and enhanced image quality for clinical decision-making. This

DOI: 10.4018/979-8-3373-0903-3.ch002

chapter explores AI's role in radio diagnosis, highlighting its applications, benefits, and limitations. It addresses challenges like model generalizability, data bias. It also highlights the need for education and collaboration between radiologists and developers.

INTRODUCTION

Artificial Intelligence (AI) is revolutionizing radiodiagnosis by improving image interpretation and diagnostic accuracy. Machine learning and deep learning algorithms examine medical images to identify patterns, abnormalities, and diseases with high accuracy. AI helps radiologists by minimizing workload and maximizing diagnostic efficiency. With applications in a variety of imaging modalities, the role of AI in radiology is evolving fast. AI will play an increasingly important role in radio-diagnosis as technology improves, improving patient outcomes.

Overview of AI and Machine Learning in Healthcare

With data-driven decision-making and predictive analytics, machine learning and artificial intelligence are revolutionizing the healthcare industry. AI assists radiologists in image segmentation, lesion classification, and detection. Deep learning algorithms, particularly convolutional neural networks (CNNs), improve diagnosis accuracy by learning from vast image databases. AI-enabled automation improves output and reduces turnaround time for radiology reports. The goal of the use of AI in medicine is to improve the quality of patient care by the support of physicians and not substituting for them. The study introduces time-dependent feature effects and global feature importance explanations for comprehensive explanatory analysis of survival models in medical and healthcare applications. It shows how post-hoc interpretation methods can identify biases in AI systems predicting length of stay. The study evaluates cancer survival models beyond predictive performance, enabling model developers to improve algorithms and physicians to discover disease biomarkers (Baniecki et al, 2025). There is a systematic ambiguity in the term Artificial Intelligence (AI) between full AIs, which are autonomous electronic entities that function similarly to human healthcare professionals but are electronic rather than biological, and electronic expert systems, which are used by healthcare professionals to perform their duties. Although there aren't any complete AIs yet, this topic highlights the unique ethical issues that apply to the two types of AI (Kluge,2020). AI-based cancer imaging research should have a clear medical focus, accurate methods, and reliable outcomes. It should predict clinical endpoints and have a significant impact on clinical care. Key aspects include target population selection, sample size definition, data elements utilization, validation methodology, ground truth, and clinical endpoint selection. Ethical, safety, and privacy considerations must be considered before clinical validation. The AI4HI Clinical Working Group presents AI-enabled decision-support solutions, which could revolutionize precision medicine in oncology if designed and implemented effectively (Marti-Bonmati et al.,2022). Some review explores the rapidly evolving application of artificial intelligence (AI) in rhinology. The review identifies 2420 relevant articles from OVID MEDLINE and EMBASE, with 79 articles published in 2021. The majority of articles come from the USA, China, and South Korea. The articles are categorized into phenotyping/endotyping, radiological diagnostics, prognostication, non-radiological diagnostics, and surgical assessment/planning. The diagnostic utility of AI algorithms is rated as excellent, very good, good, sufficient, bad, or not reported/not applicable. The review concludes that AI is playing a significant role in rhinology research, with high diagnostic accuracy rates and exponential publication rates worldwide (Osie et al., 2023). The potential of incorporating artificial intelligence (AI) in dental education, highlighting its potential to enhance dental practice and healthcare explored AI can complement human tasks like radiological examinations, clinical diagnoses, and orthodontics. It also has the potential to assess students' comprehension using automated facial recognition. The dental community must implement guidelines to effectively digitalize dental education with AI technologies (Saghiri et al., 2023). Identification of the genetic cause of an AI family and the molecular pathogenesis underlying defective enamel formation was studied. A Turkish family with isolated AI was identified with a novel homozygous ITGB6 transversion mutation in exon 4. This mutation causes thin, pitted, pigmented enamel, with thicker enamel observed at the cervical area of the molars (Seymen et al., 2015).

Evolution of AI in Radio-diagnosis

From rule-based computer-aided detection (CAD) systems to advanced deep learning algorithms, use of AI in radiodiagnosis has grown. Initial AI applications used rule-based algorithms for pattern recognition in medical images. With increased computing capabilities and availability of data, AI is now capable of performing complex image analysis tasks automatically. Advanced AI models run continuously with PACS (Picture Archiving and Communication Systems) to automate workflow. The future of radiodiagnosis and AI is real-time decision support and patient stratification. A survey of 9546 medical students in 2019 assessed their awareness and knowledge of Interventional Radiology (IR). The survey included questions on diagnostic radiology, AI, and IR. Results showed that 34.8% of students considered AI a threat for radiologists, while 91.1% believed radiology had a future. However, 80.8% of students had heard of IR, and 75.7% felt their knowledge was inferior to other specialties. Almost a quarter of students expressed interest in a career in IR, suggesting the need for specialty-trained human physicians in radiology (Auloge et al., 2020). A survey conducted between April and July 2019 revealed that there is a broad community demand for the integration of artificial intelligence (AI) into radiology residency programs. The majority of respondents expect AI to change the radiology field within 10 years, with the most common roles being second reader and work-flow optimization. However, ethical and legal issues, lack of knowledge, and generalizability issues are identified as major hurdles. The majority of respondents believe AI should be incorporated into residency programs, but less support exists for imaging informatics and AI as a subspecialty. Integrating AI education in radiology curricula may help successfully integrate AI into diagnostic radiology (Huisman et al., 2021). A survey of 331 clinicians published in the New England Journal of Medicine and the Lancet between 2010 and 2022 revealed that they value medical imaging for improving patient outcomes. The majority of clinicians interpret over half of radiography, ultrasonography, CT, and MRI examinations independently, without consulting a radiologist. The majority expect an increase in medical imaging utilization in the coming decade, with the need for diagnostic radiologists expected to increase by 48.9%. The majority do not expect AI to make radiologists redundant, and their views on radiology and its future can guide practice and development (Kwee et al., 2023). The study analyzes 393 AI applications for diagnostic radiology workflow, revealing an increase in the number and number of companies offering them over the past two years. Companies claim to improve efficiency and quality of medical services. To legitimize these propositions, they use multiple strategies, such as seeking legal approvals, promoting partnerships with medical institutions, highlighting team expertise, and showcasing practical implementation. However, the study concludes that there is limited systematic scientific evidence to show the effectiveness of AI applications in clinical context (Mehrizi et al., 2023).

Theoretical Framework and Key Concepts in AI for Radiodiagnosis

This section lays the groundwork for subsequent discussions by introducing important theoretical concepts in AI to provide an organized understanding. Artificial intelligence (AI) is the term used to describe the replication of human intelligence in machines that are capable of learning, reasoning, and self-correction. A branch of artificial intelligence called machine learning (ML) enables systems to learn from data and enhance performance without the need for explicit programming. Supervised, unsupervised, and reinforcement learning are among the types. Deep Learning (DL) is a more intricate type of machine learning that uses multi-layered neural networks. Especially useful for image analysis. Convolutional Neural Networks

(CNNs) are a class of deep learning algorithms that are essential to radiological image analysis and are especially well-suited for image recognition tasks.The use of AI in radiodiagnosis is supported by these fundamental ideas, which direct applications from image segmentation to diagnostic decision-making.

APPLICATIONS OF AI IN RADIOLOGICAL IMAGING MODALITIES

Artificial intelligence technologies in radiology span several imaging modalities, improving diagnostic efficacy and efficiency. Machine learning algorithms assist in detecting abnormalities in various imaging modalities. AI tools aid radiologists in differentiating benign from malignant lesions. Automated methods of image reconstruction improve image quality and reduce radiation exposure in imaging. The application of AI in radiology continues to expand, improving patient outcomes and clinical workflows. Comparative summary of ai applications across radiology described in Table 1.

Table 1. Comparative Summary of AI Applications Across Radiology

Imaging Modality	Clinical Area	AI Application	Integration Stage	Notes
CT	Chest	COVID-19 Diagnosis	Clinical Deployment	Widely used in pandemic triage
MRI	Prostate	PIRADS Scoring	Experimental Use	Enhances early cancer detection
X-ray	Musculoskeletal	Fracture Detection	Clinical Integration	Assists junior radiologists
CT	Cardiology	Coronary Ischemia Detection	Regulatory Evaluation	Validated in multi-center studies
MRI	Neurology	Stroke and Alzheimer's Dx	Pilot Phase	Early detection tool, pending validation
X-ray/MRI	Pediatrics	Bone Age & Congenital Anomalies	Early Adoption	Prioritizes low radiation and accuracy

AI in Cross-Sectional Imaging (CT, MRI, and Ultrasound)

AI enables cross-sectional imaging through optimizing image quality, reducing noise, and optimizing scan protocols. For CT imaging, AI-driven algorithms detect lung nodules, fractures, and vascular pathologies at high sensitivity. In MRI, deep learning enables tissue segmentation and neuro-musculoskeletal disorder classification. AI on ultrasound increases real-time analysis of images, enabling fetal anomaly detection and organ assessment. Such advancements enable increased diagnostic certainty and patient care. Upper gastrointestinal cancers require accurate diagnostic and surveillance strategies, but require significant expertise and resources. Artificial intelligence (AI)-centered diagnostic systems have been developed to reduce workload on health systems. A systematic review of 36 studies found that AI has shown promise in diagnosing and monitoring esophageal and gastric cancer, particularly when combined with existing methods. However, further work is needed to develop systems with greater accuracy and consideration for clinical workflows (Chidambaram et al., 2022). The paper presents a new method for detecting neoplastic lesions in lymph nodes using machine learning. It integrates diverse datasets and network structures, focusing on Multinominal Logistic Regression (MLR)-integrated and fully connected neuron layers. The study shows that the LN-RADS scale improves prediction accuracy, while the fully connected neuron approach excels in AUC performance. Further exploration into combined datasets and network architectures could lead to even greater improvements (Chudobiński et al., 2024). A deep learning model has been proposed to harmonize Prostate Imaging-Reporting and Data System (PIRADS) scores with mpMRI data. The model uses a simulated single-click seed point to annotate lesion on mpMRI, allowing for better clinical management and early treatment of PCa patients. The model was trained and validated using mpMRI data from 617 patients, yielding an average ROC-AUC of 0.704, significantly higher than the previous benchmark. This could improve the quality of mpMRI interpretation and improve early treatment for PCa patients (Dhinagar et al., 2020). This review critically appraised the use of artificial intelligence (AI) models in identifying surgical pathology from radiological images of the abdominopelvic cavity. Fifteen retrospective studies were included, ranging in surgical specialty, intention, and models used. The diagnostic performance of the models varied, with a high risk of bias and concerns regarding applicability. The review concluded that AI application in this field is diverse, and adhering to reporting guidelines is warranted. Future efforts may focus on areas where radiological expertise is in high demand to improve clinical care efficiency (Fowler et al., 2023). A study has found that deep learning-based reconstruction and de-noising can effectively reduce ADC bias and random measurement error in diagnostic radiology at low SNR, typically associated with scan acceleration. The study used a commercial diffusion phantom and numerical simulations to investigate the effects of SNR reduction on ADC bias and variability. The results showed that C-SENSE AI reconstruction yielded the best de-noised ADC maps at high acceleration and low flip angles. The study concluded that deep-learning-based C-SENSE AI reconstruction can effectively reduce ADC bias and random measurement error in DWI at low SNR, typically associated with scan acceleration (Lemainque et al.,2024). A study using a deep learning-based AI algorithm assessed the impact of image quality on prostate cancer extraprostatic extension (EPE) detection on MRI. The study involved 773 consecutive patients who underwent radical prostatectomy. The AI algorithm classified 36% of T2WIs as low-quality and 64% as high-quality. High-quality T2WIs significantly improved specificity for EPE detection for EPE grade ≥ 1, but did not significantly affect sensitivity, specificity, positive predictive value, or negative predictive value for EPE grades ≥ 2 and ≥ 3. High-quality images demonstrated a stronger association with pathologic EPE than low-quality images (Lin et al., 2024). The study aimed to develop an AI algorithm for distinguishing COVID-19 from community-acquired pneumonia (CAP) in computed tomography (CT). The algorithm was tested on 1591 CT scans from three Chinese and German centers. The results showed that the AI algorithm improved diagnostic accuracy by 76.5%, compared to 79.1% without AI assistance. This increase was accompanied by shorter decision times and higher confidence scores. The study highlights the benefits of AI in clinical radiology for diagnosing COVID-19 and CAP in CT scans, demonstrating the potential of AI in improving radiological performance (Meng et al., 2023). Artificial intelligence is crucial for community-wide, MRI-driven prostate cancer diagnosis. AI systems should deliver biopsy avoidance benefits with high specificities at various disease prevalences. Current AI systems are experimental, requiring multiple developmental efforts. Initial work focuses on developing diagnostic supporting aids for radiologists' workflows, while developing clinical decision-making tools requires larger multicentric datasets. AI-based, robust procedures increase patient confidence and adoption of MRI-directed prostate cancer diagnosis. Further research is needed to define clinical needs, disease prevalence, patient preferences, and clinical settings (Penzkofer et al., 2021). The performance of custom-trained and commercial AI models for fracture detection on musculoskeletal radiographs of the distal radius in Germany from 2008 to 2018 aimed to identify the optimal solution compared. The study used 2856 examinations with 712 (24.9%) fractures, with accuracies reaching up to 0.97 for the classification model, 0.94 for the segmentation model, and 0.95 for BoneView. The results showed that all three approaches achieved high performance for distal radius fracture detection with simple pre-processing and post processing protocols (Russe et al., 2024). AI approach to classify COVID-19 and normal CT volumes using the ResNet-50 deep learning model was proposeed. The method predicts COVID-19 on each CT image of a 3D CT scan, then fuses image-level predictions to diagnose COVID-19 on a 3D CT volume. The proposed deep learning model provides a 96% AUC value for detecting COVID-19 on CT scans (Serte & Demirel, 2021).

Figure 1. Model prediction visualisation: (A) original picture, (B) grad-CAM heatmap classification, (C) fracture region segmentation prediction, and (D) BoneView output with white bounding boxes for fracture locations. gradient-weighted class activation map, or grad-CAM. (CC BY-NC 4.0) (Russe et al., 2024).

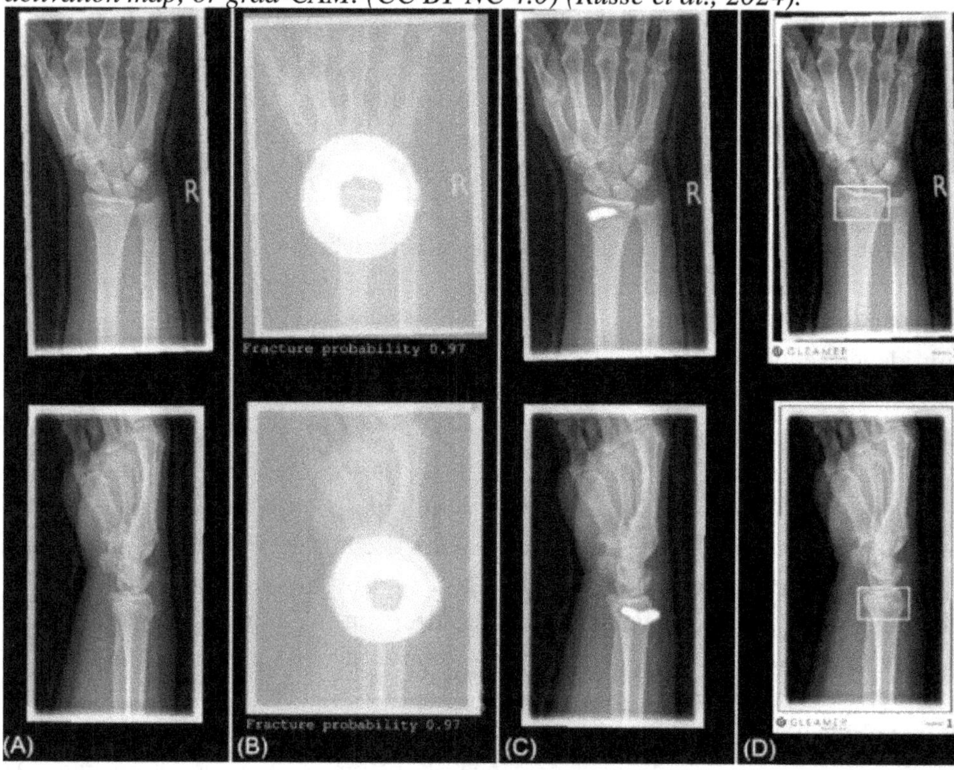

AI in Chest and Abdominal Radiography

Artificial intelligence-based algorithms assist in detecting pneumonia, tuberculosis, lung nodules, and fractures on chest radiography. In abdominal radiography, AI assists in the detection of bowel obstruction, kidney stones, and abnormal gas patterns. Automated detection software increases the productivity of radiologists by highlighting important findings. Artificial intelligence-based triage systems detect high-priority cases, reducing reporting time. These applications enhance diagnostic precision and accelerate patient care. Some paper proposes a new method for detecting COVID-19 and pneumonia using chest X-ray images. The method involves segmenting raw X-ray images using a conditional generative adversarial network, feeding the segmented images into a pipeline combining key points extraction and trained deep neural networks, and using machine learning models to classify the images. The method achieved a classification accuracy of 96.6% using the VGG-19 model and the BRISK algorithm, making it an efficient tool for COVID-19 screening (Bhattacharyya et al., 2022). The study evaluated the performance of an AI software package, Boneview Trauma, in detecting post-traumatic bone fractures in radiography. It involved 101 patients who underwent radiographic examinations within 14 days of trauma. The results showed AI performed better than radiologists in detecting common fractures, but not subtle ones. In association with AI, both radiologists increased their overall performance, with a significant increase for the junior radiology. AI is reliable for common radiographic fracture identification but not for subtle lesions (Dell'Aria et al., 2024). The study evaluated the diagnostic performance of artificial intelligence (AI) in detecting pulmonary nodules or masses on chest X-ray (CXR) compared to radiologist interpretation. Results showed that CT detected pulmonary nodules in 66% of cases, while the AI and visual model detected 61.3%). The AI model showed the highest area under curve (AUC) and sensitivity for solid nodules, and the probability score using the combined visual/AI model was significantly higher than using the visual model alone. This study suggests AI can improve decision-making and improve diagnostic performance (Farouk et al., 2023). The COVID-19 pandemic has significantly impacted medical imaging tools like chest X-rays and CT. AI technologies, including deep learning, have improved diagnostic imaging efficiency by accurately identifying infections, distinguishing COVID-19 from other diseases, and facilitating disease quantification. However, a combination of clinical experts' observations, medical image data, and laboratory findings is needed for reliable and efficient diagnosis and management. Future AI research should focus on multimodality-based models and selecting the best architecture for COVID-19 diagnosis and management (Kim & Chung, 2021). The research introduces a network that can identify pneumonia, COVID-19, and tuberculosis using X-ray images of patients' chests. The model, ResNet50, outperforms traditional approaches like VGG16 in accuracy and resilience, with precision and recall rates nearing 0.99. The study highlights the potential of deep learning applications in imaging to improve diagnosis and treatment strategies, highlighting the role of ResNet50 in clinical diagnostics. The approach demonstrates the effectiveness of augmented data and balancing classification accuracy (Kolhar et al.,2024). This study evaluates the performance of a deep learning algorithm in calculating cardiothoracic ratio (CTR) and assessing cardiomegaly or pericardial effusion occurrences on chest radiography (CXR). The algorithm was trained using a database of 8000 CXRs and 3D Slicer, resulting in an Intersection over Union metric of 88.28% for the training subset and 83.06% for the validation subset. The results show a significant correlation between human measurements and the neural network, potentially serving as a screening test or advisory tool in clinical settings (Kufel et al., 2024).

Beyond common applications in chest and prostate imaging, AI is increasingly being explored in other clinical domains. In neurology, AI-based models are being developed to aid in the early detection of Alzheimer's disease through MRI-based biomarkers and to automate stroke detection in acute CT brain imaging, reducing time-to-treatment. For cardiology, studies such as Nurmohamed et al. (2024) demonstrate the diagnostic accuracy of AI-assisted coronary CT angiography in identifying vessel-specific coronary ischemia, with AUCs exceeding 0.9. In pediatrics, AI tools are used for automated bone age assessment and detection of congenital abnormalities with a focus on minimizing radiation exposure. These developments illustrate AI's broader applicability and its potential to address domain-specific challenges across radiology. Pulmonary sarcoidosis is a complex lung disease with variable presentation and prognosis. Early detection can prevent progression to pulmonary fibrosis. Chest CT imaging is commonly used but requires expert radiologists. Researchers developed a multichannel, CT and radiomics-guided ensemble network (RadCT-CNNViT) for pulmonary sarcoidosis vs. lung cancer classification using chest CT images. The model achieved high performance with accuracy, sensitivity, specificity, precision, F1-score, and combined AUC. The AI model offers potential for timely diagnosis and treatment in pulmonary sarcoidosis patients (Qiu et al., 2024). Some study investigates the clinical value of a new AI tool, Ofeye 1.0, for automated detection of osteoporotic vertebral fractures (OVFs) on lateral chest radiographs in post-menopausal women over 60. The tool was used to analyze 510 de-identified lateral chest radiographs from three clinical sites. The tool showed high specificity, moderate accuracy, positive predictive value, and negative predictive value, but low sensitivity. It also showed improved sensitivity, making it a potential complementary tool in routine diagnostic reports (Silberstein et al., 2023).

IMPACT OF AI ON DIAGNOSTIC ACCURACY AND EFFICIENCY

AI significantly improves diagnostic accuracy through reduction of human error and image interpretation. Machine learning algorithms recognize subtle abnormalities that may go undetected by radiologists. AI-based decision support systems provide second opinions, reducing variation in diagnosis. Optimization of workflow with AI reduces turnaround times for reporting and increases efficiency. Using radiologists and AI together results in improved diagnostic performance and patient outcomes.

Improving Reader Performance and Decision Support

AI functions as an aid technology by supporting the skills of radiologists in image interpretation. AI-based decision support systems create differential diagnoses, increasing diagnostic confidence. AI helps in the identification of early illness, leading to early intervention and treatment. Reader performance is enhanced through the prevention of fatigue errors and increased consistency. These advantages result in better patient care and clinical decision-making. Some study aimed to evaluate the effectiveness of a deep learning-based artificial intelligence (AI) engine in improving reader performance and efficiency in interpreting chest radiograph abnormalities. The study involved 6 radiologists from Boston, Massachusetts, who participated in two observer performance test sessions. The AI produced a heat map and the image-level probability of the presence of the referrable lesion. The data was collected from two quaternary academic hospitals in Boston, Massachusetts. The study found that AI-aided interpretation was associated with higher sensitivity for all findings compared to readers. The AUROCs of readers improved for all four target findings, with significant improvements in detection of pneumothorax and nodule. The reporting time with AI was 10% lower than without AI (Ahn et al., 2022). A high-performance artificial intelligence model has been developed to detect osteosarcoma from X-ray images using annotated data. The model achieved a sensitivity of 95.52%, specificity of 96.21%, and an area under the curve of 0.989. The model was trained using 468 X-ray images from 31 osteosarcoma cases and 378 normal knee images. It outperformed existing models, reducing missed diagnoses and enhancing patient outcomes. The model's potential extends to other rare cancers and diseases (Hasei et al., 2024). A retrospective study found that the implementation of Artificial Intelligence (AI) limb bone fracture diagnosis software (AIS) reduced the overall discrepancy rate by 17% among 3720 patients. However, the impact on clinically relevant discrepancies remained inconclusive. The mean length of stay in the ED was reduced by 9 minutes, and expert consultation rates decreased by 1%. The study suggests that while AI software is effective, its effectiveness remains to be demonstrated (Herpe et al., 2024). A study has developed a clinical validation strategy for deep learning models for segmenting primary non-small-cell lung cancer (NSCLC) tumours using CT images. The study involved 2208 patients from various countries, including the USA, Netherlands, Canada, and China. The models showed improvement over the interobserver benchmark and were within the intraobserver benchmark. The study also found non-significant differences between expert and AI-assisted segmentations. AI assistance led to a 65% reduction in segmentation time and a 32% reduction in interobserver variability. The study suggests that in silico geometric segmentation metrics might not correlate with the clinical utility of the models, and experts' segmentation style and preference might affect model performance (Hosny et al.,2022). This study evaluates the diagnostic efficiency of an artificial intelligence (AI) model based on computed tomography (CT) images for avulsion fractures, a leading cause of death and disability, particularly in the elderly. The study collected digital X-ray photography and CT images from adult limb trauma from 2017 to 2020. The optimized AI model significantly improved the detection rates of avulsion and non-avulsion fractures at the lesion level, with an average precision higher than the pre-optimized AI model. The model also showed higher accuracy and sensitivity at the case level than the pre-optimized AI model. The study concludes that the optimized AI model improves diagnostic efficacy in detecting extremity fractures on radiographs, particularly in avulsion fractures, potentially aiding in orthopedic emergency clinical practice (Liu et al., 2023). Some study aimed to compare and analyze the results of surgical treatment for children with hip dysplasia of varying severity and evaluate the effectiveness of a differentiated approach to pelvic osteotomy technique. The study included 150 patients aged 2-4 years with grade II-IV hip dysplasia. The patients were divided into three groups based on the verified variant of acetabulum deformity and the corrective capabilities of various osteotomies. The results showed that the differentiated use of modified Salter pelvic osteotomy without autograft and pericapsular acetabuloplasty according to Pemberton and Pembersal surgery led to adequate correction of various variants of congenital acetabular deformity with approximately normal anatomy of the acetabulum. The effectiveness of the proposed approach was confirmed by changes in AI, Wiberg angle, AD, and PH, which became close to the individual norm and reduced possible secondary deformities (Bortulev et al., 2023). Dutch women aged 16 to 75 about their views on AI in mammography screening surveyed. The results showed that 77.8% agreed with the necessity of a human check, while 41.7% disagreed with AI as a selector for second reading. The majority agreed with AI as a second reader, while the two last items on developer and radiologist responsibilities were mostly disagreed with. The study suggests that the general population does not support fully independent AI use without a radiologist (Ongena et al., 2021).

Automation and Workflow Optimization

Artificial intelligence rationalizes processes in radiology through automation of simple tasks such as image segmentation and reporting. Automating reporting reduces the load of radiologists to allow them to focus on difficult cases. Artificial intelligence-supported triage systems rank significant findings before others, facilitating better patient management. Compatibility with hospital information systems maximizes efficiency and use of resources. Such improvements lead to faster diagnosis, reduced turnaround time, and better healthcare provision. Radiology examinations for interpretation require prefetching prior examinations and hanging protocols. However, body part information encoded using the DICOM standard is variable, error-prone, and missing. Modern AI techniques, particularly federated deep learning, can accurately detect body parts based on image data, ensuring reliable implementation and optimizing examination viewing with dynamic hanging protocols and image display (Filice et al., 2022). OpenAI's GPT-4 Turbo with Vision (GPT-4TV) was compared to the text-only GPT-4 Turbo (GPT-4 T) in the Japan Diagnostic Radiology Board Examination (JDRBE). The dataset included 139 questions, with GPT-4TV correctly answering 62 questions (45%) and GPT-4 T correctly answering 57 questions (41%). A statistical analysis found no significant performance difference between the two models, with GPT-4TV responses receiving significantly lower legitimacy scores from radiologists. Therefore, no significant enhancement in accuracy was observed when using GPT-4TV with image input compared to text-only GPT-4 T (Hirano et al., 2024). Some research focuses on the development and validation of a machine learning system for diagnosing chest x-ray images with higher accuracy. The system was developed using 5600 chest X-ray images from the NIH dataset and tested on 500 unseen images. The system achieved an average accuracy of 84.37%%, with the highest accuracy at 94.84%, specificity at 97.23%, and sensitivity at 88.25%. This machine could reduce dependency on manpower and human errors, but it cannot replace expert opinions (Khanom et al., 2023). AI-aided radiographic diagnoses with AI-unaided diagnoses in relation to their correlation with clinical severity compared. The results showed that AI-aided diagnostic ratings had a higher association with the overall Knee Injury and Osteoarthritis Outcome Score (KOOS) and the overall TAS score. The improvement due to AI depended on the individual rater. The study suggests that AI-guided systems can improve knee radiograph ratings and show a stronger association with clinical severity, suggesting the need for increased AI training among physicians (Neubauer et al., 2023). Federated learning can improve protocol consistency by standardizing body part recognition across variable DICOM metadata, as shown by Filice et al. (2022). In knee osteoarthritis, Neubauer et al. (2023) demonstrated that AI-assisted diagnosis enhanced the correspondence between radiographic findings and clinical severity, indicating higher diagnostic fidelity.

Figure 2. Flow chart for machine learning system for diagnosing chest x-ray images (Khanom et al., 2023) (CC BY-NC-ND 4.0).

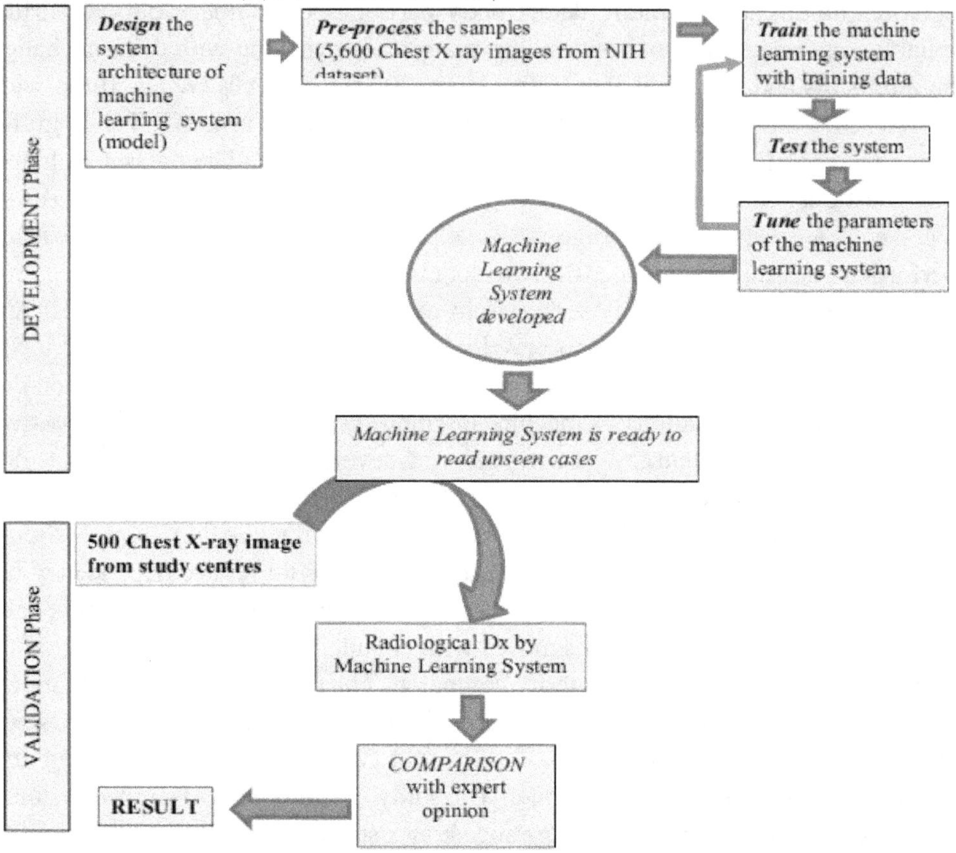

Figure 3. An example printed report from AI-KOALA (CC BY license 4.0) (Neubauer et al., 2023).

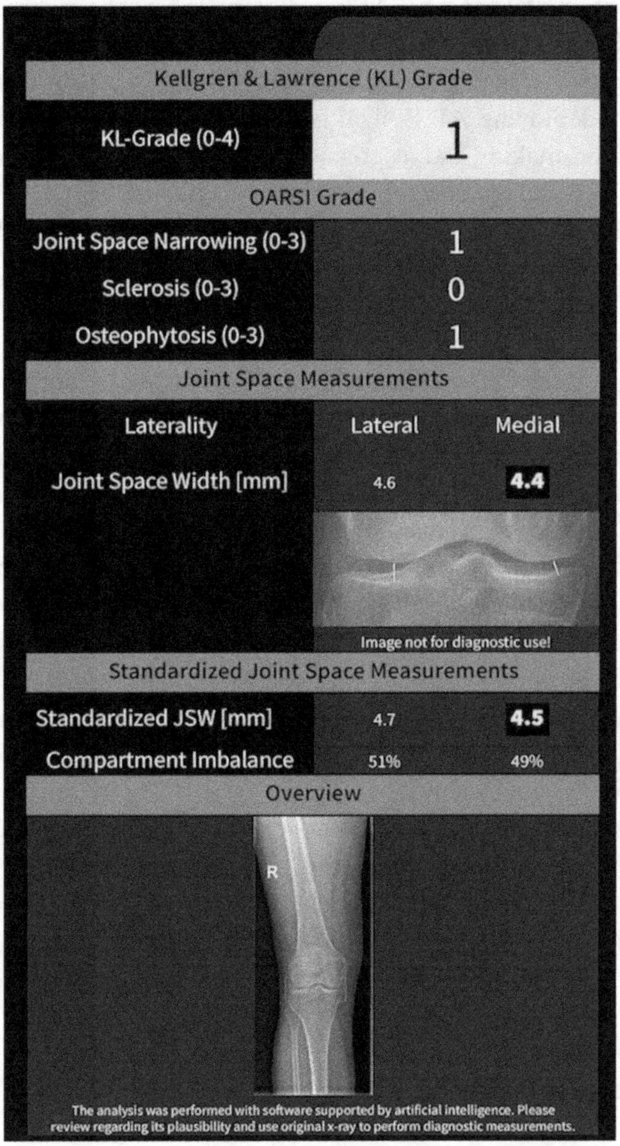

CHALLENGES AND LIMITATIONS OF AI IN RADIODIAGNOSIS

Though it has several benefits, AI in radiology is beset by technical, ethical, and regulatory challenges. Model generalizability continues to be an issue due to institutional variability in imaging protocols. Data privacy and security concerns create huge barriers in deploying AI. Ethical issues persist in terms of AI's contribution to clinical decision-making and responsibility in the event of a mistake. Regulatory standards need to be adapted to support safe and effective deployment of AI. Solving these issues is essential for the successful implementation of AI in radiology.

Regulatory Frameworks for AI in Clinical Practice

Clinical deployment also depends heavily on seamless workflow integration. AI tools must be interoperable with Picture Archiving and Communication Systems (PACS), Radiology Information Systems (RIS), and adhere to standards like DICOM and HL7. However, inconsistent imaging protocols and lack of universal data standards present integration challenges. Furthermore, institutional readiness, IT infrastructure, and user training are often limiting factors, even after regulatory approval. Addressing these workflow barriers is critical for the successful scaling of AI in clinical practice. AI deployment in radiology requires navigating complex regulatory landscapes:

FDA (U.S.): The FDA's Digital Health Center of Excellence outlines pathways including De Novo, 510(k), and Breakthrough Device Designation. Tools must show clinical effectiveness and safety.

EMA (EU): The European Medicines Agency aligns with the Medical Device Regulation (MDR), requiring CE marking and clinical evaluation.

Asia-Pacific (e.g., Japan, South Korea): Frameworks are evolving to align with global standards but vary widely in approval timeframes and data privacy stipulations.

Understanding these pathways facilitates clinical adoption and international deployment of AI tools.

Critical Appraisal of the Literature

Numerous limitations that temper the encouraging results presented in AI-based radiodiagnosis research are revealed by a critical review of the literature. Numerous studies have a retrospective design and only use data from one center, which limits how broadly their findings can be applied. There are frequently insufficient external validation cohorts and small or underpowered sample sizes. Reproducibility is further hampered by the fact that few studies reveal important information like model architectures, hyper parameter settings, and algorithm training data. Direct comparison between studies is made even more difficult by the lack of standardized evaluation metrics. For instance, although Dhinagar et al. (2020) report improved diagnostic accuracy with mpMRI, its clinical applicability to a variety of populations and imaging systems is still unknown. To create reliable and clinically useful AI models, these gaps must be filled by prospective multicentre trials, open reporting guidelines, and benchmark datasets.

Technical and Algorithmic Limitations

AI models need extensive, high-quality training data, which can be difficult to access. AI model performance is influenced by variability in imaging protocols and patient populations. Algorithmic bias can cause differences in diagnostic accuracy for different populations. AI's present "black box" nature creates difficulty in interpreting decision-making. Ongoing validation and updating of AI models are required for safe clinical use. Some study evaluated the diagnostic reliability of a web-based Artificial Intelligence program for detecting and classifying dental structures and treatments on panoramic radiographs. 300 orthopantomographies were selected and visually evaluated by two radiodiagnosis experts. Results showed the software performed well in detecting implants, crowns, metal fillings, and endodontic treatments, but not in classifying dental structures or resin-based restorations. The study suggests that web-based AI tools can improve general diagnostic and treatment decisions using orthopantomographies, avoiding clinician subjectivity and lapses (Bonfanti-Gris et al., 2022).

In addition to known technical challenges, AI models often suffer from data homogeneity, leading to bias in predictive accuracy across ethnicities, genders, and age groups. Underrepresentation of minority populations in training datasets can cause misdiagnoses or reduced sensitivity. Mitigation strategies include curating diverse training datasets, employing federated learning to access global data without sharing patient records, and adopting domain adaptation techniques to improve generalizability. Institutions and developers must prioritize inclusivity and fairness in model design and validation. A denoising convolutional neural network (DnCNN-MARHR) algorithm for reducing metal objects in digital tomosynthesis for arthroplasty developed. The algorithm uses projection data to estimate residual reference and object images, involving hybrid and subjectively reconstructed image usage. The DnCNN-MARHR algorithm was compared with other methods, including DEMDRA, VM, MLEM, FBP, and SARTTV. The algorithm showed adequate performance in reducing artifacts, generated better MAR, and showed the best image homogeneity in texture analysis. It is particularly useful for reducing artifacts in the longitudinal direction and is not affected by tissue misclassification (Gomi et al., 2019). The diagnostic performance of large language artificial intelligence (AI) models, Claude 3 Opus and Claude 3.5 Sonnet, in response to radiological images investigated. The models were tasked with listing primary diagnoses and differential diagnoses for 322 quiz questions from Radiology's "Diagnosis Please" cases. The models showed significantly improved diagnostic performance when inputting both key images and clinical history. Claude 3.5 Sonnet outperformed in all conditions, but a statistically significant difference was observed only in the comparison for Condition 3. The models' ability to identify important differential diagnoses under these conditions was confirmed (Kurokawa et al., 2024). Artificial intelligence (AI) used to identify, segment, and quantify COVID-19 pulmonary lesions. The LungQuant system, based on two U-nets, was developed using multiple datasets with different annotation criteria. The system's accuracy in predicting CT-Severity Score (CT-SS) was evaluated using Dice Similarity Coefficients. Results showed that the U-net segmentation and accuracy depended on the quality of the lesion annotations. The system achieved an accuracy of 90% in CT-SS identification on an independent dataset. The study highlights the system's generalization ability (Lizzi et al., 2022). An AI-guided quantitative coronary computed tomography angiography (AI-QCTISCHEMIA) model for diagnosing coronary ischemia developed. The model integrates atherosclerosis and vascular morphology measures and evaluates its prognostic utility for major adverse cardiovascular events (MACE). The model was developed in the CREDENCE and PACIFIC-1 studies, and its diagnostic performance was evaluated in both cohorts. The results showed that the AI-QCTISCHEMIA model accurately diagnoses coronary ischemia by invasive FFR and provides robust prognostic utility for MACE beyond the presence of stenosis. The model's prognostic value was also investigated in PACIFIC-1 (Nurmohamed et al., 2024). A digital twin is a virtual model that accurately reflects a physical thing or system, such as a radiological device. It allows developers to test characteristics, make modifications, and test the success or failure of these changes. Innovative technologies like AI and -omics sciences can create continuously adjustable virtual models for patients, improving personalized medicine and revolutionizing disease detection and management (Pesapane et al.,2022). A significant gap between AI's promises and its applications in diagnostic radiology revealed. It analyzed 269 AI applications from 99 companies, revealing that most are narrow in terms of tasks, modality, and anatomic region, and primarily focus on "perception" and "reasoning" tasks. A systematic framework for analyzing technological developments in radiology, empirical evidence on AI applications, and insights into the current state of AI applications studied (Rezazade Mehrizi et al., 2021). A deep-learning-based vertebral fracture diagnostic system has been developed and validated to improve diagnosis and treatment outcomes. The system uses area loss ratio to detect and grade vertebral fractures using plain radiographs. The system was tested on 11,397 plain radiographs from six community centers in Shanghai and 1276 participants from the Shanghai Sixth People's Hospital. The results showed high accuracy and computational speed in skeletal position detection and segmentation. The AI_OVF_SH system is an efficient tool for radiologists and clinicians to improve the diagnosis of vertebral fractures (Shen et al., 2023). Lung cancer screening (LCS) using low-dose computed tomography (LDCT) can detect small pulmonary nodules, known as ground-glass nodules (GGNs) and part-solid nodules (PSNs). Artificial intelligence (AI)-based vessel suppression (AI-VS) and automatic detection (AI-AD) algorithms can improve the detection of SSNs on LDCT. A study involving 123 LDCT examinations found that AI-VS improved the detection and classification of SSNs into GGN and PSN on LDCT. The accuracy of AI-AD was lower than both radiologists, suggesting that AI-VS can improve early detection of SSNs (Singh et al., 2021). The BlackBox Counterfactual Explainer is a new framework designed to explain image classification models in medical applications. It uses a Generative Adversarial Network (GAN) to generate perturbations to a query image, causing the classification decision to change from its original class to its negation. The loss function preserves essential details in the generated images. The framework was used to audit a classifier trained on a chest X-ray dataset. Clinical evaluation was conducted using metrics like cardiothoracic ratio and healthy costophrenic recess score. The counterfactual explanation significantly improved users' understanding of the classifier's decision, making its decision-making process more transparent (Singla et al.,2023)

Ethical, Legal, and Regulatory Challenges

AI in radiology poses ethical issues of patient consent and data protection. Legal consequences are involved when AI-driven decisions result in misdiagnosis or negative outcomes. Regulatory agencies need to develop guidelines for AI validation, approval, and surveillance. The possibility of AI replacing radiologists creates workforce issues and professional opposition. Resolving these issues involves co-operation between AI developers, clinicians, and policymakers. A study assessing undergraduate medical students' knowledge, attitude, and perception of artificial intelligence (AI) in medicine found that 92.4% of students had not received formal AI training. Most (84.9%) believed AI would revolutionize medicine and radiology, with 48.9% agreeing that it could reduce the need for radiologists. Students with high AI knowledge and training were more likely to endorse AI replacing radiologists and reducing their numbers. The majority also agreed that AI would aid in the automated detection and diagnosis of pathologies. The study highlights the need for widespread AI education and training for Arab medical students, indicating its significance for healthcare systems and medical curricula (Allam et al., 2024). Cutis calcification, the deposition of calcium in skin and subcutaneous tissues, is classified into four subsets. Dystrophic calcifications are the most common type, mainly in damaged tissues or during autoimmune disease. However, the coexistence of systemic lupus erythematosus (SLE) and soft tissue calcification is rare. A 49-year-old woman with SLE developed nodular lesions in the buttock area, and the diagnosis of dystrophic calcinosis was established. The pathophysiology of calcifications in SLE patients is unclear, but a treatment algorithm should be established (Kruszewska et al., 2021).

Despite its potential, AI in radiology has a number of practical drawbacks.

- Bias Across Populations: Research indicates that AI models that have been trained on homogeneous datasets may perform poorly when applied to diverse populations. Baniecki et al. (2025) showed, for instance, that the outputs of survival models varied depending on the demographic group.
- A black-box Nature: DL models frequently have an opaque decision-making process, which raises questions about accountability and trust. To improve interpretability, strategies like counterfactual explanations and Grad-CAM are being developed (Singla et al., 2023).
- Privacy Risks: De-identification protocols and federated learning approaches mitigate patient data exposure.
- Cost Constraints: High development and integration costs delay AI deployment in resource-limited settings.
- Radiologist Acceptance: Resistance due to fear of replacement is mitigated by emphasizing AI's role as an assistive tool.
- Data Standardization: Lack of uniform imaging protocols across institutions affects model generalizability.
- Lack of Generalizability: AI tool performance may be constrained by differences in imaging protocols amongst institutions.

The safe clinical application of AI requires a committed focus on transparent model development and fair training datasets.

FUTURE DIRECTIONS AND EDUCATIONAL NEEDS

The potential of AI in radiodiagnosis lies in future advancements in deep learning, federated learning, and multimodal imaging fusion. AI-driven personalized medicine and predictive analytics will further enhance patient care. Radiologists must adopt AI-based workflows by training and educating themselves. Education in AI should be incorporated in medical curricula to educate subsequent generations of radiologists. Continual research and innovation will dictate the position of AI in radiology, leading to improved diagnostic performance and patient care. AI is shifting toward real-time diagnostic support and predictive analysis. Federated learning allows AI models to be trained on data from many institutions without exposing the data. AI-driven image reconstruction techniques reduce scan time and radiation dose in imaging. The combination of AI and molecular imaging enhances precision medicine approaches. The marriage of AI and augmented reality (AR) might revolutionize image-guided interventions. Radiologists need to acquire AI literacy to apply AI tools successfully in clinical settings. AI-related training courses and workshops need to be integrated into medical school. Exposure to practical experience with AI tools in radiology will increase the confidence of radiologists. Knowing the limitations and capabilities of AI is important for proper integration. Interactions between AI developers and radiologists will lead to future developments. A world-leading research dataset of routinely collected clinical images from the Scottish national population, including over 30 million radiological examinations, has been developed. The platform securely extracts data, links it to other datasets, removes personal data, and makes it available to researchers in a controlled Safe Haven environment. The data is valuable for training algorithms for clinical decision making, deep learning, and supporting new health research using artificial intelligence and machine learning technologies (Nind et al., 2020). Ensemble deep learning (EDL) is proposed as a superior method for lung computed tomography (CT) classification in COVID-19 ICUs. The system consists of a cascade of quality control, ResNet–UNet-based hybrid deep learning, and seven models using TL-based classification. The system was tested on unseen data and showed improvements in accuracy for both unbalanced and augmented datasets. The results confirmed EDL's superior performance over deep transfer learning (TL) systems in both seen and unseen paradigms (Dubey et al., 2023). Some study examines the prevalence and oral findings of nephrocalcinosis in patients with amelogenesis imperfecta (AI) between 2002-2007. Patients were referred to the Pediatric Dentistry Department of SDU and diagnosed with AI. Results showed suspicious radiopacity during renal ultrasonography, low calcium and normal potassium values, delayed eruption, gingival hyperplasia, pulp stones, and orthodontic problems. Early diagnosis may offer a good prognosis due to the potential risk of nephrocalcinosis (Kirzioglu et al., 2009). Chuna manual therapy (CMT) is a manual medicine practiced by Korean medical doctors in South Korea. Spinal diagnosis in CMT uses manual diagnostic and X-ray tests to detect specific vertebral malpositions. Artificial intelligence (AI) programs have been developed to assist in radiological diagnosis using X-ray images. This study aims to overcome limitations by collecting and comparing CMT diagnostic data from experts and non-experts. The study will recruit 100 non-specialist subjects and assess concordance levels between the two groups. The results will be used to test the potential use of CMT diagnostic methods and AI programs with high levels of rationality and consistency (Lee et al., 2021). A hybrid AI model to predict spinal surgical recommendations for Lumbar Spinal Stenosis (LSS), a condition affecting millions of adults in the US proposed. The model uses a random forest model and an expert Bayesian network model, combining medical vignette data and expert opinions from a multidisciplinary team. The model demonstrated high predictive accuracy, with a root mean square error of 0.0964 and an average RMSE of 0.1940. The results suggest AI can automate LSS surgical candidacy evaluations (Mourad et al., 2022). A deep learning model has been developed to diagnose subcentimetre lung nodules with a diameter of less than 1 cm. The model uses image data from the First Affiliated Hospital of Zhejiang University School of Medicine from 2016 to 2019. After data preprocessing and augmentation, the model has a diagnostic efficiency of 0.896, higher than three doctors. This system allows clinicians to create a deep learning pulmonary nodule pathology classification model without the need for deep learning experts (He et al., 2020).

Future Trends in AI for Radiodiagnosis

AI in radiology is rapidly evolving with promising frontiers:

Precision Medicine: Integration of imaging, genetics, and clinical data to tailor treatment.

Federated Learning: Enables multi-institutional model training without data exchange.

Synthetic Data Augmentation: Boosts dataset volume and diversity for rare pathologies.

Digital Twins: Virtual models of patients for simulation-based decision-making.

Multimodal AI: Combines imaging, pathology, and EMR data for holistic insights.

These innovations promise to make radiology more predictive, personalized, and participatory.

Figure 4. An outline of the architecture. The identifiable zone, which contains the raw data, the de-identified zone, which is where cohort building and data linkage occur, and the Safe Haven environment are the three zones (where a researcher carries out their analysis) (CC BY 4.0)

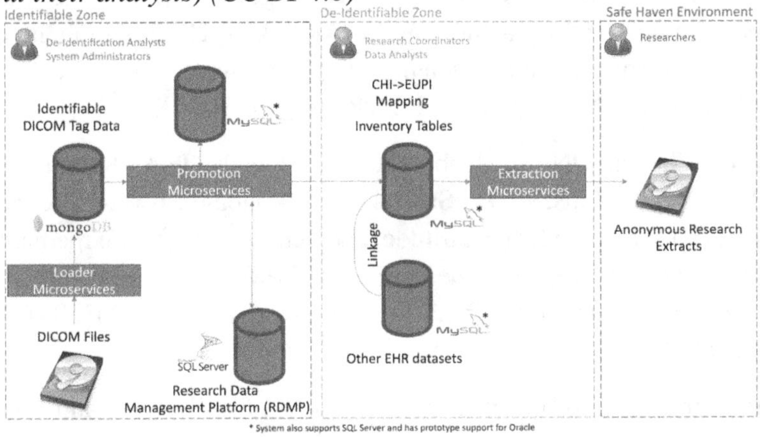

CONCLUSION

AI is transforming radiodiagnosis by improving image interpretation, diagnostic performance, and workflow efficiency. Its application across imaging modalities enhances disease detection and patient management. In spite of technical challenges, ethical considerations, and regulatory issues, the potential of AI in radiology is promising. Ongoing research, innovation, and education will determine the future of AI in radiodiagnosis. With advancement in AI, it will become an effective tool, augmenting radiologists, and enhancing healthcare outcomes. Artificial Intelligence is revolutionizing radiodiagnosis by increasing diagnostic precision, optimizing workflows, and aiding clinical decision-making. AI-based solutions are now part of multiple imaging modalities, enhancing disease detection and patient care. In spite of remarkable progress, algorithmic constraints, ethical issues, and regulatory needs need to be met for the safe integration of AI. The destiny of AI in radiology hinges on ongoing research, innovation, and collaboration among radiologists and AI developers. Ultimately, AI will become a valuable assistant, augmenting radiologists not replacing them, and defining the future of medical imaging.

REFERENCES

Ahn, J. S., Ebrahimian, S., McDermott, S., Lee, S., Naccarato, L., di Capua, J. F., Wu, M. Y., Zhang, E. W., Muse, V., Miller, B., Digumarthy, S. R., & Kalra, M. K. (2022). Association of Artificial Intelligence-Aided Chest Radiograph Interpretation with Reader Performance and Efficiency. *JAMA Network Open*, *5*(8), E2229289. DOI: 10.1001/jamanetworkopen.2022.29289 PMID: 36044215

Allam, A. H., Eltewacy, N. K., Alabdallat, Y. J., Owais, T. A., Salman, S., Ebada, M. A., Aldare, H. A., Rais, M. A., Salem, M., Al-Dabagh, J. D., Alakhrass, D. N., & Alkanj, S. (2024). Knowledge, attitude, and perception of Arab medical students towards artificial intelligence in medicine and radiology: A multi-national cross-sectional study. *European Radiology*, *34*(7), 1–14. DOI: 10.1007/s00330-023-10509-2 PMID: 38150076

Auloge, P., Garnon, J., Robinson, J. M., Dbouk, S., Sibilia, J., Braun, M., Vanpee, D., Koch, G., Cazzato, R. L., & Gangi, A. (2020). Interventional radiology and artificial intelligence in radiology: Is it time to enhance the vision of our medical students? *Insights Into Imaging*, *11*(1). Advance online publication. DOI: 10.1186/s13244-020-00942-y PMID: 33252702

Baniecki, H., Sobieski, B., Szatkowski, P., Bombinski, P., & Biecek, P. (2025). Interpretable machine learning for time-to-event prediction in medicine and healthcare. *Artificial Intelligence in Medicine*, *159*. Advance online publication. DOI: 10.1016/j.artmed.2024.103026 PMID: 39579416

Bhattacharyya, A., Bhaik, D., Kumar, S., Thakur, P., Sharma, R., & Pachori, R. B. (2022). A deep learning based approach for automatic detection of COVID-19 cases using chest X-ray images. *Biomedical Signal Processing and Control*, *71*. Advance online publication. DOI: 10.1016/j.bspc.2021.103182 PMID: 34580596

Bonfanti-Gris, M., Garcia-Cañas, A., Alonso-Calvo, R., Salido Rodriguez-Manzaneque, M. P., & Pradies Ramiro, G. (2022). Evaluation of an Artificial Intelligence web-based software to detect and classify dental structures and treatments in panoramic radiographs. *Journal of Dentistry*, *126*. Advance online publication. DOI: 10.1016/j.jdent.2022.104301 PMID: 36150430

Bortulev, P. I., Baskaeva, T. V., Vissarionov, S. V., Barsukov, D. B., Pozdnikin, I. Yu., Poznovich, M. S., Baskov, V. E., & Kornyakov, P. N. (2023). The choice of pelvic osteotomy technique in young children with hip dysplasia. Pediatric Traumatology. *Orthopaedics and Reconstructive Surgery*, *11*(1), 5–16. DOI: 10.17816/PTORS138629

Chidambaram, S., Sounderajah, V., Maynard, N., & Markar, S. R. (2022). Diagnostic Performance of Artificial Intelligence-Centred Systems in the Diagnosis and Postoperative Surveillance of Upper Gastrointestinal Malignancies Using Computed Tomography Imaging: A Systematic Review and Meta-Analysis of Diagnostic Accuracy. *Annals of Surgical Oncology*, *29*(3), 1977–1990. DOI: 10.1245/s10434-021-10882-6 PMID: 34762214

Chudobiński, C., Świderski, B., Antoniuk, I., & Kurek, J. (2024). Enhancements in Radiological Detection of Metastatic Lymph Nodes Utilizing AI-Assisted Ultrasound Imaging Data and the Lymph Node Reporting and Data System Scale. *Cancers (Basel)*, *16*(8). Advance online publication. DOI: 10.3390/cancers16081564 PMID: 38672646

Dell'Aria, A., Tack, D., Saddiki, N., Makdoud, S., Alexiou, J., de Hemptinne, F.-X., Berkenbaum, I., Neugroschl, C., & Tacelli, N. (2024). Radiographic Detection of Post-Traumatic Bone Fractures: Contribution of Artificial Intelligence Software to the Analysis of Senior and Junior Radiologists. *Journal of the Belgian Society of Radiology*, *108*(1). Advance online publication. DOI: 10.5334/jbsr.3574 PMID: 38680721

Dhinagar, N. J., Speier, W., Sarma, K. V., Raman, A., Kinnaird, A., Raman, S. S., Marks, L. S., & Arnold, C. W. (2020). Semi-automated PIRADS scoring via mpMRI analysis. *Journal of Medical Imaging (Bellingham, Wash.)*, *7*(6). Advance online publication. DOI: 10.1117/1.JMI.7.6.064501 PMID: 33392358

Dubey, A. K., Chabert, G. L., Carriero, A., Pasche, A., Danna, P. S. C., Agarwal, S., & Mohanty, L., Nillmani, Sharma, N., Yadav, S., Saba, L., & Suri, J. S. (2023). Ensemble Deep Learning Derived from Transfer Learning for Classification of COVID-19 Patients on Hybrid Deep-Learning-Based Lung Segmentation: A Data Augmentation and Balancing Framework. *Diagnostics (Basel)*, *13*(11). Advance online publication. DOI: 10.3390/diagnostics13111954 PMID: 37296806

Farouk, S., Osman, A. M., Awadallah, S. M., & Abdelrahman, A. S. (2023). The added value of using artificial intelligence in adult chest X-rays for nodules and masses detection in daily radiology practice. *The Egyptian Journal of Radiology and Nuclear Medicine*, *54*(1). Advance online publication. DOI: 10.1186/s43055-023-01093-y

Filice, R. W., Stein, A., Pan, I., & Shih, G. (2022). Federated Deep Learning to More Reliably Detect Body Part for Hanging Protocols, Relevant Priors, and Workflow Optimization. *Journal of Digital Imaging*, *35*(2), 335–339. DOI: 10.1007/s10278-021-00547-x PMID: 35018541

Fowler, G. E., Blencowe, N. S., Hardacre, C., Callaway, M. P., Smart, N. J., & MacEfield, R. (2023). Artificial intelligence as a diagnostic aid in cross-sectional radiological imaging of surgical pathology in the abdominopelvic cavity: A systematic review. *BMJ Open*, *13*(3). Advance online publication. DOI: 10.1136/bmjopen-2022-064739 PMID: 36878659

Gomi, T., Sakai, R., Hara, H., Watanabe, Y., & Mizukami, S. (2019). Development of a denoising convolutional neural network-based algorithm for metal artifact reduction in digital tomosynthesis for arthroplasty: A phantom study. *PLoS One*, *14*(9). Advance online publication. DOI: 10.1371/journal.pone.0222406 PMID: 31518374

Hasei, J., Nakahara, R., Otsuka, Y., Nakamura, Y., Hironari, T., Kahara, N., Miwa, S., Ohshika, S., Nishimura, S., Ikuta, K., Kunisada, T., & Ozaki, T. (2024). High-quality expert annotations enhance artificial intelligence model accuracy for osteosarcoma X-ray diagnosis. *Cancer Science*, *115*(11), 3695–3704. DOI: 10.1111/cas.16330 PMID: 39223070

He, Z., Lv, W., & Hu, J. (2020). A Simple Method to Train the AI Diagnosis Model of Pulmonary Nodules. *Computational and Mathematical Methods in Medicine*, *2020*. Advance online publication. DOI: 10.1155/2020/2812874 PMID: 32802147

Herpe, G., Nelken, H., Vendeuvre, T., Guenezan, J., Giraud, C., Mimoz, O., Feydy, A., Tasu, J.-P., & Guillevin, R. (2024). Effectiveness of an Artificial Intelligence Software for Limb Radiographic Fracture Recognition in an Emergency Department. *Journal of Clinical Medicine*, *13*(18). Advance online publication. DOI: 10.3390/jcm13185575 PMID: 39337062

Hirano, Y., Hanaoka, S., Nakao, T., Miki, S., Kikuchi, T., Nakamura, Y., Nomura, Y., Yoshikawa, T., & Abe, O. (2024). GPT-4 Turbo with Vision fails to outperform text-only GPT-4 Turbo in the Japan Diagnostic Radiology Board Examination. *Japanese Journal of Radiology*, *42*(8), 918–926. DOI: 10.1007/s11604-024-01561-z PMID: 38733472

Hosny, A., Bitterman, D. S., Guthier, C. V., Qian, J. M., Roberts, H., Perni, S., Saraf, A., Peng, L. C., Pashtan, I., Ye, Z., Aerts, H. J. W. L., & Mak, R. H. (2022). Clinical validation of deep learning algorithms for radiotherapy targeting of non-small-cell lung cancer: An observational study. *The Lancet. Digital Health*, *4*(9), e657–e666. DOI: 10.1016/S2589-7500(22)00129-7 PMID: 36028289

Huisman, M., Ranschaert, E., Parker, W., Mastrodicasa, D., Koci, M., Pinto de Santos, D., Coppola, F., Morozov, S., Zins, M., Bohyn, C., Leiner, T., & Willemink, M. J. (2021). An international survey on AI in radiology in 1041 radiologists and radiology residents part 2: Expectations, hurdles to implementation, and education. *European Radiology*, *31*(11), 8797–8806. DOI: 10.1007/s00330-021-07782-4 PMID: 33974148

Khanom, M., Iqbal, A., Hoque, A., Jeenia, F. T., & Uddin, M. (2023). Development and Validation of a Machine Learning System for Analysis and Radiological Diagnosis of Digital Chest X-ray Images. *Journal of Medicine (Bangladesh)*, *24*(2), 112–118. DOI: 10.3329/jom.v24i2.67273

Kim, E. Y., & Chung, M. J. (2021). Application of artificial intelligence in chest imaging for COVID-19. *Journal of the Korean Medical Association*, *64*(10), 664–670. DOI: 10.5124/jkma.2021.64.10.664

Kirzioglu, Z., Ulu, K. G., Sezer, M. T., & Yüksel, S. (2009). The relationship of amelogenesis imperfecta and nephrocalcinosis syndrome. *Medicina Oral, Patologia Oral y Cirugia Bucal*, *14*(11). Advance online publication. DOI: 10.4317/medoral.14.e579 PMID: 19680205

Kluge, E.-H. W. (2020). Artificial intelligence in healthcare: Ethical considerations. *Healthcare Management Forum*, *33*(1), 47–49. DOI: 10.1177/0840470419850438 PMID: 31340674

Kolhar, M., al Rajeh, A. M., & Kazi, R. N. A. (2024). Augmenting Radiological Diagnostics with AI for Tuberculosis and COVID-19 Disease Detection: Deep Learning Detection of Chest Radiographs. *Diagnostics (Basel)*, *14*(13). Advance online publication. DOI: 10.3390/diagnostics14131334 PMID: 39001228

Kruszewska, A., Owczarczyk-Saczonek, A., Placek, W., & Krajewska-Włodarczyk, M. (2021). Dystrophic calcifications in case of a patient with systemic lupus erythematosus – case report and literature review. *Polish Annals of Medicine*, *28*(2), 224–228. DOI: 10.29089/2020.20.00170

Kufel, J., Paszkiewicz, I., Kocot, S., Lis, A., Dudek, P., Czogalik, Ł., Janik, M., Bargieł-Łączek, K., Bartnikowska, W., Koźlik, M., Gruszczyńska, K., & Nawrat, Z. (2024). Deep Learning in Cardiothoracic Ratio Calculation and Cardiomegaly Detection. *Journal of Clinical Medicine*, *13*(14). Advance online publication. DOI: 10.3390/jcm13144180 PMID: 39064223

Kurokawa, R., Ohizumi, Y., Kanzawa, J., Kurokawa, M., Sonoda, Y., Nakamura, Y., Kiguchi, T., Gonoi, W., & Abe, O. (2024). Diagnostic performances of Claude 3 Opus and Claude 3.5 Sonnet from patient history and key images in Radiology's "Diagnosis Please" cases. *Japanese Journal of Radiology*, *42*(12), 1399–1402. DOI: 10.1007/s11604-024-01634-z PMID: 39096483

Kwee, T. C., Almaghrabi, M. T., & Kwee, R. M. (2023). Diagnostic radiology and its future: What do clinicians need and think? *European Radiology*, *33*(12), 9401–9410. DOI: 10.1007/s00330-023-09897-2 PMID: 37436504

Lee, J.-H., Woo, H.-J., Lee, J.-H., Kim, J.-I., Jang, J.-S., Na, Y. C., Kim, K.-R., & Park, T.-Y. (2021). Comparison of concordance between chuna manual therapy diagnosis methods (palpation, X-ray, artificial intelligence program) in lumbar spine: An exploratory, cross-sectional, prospective observational study protocol. *Medicine (United States)*, *100*(51), E28177. Advance online publication. DOI: 10.1097/MD.0000000000028177 PMID: 34941072

Lemainque, T., Yoneyama, M., Morsch, C., Iordanishvili, E., Barabasch, A., Schulze-Hagen, M., Peeters, J. M., Kuhl, C., & Zhang, S. (2024). Reduction of ADC bias in diffusion MRI with deep learning-based acceleration: A phantom validation study at 3.0 T. *Magnetic Resonance Imaging*, *110*, 96–103. DOI: 10.1016/j.mri.2024.04.01 PMID: 38631532

Lin, Y., Belue, M. J., Yilmaz, E. C., Law, Y. M., Merriman, K. M., Phelps, T. E., Gelikman, D. G., Ozyoruk, K. B., Lay, N. S., Merino, M. J., Pinto, P. A., & Turkbey, B. (2024). Deep learning-based image quality assessment: Impact on detection accuracy of prostate cancer extraprostatic extension on MRI. *Abdominal Radiology*, *49*(8), 2891–2901. DOI: 10.1007/s00261-024-04468-5 PMID: 38958754

Liu, Y., Liu, W., Chen, H., Xie, S., Wang, C., Liang, T., Yu, Y., & Liu, X. (2023). Artificial intelligence versus radiologist in the accuracy of fracture detection based on computed tomography images: A multidimensional, multi-region analysis. *Quantitative Imaging in Medicine and Surgery*, *13*(10), 6424–6433. DOI: 10.21037/qims-23-428 PMID: 37869340

Lizzi, F., Agosti, A., Brero, F., Cabini, R. F., Fantacci, M. E., Figini, S., Lascialfari, A., Laruina, F., Oliva, P., Piffer, S., Talamonti, C., & Retico, A. (2022). Quantification of pulmonary involvement in COVID-19 pneumonia by means of a cascade of two U-nets: Training and assessment on multiple datasets using different annotation criteria. *International Journal of Computer Assisted Radiology and Surgery*, *17*(2), 229–237. DOI: 10.1007/s11548-021-02501-2 PMID: 34698988

Marti-Bonmati, L., Koh, D.-M., Riklund, K., Bobowicz, M., Roussakis, Y., Vilanova, J. C., Fütterer, J. J., Rimola, J., Mallol, P., Ribas, G., Lekadir, K., & Tsakou, G. (2022). Considerations for artificial intelligence clinical impact in oncologic imaging: An AI4HI position paper. *Insights Into Imaging*, *13*(1). Advance online publication. DOI: 10.1186/s13244-022-01220-9 PMID: 35536446

Mehrizi, M. H. R., Gerritsen, S. H., de Klerk, W. M., Houtschild, C., Dinnessen, S. M. H., Zhao, L., van Sommeren, R., & Zerfu, A. (2023). How do providers of artificial intelligence (AI) solutions propose and legitimize the values of their solutions for supporting diagnostic radiology workflow? A technography study in 2021. *European Radiology*, *33*(2), 915–924. DOI: 10.1007/s00330-022-09090-x PMID: 35980427

Meng, F., Kottlors, J., Shahzad, R., Liu, H., Fervers, P., Jin, Y., Rinneburger, M., Le, D., Weisthoff, M., Liu, W., Zhang, H., & Persigehl, T. (2023). AI support for accurate and fast radiological diagnosis of COVID-19: An international multicenter, multivendor CT study. *European Radiology*, *33*(6), 4280–4291. DOI: 10.1007/s00330-022-09335-9 PMID: 36525088

Mourad, R., Kolisnyk, S., Baiun, Y., Falk, A., Yuriy, T., Valerii, F., Kopeev, A., Suldina, O., Pospelov, A., Kim, J., Rusakov, A., & Lebl, D. R. (2022). Performance of hybrid artificial intelligence in determining candidacy for lumbar stenosis surgery. *European Spine Journal : Official Publication of the European Spine Society, the European Spinal Deformity Society, and the European Section of the Cervical Spine Research Society*, *31*(8), 2149–2155. DOI: 10.1007/s00586-022-07307-7 PMID: 35802195

Neubauer, M., Moser, L., Neugebauer, J., Raudner, M., Wondrasch, B., Führer, M., Emprechtinger, R., Dammerer, D., Ljuhar, R., Salzlechner, C., Salzlechner, C., & Nehrer, S. (2023). Artificial-Intelligence-Aided Radiographic Diagnostic of Knee Osteoarthritis Leads to a Higher Association of Clinical Findings with Diagnostic Ratings. *Journal of Clinical Medicine*, *12*(3). Advance online publication. DOI: 10.3390/jcm12030744 PMID: 36769394

Nind, T., Sutherland, J., McAllister, G., Hardy, D., Hume, A., MacLeod, R., Caldwell, J., Krueger, S., Tramma, L., Teviotdale, R., Morris, A., & Jefferson, E. (2020). An extensible big data software architecture managing a research resource of real-world clinical radiology data linked to other health data from the whole Scottish population. *GigaScience*, *9*(10). Advance online publication. DOI: 10.1093/gigascience/giaa095 PMID: 32990744

Nurmohamed, N. S., Danad, I., Jukema, R. A., de Winter, R. W., de Groot, R. J., Driessen, R. S., Bom, M. J., van Diemen, P., Pontone, G., Andreini, D., Sprengers, R. W., & Raijmakers, P. G. (2024). Development and Validation of a Quantitative Coronary CT Angiography Model for Diagnosis of Vessel-Specific Coronary Ischemia. *JACC: Cardiovascular Imaging*, *17*(8), 894–906. DOI: 10.1016/j.jcmg.2024.01.007 PMID: 38483420

Ongena, Y. P., Yakar, D., Haan, M., & Kwee, T. C. (2021). Artificial Intelligence in Screening Mammography: A Population Survey of Women's Preferences. *Journal of the American College of Radiology*, *18*(1), 79–86. DOI: 10.1016/j.jacr.2020.09.042 PMID: 33058789

Osie, G., Darbari Kaul, R., Alvarado, R., Katsoulotos, G., Rimmer, J., Kalish, L., Campbell, R. G., Sacks, R., & Harvey, R. J. (2023). A Scoping Review of Artificial Intelligence Research in Rhinology. *American Journal of Rhinology & Allergy*, *37*(4), 438–448. DOI: 10.1177/19458924231162437 PMID: 36895144

Penzkofer, T., Padhani, A. R., Turkbey, B., Haider, M. A., Huisman, H., Walz, J., Salomon, G., Schoots, I. G., Richenberg, J., Villeirs, G., Logager, V. B., & Barentsz, J. (2021). ESUR/ESUI position paper: Developing artificial intelligence for precision diagnosis of prostate cancer using magnetic resonance imaging. *European Radiology*, *31*(12), 9567–9578. DOI: 10.1007/s00330-021-08021-6 PMID: 33991226

Pesapane, F., Rotili, A., Penco, S., Nicosia, L., & Cassano, E. (2022). Digital Twins in Radiology. *Journal of Clinical Medicine*, *11*(21). Advance online publication. DOI: 10.3390/jcm11216553 PMID: 36362781

Qiu, J., Mitra, J., Ghose, S., Dumas, C., Yang, J., Sarachan, B., & Judson, M. A. (2024). A Multichannel CT and Radiomics-Guided CNN-ViT (RadCT-CNNViT) Ensemble Network for Diagnosis of Pulmonary Sarcoidosis. *Diagnostics (Basel)*, *14*(10). Advance online publication. DOI: 10.3390/diagnostics14101049 PMID: 38786347

Rezazade Mehrizi, M. H., van Ooijen, P., & Homan, M. (2021). Applications of artificial intelligence (AI) in diagnostic radiology: A technography study. *European Radiology*, *31*(4), 1805–1811. DOI: 10.1007/s00330-020-07230-9 PMID: 32945967

Russe, M. F., Rebmann, P., Tran, P. H., Kellner, E., Reisert, M., Bamberg, F., Kotter, E., & Kim, S. (2024). AI-based X-ray fracture analysis of the distal radius: Accuracy between representative classification, detection and segmentation deep learning models for clinical practice. *BMJ Open*, *14*(1). Advance online publication. DOI: 10.1136/bmjopen-2023-076954 PMID: 38262641

Saghiri, M. A., Vakhnovetsky, J., Samadi, E., Amanabi, M., & Morgano, S. M. (2023). C.E. Credit. Innovating Dental Education with Artificial Intelligence. *Journal of the California Dental Association, 51*(1). Advance online publication. DOI: 10.1080/19424396.2023.2217692

Serte, S., & Demirel, H. (2021). Deep learning for diagnosis of COVID-19 using 3D CT scans. *Computers in Biology and Medicine, 132*. Advance online publication. DOI: 10.1016/j.compbiomed.2021.104306 PMID: 33780867

Seymen, F., Lee, K.-E., Koruyucu, M., Gencay, K., Bayram, M., Tuna, E., Lee, Z., & Kim, J.-W. (2015). Novel ITGB6 mutation in autosomal recessive amelogenesis imperfecta. *Oral Diseases, 21*(4), 456–461. DOI: 10.1111/odi.12303 PMID: 25431241

Shen, L., Gao, C., Hu, S., Kang, D., Zhang, Z., Xia, D., Xu, Y., Xiang, S., Zhu, Q., Xu, G., Yu, W., & Zhang, Z. (2023). Using Artificial Intelligence to Diagnose Osteoporotic Vertebral Fractures on Plain Radiographs. *Journal of Bone and Mineral Research : the Official Journal of the American Society for Bone and Mineral Research, 38*(9), 1278–1287. DOI: 10.1002/jbmr.4879 PMID: 37449775

Silberstein, J., Wee, C., Gupta, A., Seymour, H., Ghotra, S. S., Sá dos Reis, C., Zhang, G., & Sun, Z. (2023). Artificial Intelligence-Assisted Detection of Osteoporotic Vertebral Fractures on Lateral Chest Radiographs in Post-Menopausal Women. *Journal of Clinical Medicine, 12*(24). Advance online publication. DOI: 10.3390/jcm12247730 PMID: 38137799

Singh, R., Kalra, M. K., Homayounieh, F., Nitiwarangkul, C., McDermott, S., Little, B. P., Lennes, I. T., Shepard, J.-A. O., & Digumarthy, S. R. (2021). Artificial intelligence-based vessel suppression for detection of sub-solid nodules in lung cancer screening computed tomography. *Quantitative Imaging in Medicine and Surgery, 11*(4), 1134–1143. DOI: 10.21037/qims-20-630 PMID: 33816155

Singla, S., Eslami, M., Pollack, B., Wallace, S., & Batmanghelich, K. (2023). Explaining the black-box smoothly—A counterfactual approach. *Medical Image Analysis, 84*. Advance online publication. DOI: 10.1016/j.media.2022.102721 PMID: 36571975

KEY TERMS AND DEFINITIONS

Artificial Intelligence (AI): The simulation of human intelligence processes by machines, especially computer systems, to perform tasks such as learning, reasoning, and decision-making.

Machine Learning (ML): A subset of AI that enables computers to learn from data and improve performance without being explicitly programmed. Includes supervised, unsupervised, and reinforcement learning.

Deep Learning (DL): A specialized area of machine learning involving neural networks with many layers, particularly effective for complex tasks like image and speech recognition.

Convolutional Neural Networks (CNNs): A class of deep learning models particularly suited for image analysis, using convolutional layers to detect spatial hierarchies in data such as radiological images.

DICOM (Digital Imaging and Communications in Medicine): A standard for handling, storing, and transmitting information in medical imaging.

FDA (Food and Drug Administration): The U.S. regulatory body responsible for approving medical devices, including AI software, for clinical use.

EMA (European Medicines Agency): The EU counterpart to the FDA, responsible for the evaluation and supervision of medical products including AI tools.

Chapter 3
AI-Enhanced Image Analysis and Interpretation

S. Abhijith
https://orcid.org/0000-0003-2726-1721
Manipal Academy of Higher Education, India

P. Saikiran
https://orcid.org/0000-0001-7933-1192
Manipal Academy of Higher Education, India

P. Aswathi
https://orcid.org/0009-0006-7702-3229
REVA University, Bangalore, India & Srinivas University, Mangalore, India

Priyanka
https://orcid.org/0000-0002-9792-6242
Manipal Academy of Higher Education, India

Tancia Pires
https://orcid.org/0009-0002-8838-8953
Manipal Academy of Higher Education, India

M. Obhuli Chandran
Manipal Academy of Higher Education, India

ABSTRACT

Artificial Intelligence (AI) is transforming medical imaging by improving accuracy, efficiency, and interpretability in diagnostics and treatment. This chapter examines AI's role in image analysis across medical domains using machine learning (ML), deep learning (DL), and radiomics. AI has demonstrated effectiveness in various applications, often matching or surpassing clinicians. It enhances diagnostic and predictive capabilities, streamlines workflows, and aids in early detection, disease characterization, and treatment planning. However, challenges like robustness, bias reduction, and generalizability across datasets hinder adoption. Addressing these issues is key to seamless clinical integration. Emerging trends focus on multimodal data and generalized models to broaden AI's applicability. While promising, these

DOI: 10.4018/979-8-3373-0903-3.ch003

technologies require validation through multicenter studies, larger datasets, and strong algorithmic frameworks. Through collaboration, AI-driven imaging can advance precision medicine, improve patient outcomes, and redefine medical diagnostics.

INTRODUCTION

Traditional methods of medical image interpretation often rely heavily on the expertise of radiologists, which can be time-consuming and subject to human error, fatigue, and inter-observer variability. These limitations may result in missed subtle pathologies, delayed diagnoses, and inconsistencies in clinical decision-making (Khalifa & Albadawy, 2024). Artificial Intelligence (AI) is increasingly addressing these challenges by transforming the landscape of medical image analysis. With advanced techniques such as machine learning (ML) and deep learning (DL), AI systems can rapidly process large volumes of imaging data, identify complex patterns, and detect features that may be imperceptible to the human eye (Pinto-Coelho, 2023). AI has been used in imaging modalities like MRI, CT, ultrasound, and X-ray to improve accuracy and efficiency. In particular, AI-driven voxel-based feature extraction from multimodal images shows promise for early disease detection and classification by severity or aggressiveness.(Rana & Bhushan, 2023).

AI in medical imaging has evolved significantly, starting with foundational ideas in the 1940s and progressing through major technological advances. In the 1970s and 1980s, expert systems using rule-based logic aided clinical decisions but lacked adaptability(Avanzo et al., 2024). The introduction of artificial neural networks and computer-aided detection (CAD) tools during the 1980s marked a significant breakthrough, enabling machines to assist radiologists particularly in tasks like lesion detection in mammography (Fazal et al., 2018). Recently, advances in deep learning, powered by better computing, large datasets, and convolutional neural networks (CNNs), have transformed medical imaging. AI now matches or surpasses human performance in image classification, segmentation, and lesion detection.(Avanzo et al., 2024). However, challenges related to interpretability, workflow integration, and ethical concerns such as fairness and accountability remain central to ongoing development and adoption.

This chapter aims to outline the steps involved in the training and assessment of ML and DL models along with applying AI enhanced diagnosis of various diseases and prediction of their phenotype and prognosis and planning personalized treatment planning and monitoring the treatment responses across various imaging modalities.

METHODOLOGY USED FOR IMAGE ANALYSIS

Image Pre-Processing

Medical image preprocessing standardizes and enhances image quality for analysis. Images are first converted to a uniform format and resampled for consistent voxel size. Registration aligns multimodal images spatially. Background removal, intensity normalization, and bias-field correction reduce scanner and acquisition variability. Gaussian smoothing, non-local means filtering, and data augmentation (flipping, rotation, intensity scaling) further improve quality and analysis reliability. (Masoudi et al., 2021; Preim & Botha, 2014).

Segmentation

Segmentation is crucial in medical imaging to isolate regions of interest. It can be manual, semi-automated, or fully automated based on complexity and precision needs. Traditional methods like thresholding, edge detection, and clustering work well for simple regions. Advanced approaches, such as active contours and Markov Random Fields, use spatial and texture data for better results. Recently, deep learning models like CNNs and U-Nets have improved accuracy, consistency, and reduced observer variability in complex segmentation tasks.(Chowdhary & Acharjya, 2020; L. Huang et al., 2023; Preim & Botha, 2014).

Machine Learning

Feature Extraction

Feature extraction from segmented medical images quantifies ROI characteristics for analysis. It includes first-order statistics (intensity), shape features (geometry), and texture (spatial intensity patterns). Advanced methods use wavelets and higher-order statistics for multi-scale details. Tools like PyRadiomics follow IBSI standards for consistency, while normalization methods like Z-score standardization ensure comparability across modalities(Chowdhary & Acharjya, 2020; Collewet et al., 2004).

In segmentation-based radiomics, feature extraction is tailored to imaging modalities and study goals. Statistical and texture features like GLCM, GLRLM, and GLSZM capture heterogeneity within segmented areas. Higher-order methods, such as wavelet filtering, improve sensitivity to subtle texture and intensity changes. These features are combined with clinical data to create structured inputs for predictive modeling and decision support.(Chowdhary & Acharjya, 2020).

Feature Reduction

Feature reduction manages high-dimensional data by removing redundant and uninformative variables while keeping key features. Common methods include variance thresholding, correlation analysis, and recursive feature elimination (RFE). Advanced techniques like Maximum Relevance–Minimum Redundancy (MRMR) balance relevance and redundancy. These improve model interpretability, reduce overfitting, and enhance computational efficiency.(Popov, 2023; Velliangiri et al., 2019).

Feature Selection

Feature selection identifies the most relevant attributes to boost predictive accuracy. Common methods include SelectKBest, Lasso regression, and Variance Inflation Factor (VIF) analysis. SelectKBest ranks features by mutual information, while Lasso shrinks irrelevant coefficients to zero, reducing multicollinearity and dimensionality. Cross-validation finds the optimal feature set, and Intraclass Correlation Coefficient (ICC) checks feature stability across datasets.Feature selection methods fall into two categories: supervised (e.g., RFE, SelectKBest), which use class labels, and unsupervised (e.g., variance thresholding, correlation analysis), which do not—making them ideal for exploratory analysis. Combining these approaches improves model performance while balancing complexity and interpretability.

Feature selection aims to identify the most relevant attributes that improve predictive accuracy. Common methods include SelectKBest, Lasso regression, and Variance Inflation Factor (VIF) analysis. SelectKBest ranks features by relevance using mutual information, while Lasso performs selection and regularization by shrinking irrelevant feature coefficients to zero, helping reduce multicollinearity and dimensionality. Cross-validation helps determine the optimal feature set, and reproducibility checks like the Intraclass Correlation Coefficient (ICC) ensure feature stability across datasets.

Feature selection methods fall into two categories: supervised (e.g., RFE, SelectKBest), which use class labels, and unsupervised (e.g., variance thresholding, correlation analysis), which do not—making them ideal for exploratory analysis. Combining these approaches improves model performance while balancing complexity and interpretability(J. Cai et al., 2018; Popov, 2023).

Classifiers

Machine learning classifiers are key to predictive modeling in medical imaging and radiomics. Common algorithms include SVC, Logistic Regression, Decision Tree, KNN, Random Forest, AdaBoost, XGBoost, LGBM, and Extra Trees. Ensemble methods like stacking and voting combine multiple models to improve accuracy (Sarker, 2021). Hyperparameter tuning, often performed through grid search cross-validation, optimizes model parameters for improved accuracy, precision, recall, F1-score, and the area under the receiver operating characteristic (ROC) curve (AUC) To address class imbalance, techniques like the synthetic minority over-sampling technique (SMOTE) are implemented. Bootstrap methods are used to estimate confidence intervals for both accuracy and AUC.while additional performance metrics such as the Brier score provide further insights into model calibration. One-vs-one and one-vs-rest strategies are frequently employed to refine multi-class classification outcomes. Supervised learning models remain the dominant choice in radiomics due to their ability to analyze labeled data, while unsupervised and semi-supervised approaches offer alternative methodologies for pattern recognition. Shallow models, preferred over deep learning methods in certain radiomics applications, effectively capture complex relationships within imaging data (Perniciano et al., 2024; Sarker, 2021). The ultimate goal of ML classifiers is to facilitate accurate and reliable decision-making by leveraging discriminative radiomic features extracted from medical images.

Figure 1. Illustration of Machine learning-based image analysis workflow

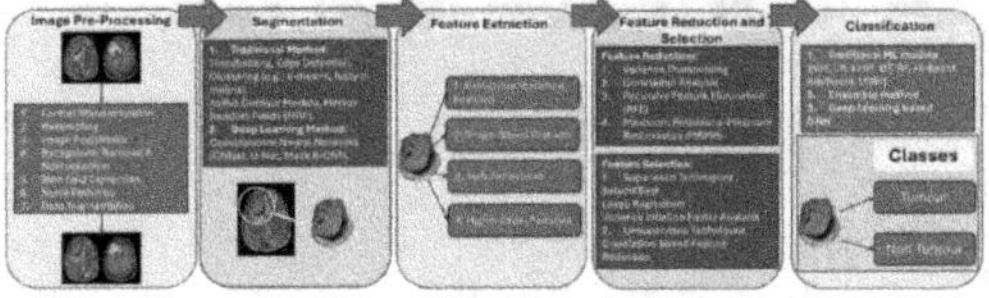

Deep Learning

Deep learning-based medical image analysis has revolutionized the field of diagnostics radiology by enabling automated, accurate, and efficient analysis of complex medical images. Convolutional Neural Networks (CNNs) are at the core of this revolution, since they are capable of automatically learning and extracting hierarchical features from raw medical images without requiring manual feature selection (X. Zhao et al., 2024). CNN architectures such as AlexNet, VGGNet, ResNet, and GoogLeNet have been extensively used for medical imaging tasks like disease classification, tumor detection, and organ segmentation (Kora et al., 2022). These models are effective in analyzing data from any modalities like MRI, CT, PET, and X-rays, offering significant improvements over traditional machine learning techniques.

Deep learning enables end-to-end learning in medical imaging, where CNNs directly analyze raw images to detect pathologies. Transfer learning, using pre-trained models like those from ImageNet, helps overcome limited annotated data by fine-tuning for medical tasks. However, challenges remain, including data scarcity, interpretability, and domain adaptation. (Kora et al., 2022; X. Zhao et al., 2024). Medical image datasets are often small and heterogeneous, posing a challenge for CNNs to generalize well across different populations. Researchers are actively working on solutions such as explainable AI (XAI) techniques, data augmentation, and federated learning to address these challenges and enhance the robustness of deep learning models in medical imaging (Borys et al., 2023).

Figure 2. Illustration of Deep learning-based image analysis workflow

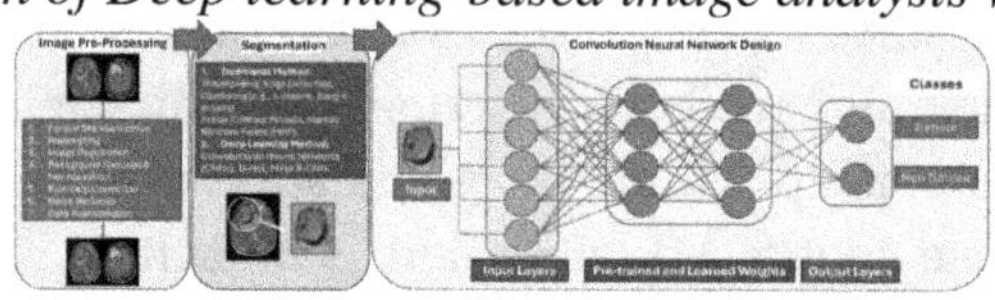

APPLICATIONS OF AI IN IMAGE ANALYSIS

Neuro Imaging

Advanced imaging analysis and predictive modeling have been enabled by ML and DL, revolutionizing diagnosis and management of head and neck tumors. Radiomics-based ML models have shown high accuracy in tumor classification by extracting and analyzing quantitative imaging features that extend beyond conventional radiological assessment. For example, radiomic features derived from MRI, PET/CT, and advanced imaging techniques such as DTI, ASL have been employed to train ML algorithms, including SVM, RF for differentiation between grades, accurate glioma subtype classification (Nayak et al., 2024; Zachariah et al., 2023). Furthermore, ML models incorporating radiomic workflows—comprising tumor segmentation, feature extraction, and predictive modeling with CNNs have enhanced diagnostic accuracy and prognosis prediction in pediatric neuro-oncology (Pacchiano et al., 2024).

DL-based segmentation has greatly improved the accuracy and efficiency of brain tumor assessment. CNN-driven tumor segmentation, combined with radiomic features, shows strong potential in predicting overall survival in high-grade glioma patients receiving immunotherapy, outperforming traditional radiomics methods. (Q. Wan et al., 2025). ML models using radiomic features from ADC maps have effectively distinguished tuberculomas from gliomas and metastases with high accuracy (Indoria et al., 2024). Hybrid models combining clinical, radiomic, and DL features further improve predictions of local tumor control after stereotactic radiotherapy for brain metastases. (Kanakarajan et al., 2024). These multimodal approaches improve decision-making by combining imaging-based insights with clinical parameters, thereby enhancing treatment planning and patient outcomes. Despite these promising advancements, challenges such as data standardization, model interpretability, and generalizability remain critical areas for future research. For further insights into radiomics applications in skull base oncology, readers may refer to the following reference (Patel et al., 2024).

Beyond oncology, DL and ML have demonstrated remarkable applications in lots of domains of neuroimaging, these techniques have been employed for the early diagnosis and classification of neurodegenerative disorders like Alzheimer's disease, Parkinson's disease, leveraging AI-based segmentation and radiomics biomarkers to improve diagnostic accuracy (Panahi & Hosseini, 2024; Yoon et al., 2024; Zarei et al., 2024). In stroke imaging, DL and ML have been integrated with radiomics to enhance ischemic stroke assessment, including automated ASPECTS scoring and posterior circulation stroke onset time estimation, identifying vulnerable carotid artery plaques reducing observer variability and improving decision-making for acute management (Fang et al., 2024; Z. Liu et al., 2024; Meddings et al., 2024). In the context of intracerebral hemorrhage, non-contrast CT-based radiomics approaches have been explored for predicting hematoma expansion, potentially guiding early intervention and prognosis (Q. Chen et al., 2024).

Breast Imaging

Breast cancer is the most diagnosed cancer among women globally, making early detection crucial for improving survival rates. Imaging techniques like mammography, ultrasound, and MRI play a great role in early diagnosis and management. However, the interpretation of breast images is complex and subject to variability among radiologists. In recent years, AI has emerged as a transformative tool in breast image analysis, offering automated, accurate, and efficient diagnostic support.

Breast density is classified into four ACR BI-RADS categories: A (fatty), B (scattered fibro-glandular), C (heterogeneously dense), and D (highly dense). Accurate assessment is vital for risk but varies among radiologists. AI enables automated breast density detection using T1 fat-sat MRI with 3D segmentation and a 3D EfficientNet CNN in PyTorch, alongside RF, SVM, and LR models. Deep learning and radiomics improve assessment accuracy and inter-observer agreement. (Jing et al., 2024).

Faster MRI acquisition and distinction between benign and malignant breast lesions is now made possible by radiomics model based on T2W and DW images. The model shows good diagnostic performance using Gaussian Process classifiers, achieving high AUC and F1 scores (Y. Liu, Jia, et al., 2024; Maiti et al., 2024). Identifying molecular subtypes of malignant lesions is crucial for tailored treatment. CORONet, a novel approach using incomplete DCE-MRI scans, enables this classification. It employs a Cross-Sequence Joint Representation (COR) module to enhance image quality and extract key features, then fuses multiple COR features while eliminating redundancy. Hypergraph Convolution Networks are used to capture complex patient relationships. (Xie et al., 2024). Similarly, CNNs have demonstrated robust classification capabilities in histopathological image analysis, playing a crucial role in distinguishing tumor characteristics and aiding in precise diagnosis . By integrating DL techniques like CNNs with radiomics and multi-source data, AI-driven models further enhance diagnostic accuracy, improve risk prediction, and optimize personalized treatment strategies (Darbandi et al., 2024).

After malignancy detection, predicting treatment response—especially to neoadjuvant chemotherapy (NAC)—is vital. AI-driven models across imaging modalities have shown strong results. Mammography-based deep learning models using DETR, contrast enhancement, and dual-path ResNet-18 performed well in classification. Ultrasound CAD systems using RNNs, dual-branch CNNs, and DenseNet201-CNN nomograms achieved AUCs above 0.7. MRI-based models further improved predictions; DCE-MRI with feature fusion and ANN reached an AUC of 0.96. The I-SPY 1 TRIAL combined imaging and biomarkers with ensemble learning (Logistic Regression, AdaBoost, Adabag), achieving 99.1% accuracy. Multi-modal MRI CAD tools integrated contrast-enhanced and diffusion-weighted imaging with clinical features via HITON-Markov Blanket selection. Key predictors varied—some models focused on enhancement fraction and tumor volume; others on HER2, Ki-67, TNM stage, or pathology. AI-powered radiomics systems also predicted partial response by combining MRI texture, diffusion metrics, and clinical data using stacking ensembles, genetic feature selection, and a two-stage classifier to distinguish responders and subtypes of non-response (pCR vs. SD).(Gamal et al., 2024; Jiang et al., 2024).

Lymphovascular invasion (LVI), a key factor in breast cancer metastasis, involves cancer cells in lymphovascular channels. While MRI aids in LVI detection, its accuracy is limited by physician interpretation. Radiomics offers a quantitative alternative by extracting tumor heterogeneity features. Combining multimodal preoperative MRI radiomics with deep learning improves performance. A logistic regression model using gross and peritumoral volumes from post-contrast T1-weighted MRI, with features selected via LASSO, showed strong results. Additionally, ResMM-Net, a novel end-to-end deep learning model, further enhanced LVI classification. (W. Liu et al., 2024). With DenseNet-201-based feature extraction from ultrasound images along with around 480 radiomics feature extraction using LASSO, A hybrid model created improved Axillary Lymph node metastasis prediction (L. Qian et al., 2024).

Volumetric Modulated Arc Therapy (VMAT), an advanced IMRT technique, delivers precise radiation to breast tumors while sparing healthy tissue. Radiation dermatitis (RD) is a common side effect, but AI prediction improves by combining clinical, radiomic, and dosiomic features. Extracting these features from CT ROI analysis, selecting key ones via ANOVA and LASSO, and using logistic regression yields strong predictive accuracy, enhancing therapy planning and patient care.(T. F. Lee et al., 2024).

Lung Imaging

AI has revolutionized lung image analysis, enhancing detection and diagnosis of lung cancer, COPD, fibrosis, and infections like COVID-19. CNNs such as ResNet, VGGNet, and U-Net have improved lung nodule detection and classification on CT scans, surpassing traditional methods.(Alahmari et al., 2018; Ebrahimpour et al., 2024; Yan et al., 2024). AI-powered radiomics, utilizing ML algorithms such as SVM and RF, has demonstrated efficacy in characterizing tumor heterogeneity and predicting patient outcomes in lung cancer cases (Kuang et al., 2024; Liang et al., 2024). Additionally, transformer-based deep learning models have been explored for classifying interstitial lung diseases (ILDs), providing high diagnostic accuracy and aiding in disease stratification (M. Wang et al., 2024; J. Zhang et al., 2024).

For infectious and inflammatory lung conditions, AI played a crucial role in differentiating bacterial pneumonia, viral pneumonia, and COVID-19 using deep learning-based classification models like DenseNet and EfficientNet (Deng et al., 2024; M. Wang et al., 2024). In COPD and pulmonary fibrosis, ML models, including KNN and gradient boosting, have been employed to quantify lung texture abnormalities from high-resolution CT (HRCT) and functional MRI scans (Ebrahimpour et al., 2024; Selvam et al., 2024). Furthermore, diffusion-weighted MRI, coupled with AI-driven segmentation algorithms, has enabled the extraction of functional lung parameters, improving early disease detection and treatment monitoring (Deng et al., 2024; Kuang et al., 2024). Despite these advancements, challenges such as model generalization across diverse patient populations, data standardization, and regulatory compliance must be addressed to ensure AI's seamless integration into clinical workflows (Selvam et al., 2024; Yan et al., 2024).

Furthermore, Advanced segmentation models, such as the transformer-based U-NETR, have demonstrated efficacy in automatically extracting radiomic features from lung tumors, facilitating persistence and reappearance prediction following the image-guided thermal ablation (Zaki et al., 2025). Similarly, ML models leveraging PET- and CT-derived radiomic features have been employed to predict recurrence patterns in non-small cell lung cancer (NSCLC) patients treated with stereotactic body radiotherapy, with SVMs and Naïve Bayes classifiers showing promising performance (Nemoto et al., 2024). Hybrid approaches, like genotype-guided radiomics, further improve prediction accuracy by integrating handcrafted and DL-based features to estimate gene expression from CT images, enabling cost-effective yet high-accuracy recurrence prediction (Aonpong et al., 2021). In the realm of immunotherapy response assessment, DeepSurv models combining intratumoral and peritumoral-vasculature radiomics with clinical features have enhanced progression-free survival predictions, supporting the development of personalized treatment strategies (Liao et al., 2024). The application of ML-based radiogenomics has also proven instrumental in linking imaging biomarkers with gene expression profiles, uncovering biological processes relevant to NSCLC and potential drug resistance mechanisms (Sukhadia et al., 2024). These advancements illustrate how AI-driven radiologic analysis extends beyond conventional diagnostic applications, offering predictive insights into treatment response, tumor biology, and personalized therapy planning.

Liver Imaging

Liver pathologies are traditionally diagnosed using imaging modalities like Ultrasound, CT, and MRI, relying on visual assessment and radiologist expertise. With AI, interpretation has become faster, more objective, and accurate. In liver imaging, the first diagnostic step is lesion characterization. Deep learning models can accurately detect and classify liver tumors, distinguishing benign (e.g., hemangiomas) from malignant ones (e.g., HCC, cholangiocarcinoma). AI also aids in early detection of fibrosis and cirrhosis by extracting quantitative biomarkers. Additionally, 3D radiomic features from CT images provide stable, noninvasive insights into tumor traits like cellularity, vascularity, and necrosis—helping assess tumor heterogeneity and aggressiveness. (Nam et al., 2022).

Accurate liver diagnosis requires precise segmentation for volumetry, anatomical localization, and biomarker extraction. While manual segmentation and radiomic feature extraction are time-consuming, deep learning models streamline this process. CNN-based image conversion also enhances consistency across different CT reconstruction algorithms. (H. Lee et al., 2024). CNN-based models have proven effective for MRI breast density assessment using features from T1-weighted contrast-enhanced images (Gross et al., 2024). n diagnosis, ruling out mimics, accurate grading, classification, and identifying primary sources in secondary lesions are crucial. Deep Learning Radiomics (DLR) models combining DL and radiomics on contrast-enhanced CT outperform ML models in detecting primary tumors in liver metastasis cases.(Jia et al., 2024). DRL models have also shown good results in tumour gene mutations, predicting microvascular invasion (W. Zhang et al., 2024a). post-TACE prognosis, early recurrence of HCC post hepatectomy even, the recurrence-free survival of subjects can now be assessed by integrating two metastatic vascular patterns studied on pathological stains: MVI, vessels encapsulating tumor clusters (VETC) with MR deep learning radiomics (DeepSurv model), which has shown great potential (Y. Liu, Liu, et al., 2024; G. X. Qian et al., 2024; Yin et al., 2025; C. Zhang et al., 2024; W. Zhang et al., 2024b). With continuous advancements, AI-driven tools enhance diagnostic precision, risk stratification, and personalized liver disease management, ultimately leading to better patient outcomes.

Rectal imaging

An AI model combining preoperative T2-weighted MRI-based deep transfer learning, radiomics, and clinical factors using SVM enables accurate rectal cancer staging and diagnosis. (Fan et al., 2024). Rectal cancer mainly spreads via lymph node (LN) metastasis. While multiparametric MRI is commonly used for preoperative LN assessment, its diagnostic accuracy is limited. Clinical DL radiomics (CDLR) models, integrating clinical data, MRI, deep learning, and radiomics features, provide a more accurate and comprehensive approach for predicting LN involvement. (Yang et al., 2024). In addition, tumour deposits, which are isolated tumour foci in the perirectal fat without lymph node or vascular involvement, are linked to more aggressive tumours and poorer survival. Radiomics nomogram combining T2WI, ADC features, CA19-9, and mLN (metastatic lymph node) status shows strong potential for predicting TDs before surgery, helping with patient risk assessment and personalized treatment (Z. Sun et al., 2024).

In rectal cancer, deep learning enables early, noninvasive classification of patients into high- or low-risk microsatellite instability (MSI) groups before treatment. High MSI indicates a functional DNA mismatch repair system and better prognosis, while low MSI suggests the opposite. Models like KNN can predict MSI status using radiomic features from T2W and T1W CE images, supporting personalized treatment planning and clinical decision-making. (Xing et al., 2024). Neoadjuvant chemoradiotherapy, preferred over short-course radiotherapy for advanced rectal cancer, offers better long-term outcomes. Assessing treatment response is key for identifying candidates for organ preservation. Combining imaging with machine learning enables non-invasive prediction of complete response using baseline T2W MRI features aligned with tumor regression grading, along with clinical data.(Y. D. Lee et al., 2024). After treatment, or neoadjuvant therapy, the overall estimated survival time of a patient can also be predicted by using a combined model of the radiomic features extracted from the intratumoral and peritumoral regions (Guo et al., 2025).

Prostate Imaging

AI has improved prostate cancer diagnosis by automating image analysis and enhancing pattern recognition in radiology and pathology. CNNs like ResNet and U-Net are widely used in multiparametric MRI for lesion segmentation and classification, boosting tumor localization and reducing interobserver variability.

(Abdelhalim et al., 2024; Chaddad et al., 2020). Radiomics-based ML models, including SVMs and RFs, extract quantitative imaging features from multiparametric MRI to differentiate between clinically significant and indolent tumors, assisting in risk stratification (Varan et al., 2023). Additionally, DL architectures such as Vision Transformers and 3D CNNs have demonstrated superior performance in detecting prostate cancer on MRI by capturing spatial dependencies across imaging slices (W. Zhao et al., 2024). Histopathological analysis has also benefited from DL models like DeepLab and HoVer-Net, which improve the segmentation of cancerous regions in whole-slide images, aiding in automated Gleason grading and tumor microenvironment assessment (Y. Huang et al., 2024) Beyond initial diagnosis, advanced ML and DL techniques enable prostate cancer subtyping based on genetic and pathological traits. Radiomics-based models have effectively predicted TP53 mutation status using SVM and RF classifiers by integrating radiomic and clinical features. Multimodal approaches combining MRI radiomics, deep transfer learning, and pathomics also show promise in predicting bone metastases, offering valuable prognostic insights for primary prostate cancer patients.(Y. F. Zhang et al., 2024).

These classification models not only enhance risk stratification but also help guide personalized treatment strategies, such as identifying patients who may require more aggressive management due to underlying genetic mutations or metastatic potential (R. Chen et al., 2024). Integrating radiomic signatures with clinical biomarkers like PSA and PI-RADS improves differentiation of malignant prostate cancer from benign conditions, outperforming traditional screening. This highlights AI's growing role in personalized prostate cancer management using molecular and imaging data (Lu et al., 2025).

Female Reproductive System Imaging

AI-driven radiomics has shown high accuracy in distinguishing cervical cancer from normal tissue using CT, with AUCs over 0.9 (Pei et al., 2024). Dynamic MRI-based radiomics models predicted early prognosis in locally advanced cervical cancer treated with chemoradiotherapy, achieving an AUC of 0.868 when combined with clinical data (C. Cai et al., 2024). Combining radiomics and clinicopathological data improved 4-year disease-free survival prediction for cervical adenocarcinoma, reaching an AUC of 0.937 (Qiu et al., 2024). MRI-based deep learning models also predicted treatment response and aided personalized therapy (Jeong et al., 2024). In early-stage cervical squamous cell carcinoma, DL radiomics predicted pathological features for adjuvant radiotherapy, reducing complications risk (X. F. Zhang et al., 2024). Multimodal MRI ML models accurately predicted response to neoadjuvant chemoradiotherapy and survival (Z. Cai et al., 2024). Ultrasound AI using CycleGAN improved feature harmonization and lymph node metastasis prediction in early cervical cancer (Z. Zhao et al., 2024).

In endometrial cancer, DL and radiomics models using DWI features, ADC values, and clinical data have effectively predicted microsatellite instability (MSI), with top models achieving an AUC of 0.885—outperforming clinical or radiomics models alone (J. Wang, Song, et al., 2024). Hybrid models combining multiparametric MRI, DL, and multichannel image analysis have also shown strong performance in predicting MSI (AUC 0.945) and Ki-67 expression (AUC 0.888). Attention mechanisms and interpretability tools like Grad-CAM and SHAP further enhance transparency and clinical relevance. (J. Wang, Song, et al., 2024) (Z. Wang et al., 2025). AI models have been used to predict TP53 mutations in endometrial cancer, with a Gaussian process model combining DL, radiomics, and clinical features achieving an AUC of 0.914 in external validation and better risk classification than individual models(Shen et al., 2025). Radiomics research quality, assessed by RQS and METRICS, shows strong MRI and ML use for characterization and recurrence prediction, though external validation remains a key area for improvement. (Russo et al., 2024).

ML based radiomic analysis of CECT has demonstrated high efficacy in distinguishing ovarian sex cord-stromal tumors from epithelial ovarian cancers, with a mixed model outperforming traditional clinic-radiological assessment (Y. Liu et al., 2024). Similarly, DLR models applied to ultrasound imaging have been developed to assess the risk of malignancy in ovarian tumors. A DLR_Nomogram exhibited superior predictive performance and comparable efficacy to the Ovarian-Adnexal Reporting and Data System (O-RADS), offering potential for improved clinical decision-making (Du, Xiao, et al., 2024). Further, a multiclass prediction algorithm integrating radiomics and DL features has been proposed for differentiating benign, borderline, and malignant ovarian tumors. The model achieved high classification accuracy and successfully identified borderline cases, which were often misclassified by conventional methods (Du, Guo, et al., 2024).

Bone Imaging

ML models using radiomic features from lumbar spine CT, like RF and SVM, achieved strong diagnostic accuracy with AUCs near 0.9 (B. Chen et al., 2024). A hybrid transformer-CNN improved osteoporosis detection to an AUC of 0.97, while DL transfer learning with radiomics on dual-energy CT reached 0.979 (J. Wang, He, et al., 2024). AI also enhanced osteoarthritis diagnosis via T2 mapping and neural networks for early detection (Gao et al., 2024; Li et al., 2024). Additionally, radiomics from T2-weighted MRI combined with DL improved diagnosis of lower back pain (Muhaimillet al., 2024).

AI has shown strong potential in diagnosing bone tumors and malignancies. A DLR nomogram combining multimodal imaging distinguished benign from malignant sacral tumors with an AUC of 0.961 (Zheng et al., 2024). ML models using CT radiomics detected early bone metastases accurately, with a KNN-XGBoost model reaching an AUC of 0.975 (H. Wang et al., 2025). ML-based CT radiomics also effectively differentiated low-grade chondrosarcoma from enchondroma, with RF models achieving an AUC of 0.967 (Yildirim & Yildirim, 2024). X-ray radiomics using SVM classified atypical cartilaginous tumors and high-grade chondrosarcomas with expert-level accuracy (Gitto et al., 2024). Additionally, SVM-based models distinguished benign from malignant vertebral compression fractures with an AUC of 0.911 (Y. Wan et al., 2024).

Other Imaging

For vascular disease, a DL encoder-decoder with ResNet effectively segmented coronary vessels in angiography, enhancing detection by reducing background noise (Pan et al., 2019). A radiomics-clinical nomogram combining non-contrast CT and clinical data predicted unsuccessful recanalization in stroke patients with an AUC of 0.775 (T. Sun et al., 2024). In pancreatic diseases, a deep learning model integrating pathology and imaging predicted liver metastasis in panNET patients with an AUC of 0.961 (Ma et al., 2024). Similarly, an MRI-based radiomics nomogram predicted pancreatic cancer liver metastases with an AUC of 0.832, aiding early diagnosis and treatment (Yuan et al., 2024).

Table 1. Summary of AI models in Medical Image Analysis

Imaging Type	ML/DL Approach	Specific Models	Performance/Comparison
Neuro Imaging	ML, DL	SVM, RF, CNN	High accuracy in tumor classification, CNNs better for segmentation (Pacchiano et al., 2024; Q. Wan et al., 2025).
	ML	SVM, RF	ADC maps effectively differentiate tuberculomas from gliomas (Indoria et al., 2024).
Breast Imaging	ML, DL	EfficientNet-3D, Gaussian Process	High accuracy in breast density detection, lesion classification (Jing et al., 2024).
	DL	Hypergraph Convolution Networks	Improved molecular subtype detection in MRI (Xie et al., 2024).
Lung Imaging	DL	ResNet, U-Net	Superior lung nodule detection in CT scans (Alahmari et al., 2018).
	DL, Transformer	Transformer-based U-NETR	Accurate recurrence prediction in lung cancer (Zaki et al., 2025).
Liver Imaging	DL, ML	Deep Learning Radiomics, CNN	Enhanced prediction of gene mutations and survival (W. Zhang et al., 2024a; Y. Liu, 2024).
Bone Imaging	DL, ML	Transformer CNN, SVM	Effective detection of bone metastases and tumor classification (H. Wang et al., 2025; Yildirim & Yildirim, 2024).

AI at the Image Desk: Enhancing Interpretation Across Modalities

AI is increasingly integrated into the image analysis and interpretation phase of medical imaging, offering significant advancements across multiple modalities. For example, in general radiography, AI tools such as GE's Critical Care Suite 2.0 analyze chest radiographs to detect critical conditions like pneumothorax and assess endotracheal tube placement (GE HealthCare (United States)). These findings are flagged in real-time, enabling prioritization of urgent cases and reducing diagnostic delays. In CT, AI enhanced image interpretation by enabling DL based reconstruction methods that improve the quality of low-dose scans, making subtle pathologies more visible. AI also supports synthetic contrast enhancement from non-contrast

CT scans, improving tissue differentiation in patients who cannot receive contrast agents. In MRI, AI algorithms reconstruct high-quality images from accelerated scans, improving lesion detection and anatomical clarity while reducing noise and motion artifacts. Moreover, in both CT and MRI, AI is used for automated segmentation of organs and lesions, facilitating quantitative assessments, disease classification, and treatment planning. These real-world applications illustrate how AI is not only enhancing diagnostic accuracy but also helping standardize interpretation and reduce human variability in image analysis (Potočnik et al., 2023).

CURRENT CHALLENGES AND FUTURE PERSPECTIVES

The "black-box" nature of many AI systems also limits transparency and interpretability, reducing clinician trust and hindering regulatory approval. XAI has emerged as a promising response to this challenge, offering tools that make model decisions more transparent and understandable to users, particularly in high-stakes areas like medical image analysis (van der Velden et al., 2022). Still, concerns around data privacy, sharing, and standardization restrict access to diverse, high-quality datasets for training(Saw & Ng, 2022). The "black-box" nature of many AI systems also limits transparency and interpretability, reducing clinician trust and hindering regulatory approval. Additionally, unresolved concerns around data privacy, sharing, and standardization restrict access to diverse, high-quality datasets for training (Saw & Ng, 2022). The lack of unified legal frameworks and accountability further complicates ethical integration into clinical workflows. Addressing these barriers is essential for safe and effective AI-driven diagnostics.

In contrast to these challenges, the future of AI in medical image diagnosis is marked by transformative advancements that hold the potential to overcome these existing limitations. AI systems are expected to significantly enhance diagnostic accuracy, predictive analytics, and multimodal data integration, ultimately revolutionizing clinical practice (Langlotz, 2023). Leveraging large-scale imaging databases and advanced neural networks, future models will be capable of detecting subtle disease markers and predicting disease progression with unprecedented precision (Avanzo et al., 2024). The emergence of unified, cloud-based AI platforms will support the seamless integration of imaging, genomic, and clinical data, enabling more personalized and targeted treatment plans (Fazal et al., 2018). Additionally, AI-driven virtual assistants and intelligent reporting tools will help mitigate radiologist burnout by managing routine tasks, thereby reducing diagnostic errors and improving workflow efficiency (Langlotz, 2023). As these innovations continue to evolve, the role of AI is anticipated to shift from diagnostic support to proactive disease monitoring and predictive modeling, paving the way toward an era of precision health (Avanzo et al., 2024).

CONCLUSION

The incorporation of AI in medical image analysis has greatly enhanced the accuracy, efficiency, and automation of diagnostic imaging across multiple medical disciplines. Through techniques such as ML and DL, AI-driven models enable automated feature extraction, segmentation, and classification, reducing observer variability and enhancing disease detection. The methodological advancements discussed in this chapter, including preprocessing techniques, radiomics-based analysis, and classifier optimization, demonstrate the transformative potential of AI in clinical decision-making.

The applications of AI span multiple imaging domains, including neuroimaging, oncology, lung and liver imaging, and musculoskeletal assessments. AI-based radiomics and DL models have improved early detection, tumor classification, and treatment response prediction, allowing for more precise and personalized medical care. Importantly, by supporting healthcare providers with faster, more consistent, and accurate image interpretation, AI contributes to timely diagnoses and better-informed treatment decisions, ultimately improving patient care.

Despite these advances, challenges such as data standardization, model interpretability, and generalizability remain critical areas for future research. Addressing these limitations through robust validation frameworks, XAI, and federated learning approaches will be key to ensuring widespread clinical adoption. As AI continues to evolve, its integration with multimodal imaging and clinical data is poised to further revolutionize medical diagnostics, improving patient outcomes and advancing precision medicine.

REFERENCES

Abdelhalim, I., Alksas, A., Balaha, H. M., Badawy, M. A., El-Ghar, M. A., Alghamdi, N. S., Ghazal, M., Contractor, S., Van Bogaert, E., Gondim, D., Silva, S., Khalifa, F., & El-Baz, A. (2024). *Incorporating Imaging, Clinical, Pathology, and Demographic Markers for Hormonal Therapy Prediction in Prostate Cancer*. IEEE., DOI: 10.1109/ACCESS.2024.3520160

Alahmari, S. S., Cherezov, D., Goldgof, D. B., Hall, L. O., Gillies, R. J., & Schabath, M. B. (2018). Delta Radiomics Improves Pulmonary Nodule Malignancy Prediction in Lung Cancer Screening. *IEEE Access : Practical Innovations, Open Solutions*, *6*, 77796–77806. DOI: 10.1109/ACCESS.2018.2884126 PMID: 30607311

Aonpong, P., Iwamoto, Y., Han, X.-H., Lin, L., & Chen, Y.-W. (2021). Genotype-Guided Radiomics Signatures for Recurrence Prediction of Non-Small Cell Lung Cancer. *IEEE Access : Practical Innovations, Open Solutions*, *9*, 90244–90254. DOI: 10.1109/ACCESS.2021.3088234 PMID: 34892008

Avanzo, M., Stancanello, J., Pirrone, G., Drigo, A., & Retico, A. (2024). The Evolution of Artificial Intelligence in Medical Imaging: From Computer Science to Machine and Deep Learning. *Cancers (Basel)*, *16*(21), 3702. DOI: 10.3390/CANCERS16213702 PMID: 39518140

Borys, K., Schmitt, Y. A., Nauta, M., Seifert, C., Krämer, N., Friedrich, C. M., & Nensa, F. (2023). Explainable AI in medical imaging: An overview for clinical practitioners – Saliency-based XAI approaches. *European Journal of Radiology*, *162*, 110787. DOI: 10.1016/J.EJRAD.2023.110787 PMID: 37001254

Cai, C., Xiao, J. F., Cai, R., Ou, D., Wang, Y. W., Chen, J. Y., & Xu, H. P. (2024). Longitudinal dynamic MRI radiomic models for early prediction of prognosis in locally advanced cervical cancer treated with concurrent chemoradiotherapy. *Radiation Oncology (London, England)*, *19*(1), 1–12. DOI: 10.1186/S13014-024-02574-8/FIGURES/9 PMID: 39707484

Cai, J., Luo, J., Wang, S., & Yang, S. (2018). Feature selection in machine learning: A new perspective. *Neurocomputing*, *300*, 70–79. DOI: 10.1016/J.NEUCOM.2017.11.077

Cai, Z., Li, S., Xiong, Z., Lin, J., & Sun, Y. (2024). Multimodal MRI-based deep-radiomics model predicts response in cervical cancer treated with neoadjuvant chemoradiotherapy. *Scientific Reports 2024 14:1*, *14*(1), 1–11. https://doi.org/DOI: 10.1038/s41598-024-70055-9

Chaddad, A., Kucharczyk, M. J., Desrosiers, C., Okuwobi, I. P., Katib, Y., Zhang, M., Rathore, S., Sargos, P., & Niazi, T. (2020). Deep radiomic analysis to predict gleason score in prostate cancer. *IEEE Access : Practical Innovations, Open Solutions, 8*, 167767–167778. DOI: 10.1109/ACCESS.2020.3023902

Chen, B., Cui, J., Li, C., Xu, P., Xu, G., Jiang, J., Xue, P., Sun, Y., & Cui, Z. (2024). Application of radiomics model based on lumbar computed tomography in diagnosis of elderly osteoporosis. *Journal of Orthopaedic Research : Official Publication of the Orthopaedic Research Society, 42*(6), 1356–1368. DOI: 10.1002/JOR.25789 PMID: 38245854

Chen, Q., Fu, C., Qiu, X., He, J., Zhao, T., Zhang, Q., Hu, X., & Hu, H. (2024). Machine-learning-based performance comparison of two-dimensional (2D) and three-dimensional (3D) CT radiomics features for intracerebral haemorrhage expansion. *Clinical Radiology, 79*(1), e26–e33. DOI: 10.1016/J.CRAD.2023.10.002 PMID: 37926647

Chen, R., Zhou, B., Liu, W., Gan, H., Liu, X., & Zhou, L. (2024). Association of Pathological Features and Multiparametric MRI-Based Radiomics With TP53-Mutated Prostate Cancer. *Journal of Magnetic Resonance Imaging, 60*(3), 1134–1145. DOI: 10.1002/JMRI.29186 PMID: 38153859

Chowdhary, C. L., & Acharjya, D. P. (2020). Segmentation and Feature Extraction in Medical Imaging: A Systematic Review. *Procedia Computer Science, 167*, 26–36. DOI: 10.1016/J.PROCS.2020.03.179

Collewet, G., Strzelecki, M., & Mariette, F. (2004). Influence of MRI acquisition protocols and image intensity normalization methods on texture classification. *Magnetic Resonance Imaging, 22*(1), 81–91. DOI: 10.1016/J.MRI.2003.09.001 PMID: 14972397

Darbandi, M. R., Darbandi, M., Darbandi, S., Bado, I., Hadizadeh, M., & Khorram Khorshid, H. R. (2024). Artificial intelligence breakthroughs in pioneering early diagnosis and precision treatment of breast cancer: A multimethod study. *European Journal of Cancer, 209*, 114227. DOI: 10.1016/J.EJCA.2024.114227 PMID: 39053289

Deng, Z., Liu, X., Wu, R., Yan, H., Gou, L., Hu, W., Wan, J., Song, C., Chen, J., Ma, D., Zhou, H., & Tian, D. (2024). Ultrasound-based radiomics machine learning models for diagnosing cervical lymph node metastasis in patients with non-small cell lung cancer: A multicentre study. *BMC Cancer, 24*(1), 1–11. DOI: 10.1186/S12885-024-12306-6/FIGURES/5 PMID: 38678211

Du, Y., Guo, W., Xiao, Y., Chen, H., Yao, J., & Wu, J. (2024). Ultrasound-based deep learning radiomics model for differentiating benign, borderline, and malignant ovarian tumours: A multi-class classification exploratory study. *BMC Medical Imaging*, *24*(1), 1–16. DOI: 10.1186/S12880-024-01251-2/FIGURES/6 PMID: 38622546

Du, Y., Xiao, Y., Guo, W., Yao, J., Lan, T., Li, S., Wen, H., Zhu, W., He, G., Zheng, H., & Chen, H. (2024). Development and validation of an ultrasound-based deep learning radiomics nomogram for predicting the malignant risk of ovarian tumours. *Biomedical Engineering Online*, *23*(1), 1–21. DOI: 10.1186/S12938-024-01234-Y/FIGURES/8 PMID: 38594729

Ebrahimpour, L., Després, P., & Manem, V. S. K. (2024). Differential Radiomics-Based Signature Predicts Lung Cancer Risk Accounting for Imaging Parameters in NLST Cohort. *Cancer Medicine*, *13*(20). Advance online publication. DOI: 10.1002/CAM4.70359 PMID: 39463128

Fan, L., Wu, H., Wu, Y., Wu, S., Zhao, J., & Zhu, X. (2024). Preoperative prediction of rectal Cancer staging combining MRI deep transfer learning, radiomics features, and clinical factors: Accurate differentiation from stage T2 to T3. *BMC Gastroenterology*, *24*(1), 1–12. DOI: 10.1186/S12876-024-03316-6/FIGURES/7 PMID: 39103772

Fang, T., Liu, N., Nie, S., Jia, S., & Ye, X. (2024). A deep learning and radiomics based Alberta stroke program early CT score method on CTA to evaluate acute ischemic stroke. *Journal of X-Ray Science and Technology*, *32*(1), 17–30. DOI: 10.3233/XST-230119 PMID: 37980594

Fazal, M. I., Patel, M. E., Tye, J., & Gupta, Y. (2018). The past, present and future role of artificial intelligence in imaging. *European Journal of Radiology*, *105*, 246–250. DOI: 10.1016/J.EJRAD.2018.06.020 PMID: 30017288

Gamal, A., Sharafeldeen, A., Alnaghy, E., Alghandour, R., Saleh Alghamdi, N., Ali, K. M., Shamaa, S., Aboueleneen, A., Elsaid Tolba, A., Elmougy, S., Ghazal, M., Contractor, S., & El-Baz, A. (2024). A Novel Machine Learning Approach for Predicting Neoadjuvant Chemotherapy Response in Breast Cancer: Integration of Multimodal Radiomics With Clinical and Molecular Subtype Markers. *IEEE Access : Practical Innovations, Open Solutions*, *12*, 104983–105003. DOI: 10.1109/ACCESS.2024.3432459

Gao, S., Peng, C., Wang, G., Deng, C., Zhang, Z., & Liu, X. (2024). Cartilage T2 mapping-based radiomics in knee osteoarthritis research: Status, progress and future outlook. *European Journal of Radiology*, *181*. Advance online publication. DOI: 10.1016/J.EJRAD.2024.111826 PMID: 39522425

Gitto, S., Annovazzi, A., Nulle, K., Interlenghi, M., Salvatore, C., Anelli, V., Baldi, J., Messina, C., Albano, D., Di Luca, F., Armiraglio, E., Parafioriti, A., Luzzati, A., Biagini, R., Castiglioni, I., & Sconfienza, L. M. (2024). X-rays radiomics-based machine learning classification of atypical cartilaginous tumour and high-grade chondrosarcoma of long bones. *EBioMedicine*, *101*. Advance online publication. DOI: 10.1016/J.EBIOM.2024.105018 PMID: 38377797

Gross, M., Huber, S., Arora, S., Ze'evi, T., Haider, S. P., Kucukkaya, A. S., Iseke, S., Kuhn, T. N., Gebauer, B., Michallek, F., Dewey, M., Vilgrain, V., Sartoris, R., Ronot, M., Jaffe, A., Strazzabosco, M., Chapiro, J., & Onofrey, J. A. (2024). Automated MRI liver segmentation for anatomical segmentation, liver volumetry, and the extraction of radiomics. *European Radiology*, *34*(8), 5056–5065. DOI: 10.1007/S00330-023-10495-5/FIGURES/4 PMID: 38217704

Guo, X., He, Y., Yuan, Z., Nie, T., Liu, Y., & Xu, H. (2025). Association Analysis Between Intratumoral and Peritumoral MRI Radiomics Features and Overall Survival of Neoadjuvant Therapy in Rectal Cancer. *Journal of Magnetic Resonance Imaging*, *61*(1), 452–465. DOI: 10.1002/JMRI.29396 PMID: 38733601

Huang, L., Ruan, S., & Denœux, T. (2023). Application of belief functions to medical image segmentation: A review. *Information Fusion*, *91*, 737–756. DOI: 10.1016/J.INFFUS.2022.11.008

Huang, Y., Qian, H., Zheng, Y., Song, H., & Liu, X. (2024). A radiomics model based on transrectal ultrasound for predicting prostate cancer. *Medical Ultrasonography*, *26*(2), 138–146. DOI: 10.11152/MU-4329 PMID: 38537183

Indoria, A., Kulanthaivelu, K., Prasad, C., Srinivas, D., Rao, S., Sinha, N., Potluri, V., Netravathi, M., Nalini, A., & Saini, J. (2024). Radiomics features for the discrimination of tuberculomas from high grade gliomas and metastasis: A multimodal study. *Neuroradiology*, *66*(11), 1979–1992. DOI: 10.1007/S00234-024-03435-7/FIGURES/3 PMID: 39102087

Jeong, S., Yu, H., Park, S. H., Woo, D., Lee, S. J., Chong, G. O., Han, H. S., & Kim, J. C. (2024). Comparing deep learning and handcrafted radiomics to predict chemoradiotherapy response for locally advanced cervical cancer using pretreatment MRI. *Scientific Reports 2024 14:1*, *14*(1), 1–11. https://doi.org/DOI: 10.1038/s41598-024-51742-z

Jia, W., Li, F., Cui, Y., Wang, Y., Dai, Z., Yan, Q., Liu, X., Li, Y., Chang, H., & Zeng, Q. (2024). Deep Learning Radiomics Model of Contrast-Enhanced CT for Differentiating the Primary Source of Liver Metastases. *Academic Radiology*, *31*(10), 4057–4067. DOI: 10.1016/j.acra.2024.04.012 PMID: 38702214

Jiang, B., Bao, L., He, S., Chen, X., Jin, Z., & Ye, Y. (2024). Deep learning applications in breast cancer histopathological imaging: Diagnosis, treatment, and prognosis. *Breast Cancer Research : BCR*, *26*(1), 1–17. DOI: 10.1186/S13058-024-01895-6/TABLES/2 PMID: 39304962

Jing, X., Wielema, M., Monroy-Gonzalez, A. G., Stams, T. R. G., Mahesh, S. V. K., Oudkerk, M., Sijens, P. E., Dorrius, M. D., & van Ooijen, P. M. A. (2024). Automated Breast Density Assessment in MRI Using Deep Learning and Radiomics: Strategies for Reducing Inter-Observer Variability. *Journal of Magnetic Resonance Imaging*, *60*(1), 80–91. DOI: 10.1002/JMRI.29058 PMID: 37846440

Kanakarajan, H., De Baene, W., Hanssens, P., & Sitskoorn, M. (2024). Predicting local control of brain metastases after stereotactic radiotherapy with clinical, radiomics and deep learning features. *Radiation Oncology 2024 19:1, 19*(1), 1–15. https://doi.org/DOI: 10.1186/S13014-024-02573-9

Khalifa, M., & Albadawy, M. (2024). AI in diagnostic imaging: Revolutionising accuracy and efficiency. *Computer Methods and Programs in Biomedicine Update*, *5*, 100146. DOI: 10.1016/J.CMPBUP.2024.100146

Kora, P., Ooi, C. P., Faust, O., Raghavendra, U., Gudigar, A., Chan, W. Y., Meenakshi, K., Swaraja, K., Plawiak, P., & Rajendra Acharya, U. (2022). Transfer learning techniques for medical image analysis: A review. *Biocybernetics and Biomedical Engineering*, *42*(1), 79–107. DOI: 10.1016/J.BBE.2021.11.004

Kuang, Q., Feng, B., Xu, K., Chen, Y., Chen, X., Duan, X., Lei, X., Chen, X., Li, K., & Long, W. (2024). Multimodal deep learning radiomics model for predicting postoperative progression in solid stage I non-small cell lung cancer. *Cancer Imaging; the Official Publication of the International Cancer Imaging Society*, *24*(1), 1–13. DOI: 10.1186/S40644-024-00783-8/FIGURES/6 PMID: 39420411

Langlotz, C. P. (2023). The Future of AI and Informatics in Radiology: 10 Predictions. *Radiology*, *309*(1). Advance online publication. DOI: 10.1148/RADIOL.231114/ASSET/IMAGES/LARGE/RADIOL.231114.FIG1.JPEG PMID: 37874234

Lee, H., Chang, W., Kim, H. Y., Sung, P., Cho, J., Lee, Y. J., & Kim, Y. H. (2024). Improving radiomics reproducibility using deep learning-based image conversion of CT reconstruction algorithms in hepatocellular carcinoma patients. *European Radiology*, *34*(3), 2036–2047. DOI: 10.1007/S00330-023-10135-Y/TABLES/5 PMID: 37656175

Lee, T. F., Chang, C. H., Chi, C. H., Liu, Y. H., Shao, J. C., Hsieh, Y. W., Yang, P. Y., Tseng, C. D., Chiu, C. L., Hu, Y. C., Lin, Y. W., Chao, P. J., Lee, S. H., & Yeh, S. A. (2024). Utilizing radiomics and dosiomics with AI for precision prediction of radiation dermatitis in breast cancer patients. *BMC Cancer*, *24*(1), 1–17. DOI: 10.1186/S12885-024-12753-1/FIGURES/6 PMID: 39107701

Lee, Y. D., Kim, H. G., Seo, M., Moon, S. K., Park, S. J., & You, M. W. (2024). Machine learning–based response assessment in patients with rectal cancer after neoadjuvant chemoradiotherapy: Radiomics analysis for assessing tumor regression grade using T2-weighted magnetic resonance images. *International Journal of Colorectal Disease*, *39*(1), 1–14. DOI: 10.1007/S00384-024-04651-6/FIGURES/7 PMID: 38789861

Li, S., Cao, P., Li, J., Chen, T., Luo, P., Ruan, G., Zhang, Y., Wang, X., Han, W., Zhu, Z., Dang, Q., Wang, Q., Zhang, M., Bai, Q., Chai, Z., Yang, H., Chen, H., Tang, M., Akbar, A., & Ding, C. (2024). Integrating Radiomics and Neural Networks for Knee Osteoarthritis Incidence Prediction. *Arthritis & Rheumatology (Hoboken, N.J.)*, *76*(9), 1377–1386. DOI: 10.1002/ART.42915 PMID: 38751101

Liang, B., Tong, C., Nong, J., & Zhang, Y. (2024). Histological Subtype Classification of Non-Small Cell Lung Cancer with Radiomics and 3D Convolutional Neural Networks. *Journal of Imaging Informatics in Medicine*, *37*(6). Advance online publication. DOI: 10.1007/S10278-024-01152-4 PMID: 38861072

Liao, C. Y., Chen, Y. M., Te Wu, Y., Chao, H. S., Chiu, H. Y., Wang, T. W., Chen, J. R., Shiao, T. H., & Lu, C. F. (2024). Personalized prediction of immunotherapy response in lung cancer patients using advanced radiomics and deep learning. *Cancer Imaging; the Official Publication of the International Cancer Imaging Society*, *24*(1), 129. DOI: 10.1186/S40644-024-00779-4/FIGURES/6 PMID: 39350284

Liu, W., Li, L., Deng, J., & Li, W. (2024). A comprehensive approach for evaluating lymphovascular invasion in invasive breast cancer: Leveraging multimodal MRI findings, radiomics, and deep learning analysis of intra- and peritumoral regions. *Computerized Medical Imaging and Graphics*, *116*, 102415. DOI: 10.1016/J.COMPMEDIMAG.2024.102415 PMID: 39032451

Liu, Y., Jia, X., Zhao, J., Peng, Y., Yao, X., Hu, X., Cui, J., Chen, H., Chen, X., Wu, J., Hong, N., Wang, S., & Wang, Y. (2024). A Machine Learning-Based Unenhanced Radiomics Approach to Distinguishing Between Benign and Malignant Breast Lesions Using T2-Weighted and Diffusion-Weighted MRI. *Journal of Magnetic Resonance Imaging*, *60*(2), 600–612. DOI: 10.1002/JMRI.29111 PMID: 37933890

Liu, Y., Liu, Z., Li, X., Zhou, W., Lin, L., & Chen, X. (2024). Non-invasive assessment of response to transcatheter arterial chemoembolization for hepatocellular carcinoma with the deep neural networks-based radiomics nomogram. *Acta Radiologica (Stockholm, Sweden : 1987), 65*(6), 535–545. https://doi.org/DOI: 10.1177/02841851241229185

Liu, Y., Zheng, X., Fan, D., Shen, Z., Wu, Z., & Li, S. (2024). CT-based radiomic analysis for categorization of ovarian sex cord-stromal tumors and epithelial ovarian cancers. *Abdominal Radiology*, *49*(11). Advance online publication. DOI: 10.1007/S00261-024-04437-Y PMID: 38896249

Liu, Z., Zhang, S., Wang, Y., Xu, H., Gao, Y., Jin, H., Zhang, Y., Wu, H., Lu, J., Chen, P., Qiao, P. G., & Yang, Z. (2024). Posterior circulation ischemic stroke: Radiomics-based machine learning approach to identify onset time from magnetic resonance imaging. *Neuroradiology*, *66*(7), 1141–1152. DOI: 10.1007/S00234-024-03353-8 PMID: 38592454

Lu, Y., Yuan, R., Su, Y., Liang, Z., Huang, H., Leng, Q., Yang, A., Xiao, X., Lai, Z., & Zhang, Y. (2025). Biparametric MRI-based radiomics for noninvastive discrimination of benign prostatic hyperplasia nodules (BPH) and prostate cancer nodules: a bio-centric retrospective cohort study. *Scientific Reports 2025 15:1, 15*(1), 1–12. https://doi.org/DOI: 10.1038/s41598-024-84908-w

Ma, M., Gu, W., Liang, Y., Han, X., Zhang, M., Xu, M., Gao, H., Tang, W., & Huang, D. (2024). A novel model for predicting postoperative liver metastasis in R0 resected pancreatic neuroendocrine tumors: Integrating computational pathology and deep learning-radiomics. *Journal of Translational Medicine*, *22*(1), 1–14. DOI: 10.1186/S12967-024-05449-4/FIGURES/6 PMID: 39143624

Maiti, S., Nayak, S., Hebbar, K. D., & Pendem, S. (2024). Differentiation of invasive ductal and lobular carcinoma of the breast using MRI radiomic features: a pilot study. *F1000Research 2024 13:91, 13*, 91. https://doi.org/DOI: 10.12688/f1000research.146052.2

Masoudi, S., Harmon, S. A., Mehralivand, S., Walker, S. M., Raviprakash, H., Bagci, U., Choyke, P. L., & Turkbey, B. (2021). Quick guide on radiology image pre-processing for deep learning applications in prostate cancer research. *Journal of Medical Imaging (Bellingham, Wash.)*, *8*(1), 010901. DOI: 10.1117/1.JMI.8.1.010901 PMID: 33426151

Meddings, Z., Rundo, L., Sadat, U., Zhao, X., Teng, Z., & Graves, M. J. (2024). Robustness and classification capabilities of MRI radiomic features in identifying carotid plaque vulnerability. *The British Journal of Radiology*, *97*(1158), 1118–1124. DOI: 10.1093/BJR/TQAE057 PMID: 38711198

Muhaimil, A., Pendem, S., & Sampathilla, N., P S, P., Nayak, K., Chadaga, K., Goswami, A., M, O. C., & Shirlal, A. (2024). Role of Artificial intelligence model in prediction of low back pain using T2 weighted MRI of Lumbar spine. *F1000Research 2024 13:1035*, *13*, 1035. https://doi.org/DOI: 10.12688/f1000research.154680.2

Nam, D., Chapiro, J., Paradis, V., Seraphin, T. P., & Kather, J. N. (2022). Artificial intelligence in liver diseases: Improving diagnostics, prognostics and response prediction. *JHEP Reports : Innovation in Hepatology*, *4*(4), 100443. DOI: 10.1016/J.JHEPR.2022.100443 PMID: 35243281

Nayak, S. S., Pendem, S., Menon, G. R., Sampathila, N., & Koteshwar, P. (2024). Quality Assessment of MRI-Radiomics-Based Machine Learning Methods in Classification of Brain Tumors: Systematic Review. *Diagnostics (Basel)*, *14*(23), 2741. DOI: 10.3390/DIAGNOSTICS14232741/S1 PMID: 39682649

Nemoto, H., Saito, M., Satoh, Y., Komiyama, T., Marino, K., Aoki, S., Suzuki, H., Sano, N., Nonaka, H., Watanabe, H., Funayama, S., & Onishi, H. (2024). Evaluation of the performance of both machine learning models using PET and CT radiomics for predicting recurrence following lung stereotactic body radiation therapy: A single-institutional study. *Journal of Applied Clinical Medical Physics*, *25*(7). Advance online publication. DOI: 10.1002/ACM2.14322 PMID: 38436611

Pacchiano, F., Tortora, M., Doneda, C., Izzo, G., Arrigoni, F., Ugga, L., Cuocolo, R., Parazzini, C., Righini, A., & Brunetti, A. (2024). Radiomics and artificial intelligence applications in pediatric brain tumors. *World Journal of Pediatrics: WJP*, *20*(8). Advance online publication. DOI: 10.1007/S12519-024-00823-0 PMID: 38935233

Pan, S., Zhang, W., Zhang, W., Xu, L., Fan, G., Gong, J., Zhang, B., & Gu, H. (2019). Diagnostic Model of Coronary Microvascular Disease Combined with Full Convolution Deep Network with Balanced Cross-Entropy Cost Function. *IEEE Access : Practical Innovations, Open Solutions*, *7*, 177997–178006. DOI: 10.1109/ACCESS.2019.2958825

Panahi, M., & Hosseini, M. S. (2024). Multi-modality radiomics of conventional T1 weighted and diffusion tensor imaging for differentiating Parkinson's disease motor subtypes in early-stages. *Scientific Reports 2024 14:1*, *14*(1), 1–10. https://doi.org/DOI: 10.1038/s41598-024-71860-y

Patel, R. V., Groff, K. J., & Bi, W. L. (2024). Applications and Integration of Radiomics for Skull Base Oncology. *Advances in Experimental Medicine and Biology, 1462*, 285–305. DOI: 10.1007/978-3-031-64892-2_17 PMID: 39523272

Pei, J., Yu, J., Ge, P., Bao, L., Pang, H., & Zhang, H. (2024). Constructing a Classification Model for Cervical Cancer Tumor Tissue and Normal Tissue Based on CT Radiomics. *Technology in Cancer Research & Treatment, 23*. Advance online publication. DOI: 10.1177/15330338241298554 PMID: 39539120

Perniciano, A., Loddo, A., Di Ruberto, C., & Pes, B. (2024). Insights into radiomics: Impact of feature selection and classification. *Multimedia Tools and Applications, 2024*, 1–27. DOI: 10.1007/S11042-024-20388-4

Pinto-Coelho, L. (2023). How Artificial Intelligence Is Shaping Medical Imaging Technology: A Survey of Innovations and Applications. *Bioengineering (Basel, Switzerland), 10*(12), 1435. DOI: 10.3390/BIOENGINEERING10121435 PMID: 38136026

Popov, A. (2023). Feature engineering methods. *Advanced Methods in Biomedical Signal Processing and Analysis*, 1–29. https://doi.org/DOI: 10.1016/B978-0-323-85955-4.00004-1

Potočnik, J., Foley, S., & Thomas, E. (2023). Current and potential applications of artificial intelligence in medical imaging practice: A narrative review. *Journal of Medical Imaging and Radiation Sciences, 54*(2), 376–385. DOI: 10.1016/J.JMIR.2023.03.033/ATTACHMENT/7CB5D334-F035-46D6-BA09-3399D65D2920/MMC1.DOCX PMID: 37062603

Preim, B., & Botha, C. (2014). Image Analysis for Medical Visualization. *Visual Computing for Medicine*, 111–175. https://doi.org/DOI: 10.1016/B978-0-12-415873-3.00004-3

Qian, G. X., Xu, Z. L., Li, Y. H., Lu, J. L., Bu, X. Y., Wei, M. T., & Jia, W. D. (2024). Computed tomography-based radiomics to predict early recurrence of hepatocellular carcinoma post-hepatectomy in patients background on cirrhosis. https://Www.Wjgnet.Com/, *30*(15), 2128–2142. https://doi.org/DOI: 10.3748/WJG.V30.I15.2128

Qian, L., Liu, X., Zhou, S., Zhi, W., Zhang, K., Li, H., Li, J., & Chang, C. (2024). A cutting-edge deep learning-and-radiomics-based ultrasound nomogram for precise prediction of axillary lymph node metastasis in breast cancer patients ≥ 75 years. *Frontiers in Endocrinology, 15*, 1323452. DOI: 10.3389/FENDO.2024.1323452/BIBTEX PMID: 39072273

Qiu, H., Wang, M., Wang, S., Li, X., Wang, D., Qin, Y., Xu, Y., Yin, X., Hacker, M., Han, S., & Li, X. (2024). Integrating MRI-based radiomics and clinicopathological features for preoperative prognostication of early-stage cervical adenocarcinoma patients: In comparison to deep learning approach. *Cancer Imaging; the Official Publication of the International Cancer Imaging Society*, *24*(1), 1–11. DOI: 10.1186/S40644-024-00747-Y/FIGURES/6 PMID: 39090668

Rana, M., & Bhushan, M. (2023). Machine learning and deep learning approach for medical image analysis: Diagnosis to detection. *Multimedia Tools and Applications*, *82*(17), 26731–26769. DOI: 10.1007/S11042-022-14305-W/TABLES/5 PMID: 36588765

Russo, L., Bottazzi, S., Kocak, B., Zormpas-Petridis, K., Gui, B., Stanzione, A., Imbriaco, M., Sala, E., Cuocolo, R., & Ponsiglione, A. (2024). Evaluating the quality of radiomics-based studies for endometrial cancer using RQS and METRICS tools. *European Radiology*, *35*(1), 202–214. DOI: 10.1007/S00330-024-10947-6/FIGURES/6 PMID: 39014086

Sarker, I. H. (2021). Machine Learning: Algorithms, Real-World Applications and Research Directions. *SN Computer Science*, *2*(3), 1–21. DOI: 10.1007/S42979-021-00592-X/FIGURES/11 PMID: 33778771

Saw, S. N., & Ng, K. H. (2022). Current challenges of implementing artificial intelligence in medical imaging. *Physica Medica*, *100*, 12–17. DOI: 10.1016/J.EJMP.2022.06.003 PMID: 35714523

Selvam, M., Sadanandan, A., Chandrasekharan, A., Ramesh, S., Murali, A., & Krishnamurthi, G. (2024). Radiomics for differentiating adenocarcinoma and squamous cell carcinoma in non-small cell lung cancer beyond nodule morphology in chest CT. *Scientific Reports 2024 14:1*, *14*(1), 1–13. https://doi.org/DOI: 10.1038/s41598-024-83786-6

Shen, L., Dai, B., Dou, S., Yan, F., Yang, T., & Wu, Y. (2025). Estimation of TP53 mutations for endometrial cancer based on diffusion-weighted imaging deep learning and radiomics features. *BMC Cancer*, *25*(1), 45. DOI: 10.1186/S12885-025-13424-5 PMID: 39789538

Sukhadia, S. S., Sadee, C., Gevaert, O., & Nagaraj, S. H. (2024). Machine Learning Enabled Prediction of Biologically Relevant Gene Expression Using CT-Based Radiomic Features in Non-Small Cell Lung Cancer. *Cancer Medicine*, *13*(24). Advance online publication. DOI: 10.1002/CAM4.70509 PMID: 39718015

Sun, T., Yu, H. Y., Zhan, C. H., Guo, H. L., & Luo, M. Y. (2024). Non-contrast CT radiomics-clinical machine learning model for futile recanalization after endovascular treatment in anterior circulation acute ischemic stroke. *BMC Medical Imaging*, *24*(1), 1–11. DOI: 10.1186/S12880-024-01365-7/FIGURES/5 PMID: 39030494

Sun, Z., Xia, F., Lv, W., Li, J., Zou, Y., & Wu, J. (2024). Radiomics based on T2-weighted and diffusion-weighted MR imaging for preoperative prediction of tumor deposits in rectal cancer. *American Journal of Surgery*, *232*, 59–67. DOI: 10.1016/j.amjsurg.2024.01.002 PMID: 38272767

van der Velden, B. H. M., Kuijf, H. J., Gilhuijs, K. G. A., & Viergever, M. A. (2022). Explainable artificial intelligence (XAI) in deep learning-based medical image analysis. *Medical Image Analysis*, *79*, 102470. DOI: 10.1016/J.MEDIA.2022.102470 PMID: 35576821

Varan, M., Azimjonov, J., & Macal, B. (2023). Enhancing Prostate Cancer Classification by Leveraging Key Radiomics Features and Using the Fine-Tuned Linear SVM Algorithm. *IEEE Access : Practical Innovations, Open Solutions*, *11*, 88025–88039. DOI: 10.1109/ACCESS.2023.3306515

Velliangiri, S., Alagumuthukrishnan, S., & Thankumar Joseph, S. I. (2019). A Review of Dimensionality Reduction Techniques for Efficient Computation. *Procedia Computer Science*, *165*, 104–111. DOI: 10.1016/J.PROCS.2020.01.079

Wan, Q., Lindsay, C., Zhang, C., Kim, J., Chen, X., Li, J., Huang, R. Y., Reardon, D. A., Young, G. S., & Qin, L. (2025). Comparative analysis of deep learning and radiomic signatures for overall survival prediction in recurrent high-grade glioma treated with immunotherapy. *Cancer Imaging 2024 25:1*, *25*(1), 1–9. https://doi.org/DOI: 10.1186/S40644-024-00818-0

Wan, Y., Miao, L., Zhang, H. H., Wang, Y. M., Li, X., Li, M., & Zhang, L. (2024). Machine learning models based on CT radiomics features for distinguishing benign and malignant vertebral compression fractures in patients with malignant tumors. *Acta Radiologica (Stockholm, Sweden: 1987)*, *65*(11). https://doi.org/DOI: 10.1177/02841851241279896

Wang, H., Qiu, J., Lu, W., Xie, J., & Ma, J. (2025). Radiomics based on multiple machine learning methods for diagnosing early bone metastases not visible on CT images. *Skeletal Radiology*, *54*(2). Advance online publication. DOI: 10.1007/S00256-024-04752-X PMID: 39028463

Wang, J., He, Y., Yan, L., Chen, S., & Zhang, K. (2024). Predicting Osteoporosis and Osteopenia by Fusing Deep Transfer Learning Features and Classical Radiomics Features Based on Single-Source Dual-energy CT Imaging. *Academic Radiology, 31*(10). Advance online publication. DOI: 10.1016/J.ACRA.2024.04.022 PMID: 38693026

Wang, J., Song, P., Zhang, M., Liu, W., Zeng, X., Chen, N., Li, Y., & Wang, M. (2024). A prediction model based on deep learning and radiomics features of DWI for the assessment of microsatellite instability in endometrial cancer. *Cancer Medicine, 13*(16), e70046. DOI: 10.1002/CAM4.70046 PMID: 39171859

Wang, M., Wei, Y., Zhu, M., Yu, H., Guo, C., Chen, Z., Shi, W., Ren, J., Zhao, W., Yang, Z., & Chen, L. A. (2024). The Value of Topological Radiomics Analysis in Predicting Malignant Risk of Pulmonary Ground-Glass Nodules: A Multi-Center Study. *Technology in Cancer Research & Treatment, 23*. Advance online publication. DOI: 10.1177/15330338241287089 PMID: 39363876

Wang, Z., Hu, Y., Cai, J., Xie, J., Li, C., Wu, X., Li, J., Luo, H., & He, C. (2025). Potential value of novel multiparametric MRI radiomics for preoperative prediction of microsatellite instability and Ki-67 expression in endometrial cancer. *Scientific Reports 2025 15:1, 15*(1), 1–12. https://doi.org/DOI: 10.1038/s41598-025-87966-w

Xie, X., Wu, L., Su, Z., Sun, Z., Cao, X., Hou, Y., He, X., & Zhao, F. (2024). CORONet: A Cross-Sequence Joint Representation and Hypergraph Convolutional Network for Classifying Molecular Subtypes of Breast Cancer Using Incomplete DCE-MRI. *IEEE Journal of Biomedical and Health Informatics, 28*(4), 2103–2114. DOI: 10.1109/JBHI.2024.3355111 PMID: 38231805

Xing, X., Li, D., Peng, J., Shu, Z., Zhang, Y., & Song, Q. (2024). A combinatorial MRI sequence-based radiomics model for preoperative prediction of microsatellite instability status in rectal cancer. *Scientific Reports 2024 14:1, 14*(1), 1–10. https://doi.org/DOI: 10.1038/s41598-024-62584-0

Yan, H. J., Zhao, J. S., Zuo, H. D., Zhang, J. J., Deng, Z. Q., Yang, C., Luo, X., Wan, J. X., Zheng, X. Y., Chen, W. Y., Li, S. P., & Tian, D. (2024). Dual-Region Computed Tomography Radiomics-Based Machine Learning Predicts Subcarinal Lymph Node Metastasis in Patients with Non-small Cell Lung Cancer. *Annals of Surgical Oncology, 31*(8), 5011–5020. DOI: 10.1245/S10434-024-15197-W PMID: 38520581

Yang, Y., Xu, Z., Cai, Z., Zhao, H., Zhu, C., Hong, J., Lu, R., Lai, X., Guo, L., Hu, Q., & Xu, Z. (2024). Novel deep learning radiomics nomogram-based multiparametric MRI for predicting the lymph node metastasis in rectal cancer: A dual-center study. *Journal of Cancer Research and Clinical Oncology*, *150*(10), 1–12. DOI: 10.1007/S00432-024-05986-X/FIGURES/5 PMID: 39379733

Yildirim, M., & Yildirim, H. (2024). CT radiomics-based machine learning model for differentiating between enchondroma and low-grade chondrosarcoma. *Medicine*, *103*(33), e39311. DOI: 10.1097/MD.0000000000039311 PMID: 39151512

Yin, L., Liu, R., Li, W., Li, S., & Hou, X. (2025). Deep learning-based CT radiomics predicts prognosis of unresectable hepatocellular carcinoma treated with TACE-HAIC combined with PD-1 inhibitors and tyrosine kinase inhibitors. *BMC Gastroenterology 2024 25:1, 25*(1), 1–13. https://doi.org/DOI: 10.1186/S12876-024-03555-7

Yoon, J. M., Lim, C. Y., Noh, H., Nam, S. W., Jun, S. Y., Kim, M. J., Song, M. Y., Jang, H., Kim, H. J., Seo, S. W., Na, D. L., Chung, M. J., Ham, D. Il, & Kim, K. (2024). Enhancing foveal avascular zone analysis for Alzheimer's diagnosis with AI segmentation and machine learning using multiple radiomic features. *Scientific Reports 2024 14:1, 14*(1), 1–16. https://doi.org/DOI: 10.1038/s41598-024-51612-8

Yuan, Z., Shu, Z., Peng, J., Wang, W., Hou, J., Han, L., Zheng, G., Wei, Y., & Zhong, J. (2024). Prediction of postoperative liver metastasis in pancreatic ductal adenocarcinoma based on multiparametric magnetic resonance radiomics combined with serological markers: A cohort study of machine learning. *Abdominal Radiology*, *49*(1), 117–130. DOI: 10.1007/S00261-023-04047-0/FIGURES/10 PMID: 37819438

Zachariah, R. M., Priya, P. S., & Pendem, S. (2023). Classification of low- and high-grade gliomas using radiomic analysis of multiple sequences of MRI brain. *Journal of Cancer Research and Therapeutics*, *19*(2), 435–446. DOI: 10.4103/JCRT.JCRT_1581_22 PMID: 37313916

Zaki, H. A., Oueidat, K., Hsieh, C., Zhang, H., Collins, S., Jiao, Z., & Maxwell, A. W. P. (2025). Predicting Survival and Recurrence of Lung Ablation Patients Using Deep Learning-Based Automatic Segmentation and Radiomics Analysis. *Cardiovascular and Interventional Radiology*, *48*(1). Advance online publication. DOI: 10.1007/S00270-024-03912-9 PMID: 39604700

Zarei, A., Keshavarz, A., Jafari, E., Nemati, R., Farhadi, A., Gholamrezanezhad, A., Rostami, H., & Assadi, M. (2024). Automated classification of Alzheimer's disease, mild cognitive impairment, and cognitively normal patients using 3D convolutional neural network and radiomic features from T1-weighted brain MRI: A comparative study on detection accuracy. *Clinical Imaging*, *115*. Advance online publication. DOI: 10.1016/J.CLINIMAG.2024.110301 PMID: 39303405

Zhang, C., Ma, L. di, Zhang, X. lan, Lei, C., Yuan, S. sha, Li, J. peng, Geng, Z. jun, Li, X. ming, Quan, X. yue, Zheng, C., Geng, Y. yuan, Zhang, J., Zheng, Q. li, Hou, J., Xie, S. yi, Lu, L. he, & Xie, C. miao. (2024). Magnetic Resonance Deep Learning Radiomic Model Based on Distinct Metastatic Vascular Patterns for Evaluating Recurrence-Free Survival in Hepatocellular Carcinoma. *Journal of Magnetic Resonance Imaging : JMRI, 60*(1), 231–242. https://doi.org/DOI: 10.1002/JMRI.29064

Zhang, J., Hao, L., Xu, Q., & Gao, F. (2024). Radiomics and Clinical Characters Based Gaussian Naive Bayes (GNB) Model for Preoperative Differentiation of Pulmonary Pure Invasive Mucinous Adenocarcinoma From Mixed Mucinous Adenocarcinoma. *Technology in Cancer Research & Treatment*, *23*. Advance online publication. DOI: 10.1177/15330338241258415 PMID: 38819419

Zhang, W., Guo, Q., Zhu, Y., Wang, M., Zhang, T., Cheng, G., Zhang, Q., & Ding, H. (2024a). Cross-institutional evaluation of deep learning and radiomics models in predicting microvascular invasion in hepatocellular carcinoma: Validity, robustness, and ultrasound modality efficacy comparison. *Cancer Imaging; the Official Publication of the International Cancer Imaging Society*, *24*(1), 142. DOI: 10.1186/S40644-024-00790-9/TABLES/5 PMID: 39438929

Zhang, W., Guo, Q., Zhu, Y., Wang, M., Zhang, T., Cheng, G., Zhang, Q., & Ding, H. (2024b). Cross-institutional evaluation of deep learning and radiomics models in predicting microvascular invasion in hepatocellular carcinoma: Validity, robustness, and ultrasound modality efficacy comparison. *Cancer Imaging; the Official Publication of the International Cancer Imaging Society*, *24*(1), 142. DOI: 10.1186/S40644-024-00790-9/TABLES/5 PMID: 39438929

Zhang, X. F., Wu, H. Y., Liang, X. W., Chen, J. L., Li, J., Zhang, S., & Liu, Z. (2024). Deep-learning-based radiomics of intratumoral and peritumoral MRI images to predict the pathological features of adjuvant radiotherapy in early-stage cervical squamous cell carcinoma. *BMC Women's Health*, *24*(1), 1–12. DOI: 10.1186/S12905-024-03001-6/FIGURES/6 PMID: 38504245

Zhang, Y. F., Zhou, C., Guo, S., Wang, C., Yang, J., Yang, Z. J., Wang, R., Zhang, X., & Zhou, F. H. (2024). Deep learning algorithm-based multimodal MRI radiomics and pathomics data improve prediction of bone metastases in primary prostate cancer. *Journal of Cancer Research and Clinical Oncology*, *150*(2), 1–13. DOI: 10.1007/S00432-023-05574-5/FIGURES/10 PMID: 38316655

Zhao, W., Hou, M., Wang, J., Song, D., & Niu, Y. (2024). Interpretable machine learning model for predicting clinically significant prostate cancer: Integrating intratumoral and peritumoral radiomics with clinical and metabolic features. *BMC Medical Imaging*, *24*(1), 1–15. DOI: 10.1186/S12880-024-01548-2/FIGURES/6 PMID: 39736623

Zhao, X., Wang, L., Zhang, Y., Han, X., Deveci, M., & Parmar, M. (2024). A review of convolutional neural networks in computer vision. *Artificial Intelligence Review*, *57*(4), 1–43. DOI: 10.1007/S10462-024-10721-6/FIGURES/33

Zhao, Z., Qin, Y., Shao, K., Liu, Y., Zhang, Y., Li, H., Li, W., Xu, J., Zhang, J., Ning, B., Yu, X., Jin, X., & Jin, J. (2024). Radiomics Harmonization in Ultrasound Images for Cervical Cancer Lymph Node Metastasis Prediction Using Cycle-GAN. *Technology in Cancer Research & Treatment*, *23*. Advance online publication. DOI: 10.1177/15330338241302237 PMID: 39639562

Zheng, F., Yin, P., Liang, · Kewei, Liu, T., Wang, Y., Hao, W., Hao, Q., & Hong, N. (2024). Comparison of Different Fusion Radiomics for Predicting Benign and Malignant Sacral Tumors: A Pilot Study. *Journal of Imaging Informatics in Medicine 2024 37:5*, *37*(5), 2415–2427. https://doi.org/DOI: 10.1007/S10278-024-01134-6

Chapter 4
The Evolution of MRI Before and After the Introduction of AI

Shruti S. Deshmukh
https://orcid.org/0009-0001-5178-5990
Datta Meghe Institute of Higher Education and Research, India

Pranjali Deshmukh
https://orcid.org/0000-0002-6557-4334
St. Vincent Pallotti College of Engineering and Technology, Nagpur, India

Kalyani N. Satone
https://orcid.org/0009-0001-3927-352X
St. Vincent Pallotti College of Engineering and Technology, Nagpur, India

Palash Gourshettiwar
https://orcid.org/0009-0007-2184-0331
Datta Meghe Institute of Higher Education and Research, India

Meher Langote
Datta Meghe Institute of Higher Education and Research, India

ABSTRACT

Magnetic Resonance Imaging (MRI) is a perfect solution of imaging diagnostically used in medicine and its related fields. However, there has been tremendous advancement in producing MRI technology in both hardware and software besides improvements in characterization of images. This paper gives a background of MRI together with early drawbacks and the introduction of Artificial Intelligence (AI). AI has improved image acquisition, reconstruction and analysis through increased

DOI: 10.4018/979-8-3373-0903-3.ch004

speed of scans, higher and more accurate image results and thus better diagnosis. However, the use of AI in MRI encounters some hurdles, such as technical, ethical, and AI capabilities hurdles. This paper focuses on MRI history prior to and after AI incorporation, technological advancement on pre-AI MRI, roles of AI in MRI enhancement and challenges that continue to occur for enhanced achievement of desirable outcomes from AI MRI.

INTRODUCTION

Magnetic Resonance Imaging (MRI) is a diagnostic technique for acquiring images of body organs and tissues without having to perform surgery. MRI is safer as it doesn't use ionizing radiation like in X-rays or in CT scans common practices. It is based on Nuclear magnetic resonance imaging (NMRI) that hydrogen atoms of the body react to a magnetic field and to broadcast radio frequency inner signals. These signals are then picked by a computer to generate detailed images that assist in identifying the mentioned diseases and many others such as neurological disorders, orthopedics, cardiovascular diseases and cancers. MRI gives excellent contrast of soft tissues and pathological changes that can be arranged both anatomically and functionally without bioptic examinations (Katti, 2011) . MRI essentially operates using the field exhibited by hydrogen nuclei, or protons, which are prevalent in the human body as a consequence of the nature of water and fat molecules. In a state where they are under the influence of a powerful magnetic field being provided by a super conducting magnet, the protons prefer to align themselves either in parallel or an anti-parallel manner to the magnetic lines of force. The arrangement of these protons is vital to MRI procedure that will be explained under the working of MRI section (Glover, 2011).

The Radiofrequency (RF) coils in the MRI machine transmit particular radiofrequency pulses to excite the aligned protons to absorb energy and hence relocate out of t heir aligned position (Rajan, 1998). The energy absorbed by the protons during the RF pulse is released as radiofrequency signals when the pulse is switched off, by the receiving coils in the MRI machine. With the help of differences in these signals coming from various tissues, a computer generates clear and minute pictures of internal structures of the human body (Weishaupt, 2006). This process is called image reconstruction that forms the cross-sectional image based on the signal intensity, spatial distribution and other signal parameters which are very useful to doctors in diagnosis and treatment planning (Shahzad, 2020). An MRI machine consists of several essential components that work together to produce diagnostic images.

Figure 1. Components of MRI

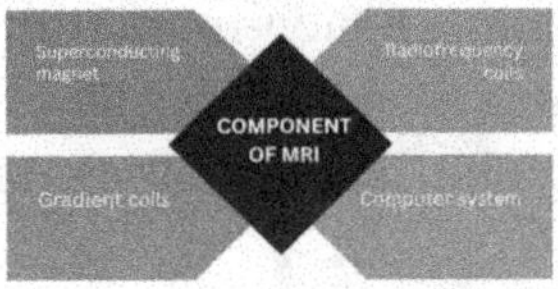

MRI techniques can be tailored to highlight different tissue characteristics and physiological processes.

T1-weighted MRI: Very good for analyzing the anatomical structure with distinction between different tissues such as fat, water, and protein content.

T2-weighted MRI: It gives distinctions in the level of water within tissues, which assists with identification of conditions such as edema or inflammation.

Functional MRI (fMRI): Determines changes in blood flow and oxygen in the brain so that one can have a map of what happens in the brain when one is performing particular tasks or perceiving sensory stimuli.

Diffusion MRI: There is the diffusion of water molecules in the tissues which helps to show the microstructure of the tissues and their integrity; helpful in the diagnosis of diseases affecting white matter and stroke (Fatahi, 2015).

MRI undoubtedly represents one of the key diagnostic tools available in the world of today's medicine, providing clients and researchers with unique opportunities to explore the human body, its structure, functions, and diseases that affect it. Because of its ability to produce high-quality image of the soft tissues including the high contrast successfully in different planes of imaging without invasive procedures used it has become a very effective tool in diagnosing and managing of different medical conditions in clinics (McCarthy, 2011). Further improvement and scientific development of MRI are still going on hence making MRI even more precise, affordable, and useful in the provision of healthcare and biomedical investigations . MRI or Magnetic Resonance Imaging first came into use in the early 1980s and has dramatically changed the way diagnostics are done. It is a noninvasive diagnostic procedure that employs powerful magnetic fields and radio waves, in conjunction with a computer system to form high quality visual images of the body's internal structures (Yan, 2007). The importance of MRI in patients' identification and further treatment cannot be overestimated, as MRI is widely used in diagnostics and therapy of numerous diseases. In this overview, all the aspects which define the necessity of MRI in the process of medical diagnostics will be discussed (Lundervold, 2019).

MRI is one of the most valuable diagnostic tools in the modern medicine due to its enhanced imaging capabilities in the vast number of diseases. Some of its advantages include better soft tissue contrast, non-intrusiveness, and non-use of ionizing radiation, thus making it the gold standard for many clinical uses. They include neurology, oncology, cardiovascular, and pediatrics imaging (Lu, 2013).

Table 1. Advantages of MRI and their examples.

Advantages of MRI	Examples
Non-invasive	No surgery or invasive procedures are required.
High contrast resolution	Excellent for imaging soft tissues like the brain, muscles, and organs.
Multiplanar imaging	Images can be taken in axial, sagittal, and coronal planes.
Functional and physiological imaging	Techniques like fMRI and DWI provide insights into brain function and tissue properties.

HISTORICAL BACKGROUND OF MRI

MRI is a modern diagnostic technique in medical imaging that has greatly impacted the medical field and especially the area of diagnostic radiology. Thus, MRI is a miracle of scientific detective work and combination of knowledge from physics, chemistry, engineering, and medicine. NMR can be said to have been the starting point or ground on which MRI was developed. NMR was discovered in 1946 by two investigators Felix Bloch and Edward Purcell, which defines that atomic nuclei in the magnetic field take up electromagnetic radiation and emit it back (Doi, 2006). There are many pioneers of other techniques in medicine, but when it comes to NMR imaging, the first person that should be named is a physician and researcher, Raymond Damadian. Dr. Damadian in the early 1970 using relaxation times (T1 and T2) of tissue to differentiate between normal and cancerous tissues using NMR.Although Damadian's work was important, it was Paul Lauterbur who Advanced an important step in converting NMR from a spectroscopic technology to an imaging instrument. In 1973, Lauterbul further expanded the notion if applying magnetic field gradients as a means to localize the signals produced. By altering the magnetic fields in this way Brinke could impress into the NMR signals the spatial information that he thus created the first two-dimensional images. Lauderbur's invention of what was then called "zeugmatography" but is now widely known as MRI was a turning point in the MRI technology (Frank, 1990). Sir Peter Mansfield the physicist from the University of Nottingham has also developed and improved MRI even more. In continuation of Lauterbur's proposals, Mansfield worked out the methods for achieving and reconstructing MRI images within a short time only (Joyce, 2008). He developed echo -planar imaging (EPI) which had a faster imaging time and better signal to noise ratio. Growth of MRI technology in its early years was as a result of the contribution of scientists and researchers who managed to make NMR theories practical and practically viable for use in imaging procedures. Other related developments and technologies in MRI have therefore pushed its use and have greatly contributed to the invaluable role in diagnosis of diseases and enhancement of patient care and results in different fields of medicine (Smith-Bindman, 2008) .

MRI has now become a very crucial and versatile examination in today's world of medical diagnosis offering very sharp picture and contrast of soft tissue. The invention of MRI therefore, presents itself as a history of many important achievements that happened over years, marked by major discoveries and innovations. MRI has advanced a lot from its genesis, however, the primitive forms of MRI had their problems. Some of the early limitations affected the resolution, the time taken to scan an image, patients' comfort and practicality of using the images in diagnostic or therapeutic procedures. This overview would present an idea of these limitations that early MRI technology had so that there could be appreciation of the difficulties that pioneers and practitioners had to go through in providing this important diagnostic tool (Sadeghi,2022).

- Image Quality and Resolution:

The first drawback of early MRI devices was the quality and detail of the image produced as compared to present day MRIs. The first MRI systems used low magnetic fields of strength, often less than one Tesla that is noted as 1T. 15 to 0. 35 Tesla which ultimately produced reduced SNR of the images acquired from the micro-MRI scans. This low SNR proved difficult for generating clear and detailed images because the NMR signals associated with these low-field magnets are often quite weak making them overshadowed by background noise. As a result, MRI image created during the early years of the technique had relatively poor spatial accuracy thereby could not provide a clear picture of smaller structures within the body and of slight changes in tissues' pathologies(Fotaki,2022). This led to a reduction of the diagnosticity of MRI in its early days since the imaging results were not detailed enough to enable clinicians to make accurate diagnoses or formulate effective treatment strategies .

- Extended Scan Times:

There was also the major problem with long scan times for early MRI systems. A single image could cost half an hour to several hours in terms of scan time, depending with the kind of scan to be done and part of the body to be scanned. These long scan times raised logistical problems within a clinical environment – thus, few patients could be scanned throughout the day, and due to the patients' ability to shift during the scan, they could become uncomfortable. Patient motion was specifically a big issue, and it was noted that even minimal movements led to the creation of erroneous movement artifacts in the image. This quite often required rescans, which extended the time it takes to conduct the examination, and the level of patient discomfort, as well as negative impacts on the operating capacities of MRI systems (Meyer-Base,2021) .

- Technological and Hardware Constraints:

It was also the problems with the hardware components in the early MRI equipment that proved to be of major concern. Early MRI use magnetic s used were basically resistive or low-field permanent magnets and they had a number of drawbacks; one was the minimal amount of magnetic field that they could produce and second they were very consumptive in terms of power and cooling systems. This made the machines large and costly to run, The limitations included; While spatial encoding and signal transmission required gradient coils and radiofrequency (RF) coils, the technology of the 1990s was much less powerful and precise than today's devices. This put a brake on the speed and efficiency of image acquisition which also hindered quick scans and less clear images. These aspects were better managed in the later years with the help of superconducting magnets and the advanced gradient and RF coils; However, these early systems were not as efficient and capable as today's machines (Kim,2023) .

- Software and Computational Challenges:

MRI also had serious software and computing issues especially when it was first introduced. Reconstruction, the process of going from raw data to actual image was a time-consuming and product-hampering step. The algorithms employed for reconstructing the images were quite rudimentary and the functional computation was also restricted. This posed a challenge in handling the immense amount of information produced during the MRI scan within a short time and turnaround time of image creation as well as the kind of imaging sequences that could be employed. These work-horse sequences of present day MRI, echo-planar imaging (EPI) and gradient echo sequences were still under developmental stage. Old MRI machines used simple sequences underlying imaging that were much slower and less sensitive, thus limiting the use of functional, dynamic imaging or any other study involving blood flow or real-time physiological processes and events (Abuzaid, 2021).

- Patient Experience and Accessibility:

One should also note that the problems concerning patient comfort and accessibility were also present in early MRI technology. Early MRI systems for instance incorporated a small, narrow tube that caused claustrophobic effects and feelings in the patients. The clinic environment turned out to be highly claustrophobic, the scans took a long time, which makes the patients uncomfortable, in addition, eight-gradient coils create a loud noise. This made some of the patients either have incomplete scans or even refused to take the scan in the first place. Also, the high cost of early MRI machines and the infrastructure necessary to support them constrained their usage to large hospitals and research centers. The latter would not be financially feasible for smaller clinics and rural healthcare centers, which means that MRI scans were still unavailable to a wider populace (Lundervold,2019).

- Technical Artifacts and Errors

Technical artefacts were this actively in first generation MRI technology. Specifically, artefacts due to differences in the local field generated as a result of the metal or air within the body were considered undesirable. These artifacts could sometimes alter the image by hiding some parts of the body thus be of less diagnostic value to the scans (Li,2022). The chemical shift artifacts because of the variation of the resonance frequencies of fat and water resulted to displacement of images and blurring across interfaces of tissues consequently made image interpretation difficult (Calivà,2022).

Figure 2. Timeline of key developments in MRI technology

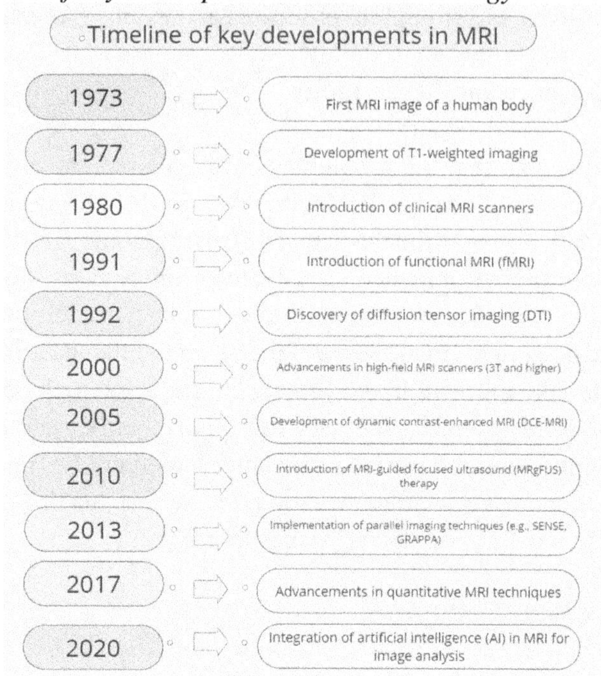

TECHNOLOGICAL ADVANCEMENT IN MRI

The technological enhancement of MRI has been received in improvement of image quality and resolution which enhances the diagnostic capabilities of MRI and horns its utility in clinical practice.An important factor in improving the visibility of structures in MRI is the indicated use of high-field and ultra-high-field magnets. The initial applicability of MRI systems was discovered in the mid 0.15 to 0.35 Tesla, generated images with low signal to noise (SNR) and this affected clarity and image definition. Superconducting magnets were introduced in the early 1980 s which eased higher magnetic fields; the initial being 1. to 5T scanners and moving to 3T and even 7T systems. These high-field magnets yield better NMR signals hence increase the SNR as compared to a superconducting magnet (Hill,2021). This improvement allows for the formation of images that are clearer and more detailed to help with the visualization of fine structures and other pathological changes essential for diagnosis and planning of treatment. Somewhat related to gradient coil technology there has also been progress in improving the image resolution. Gradient coils are used in MRI for spatial encoding and their characteristics determine the quality of the image obtained (Cau,2021) . Gradually developed coils in the past were less effective in power and precision, meaning that there were longer time taken in acquisitions and lower resolutions. The advanced gradient coils allow delivering stronger and much more accurate magnetic field gradients, which means that the corresponding imaging sequences can be performed more rapidly as well as with a higher spatial resolution. This has been especially helpful for sequences such as the echo-planar imaging (EPI) in which the prompt swapping of gradients is required for functionality and dynamics investigations (Joyce,2006). There has also been an advancement in the software and computational methods which has improved the imaging of MRI scans. Image reconstruction which is the process of reconstructing images from the acquired raw data benefitted from enhanced algorithms and enhanced computer capability. When designing the first MRI systems, multiple issues affected its usage; for example, the computers processing power was insufficient. Currently, there are superior tremendous algorithms that can quickly and accurately analyze big datasets gained from MRI. This has been made possible by today's approaches such as parallel imaging, compressed sensing as well as machine learning reconstruction algorithm (de Haën,2001).

SENSE (Sensitivity Encoding) and GRAPPA (Generalized Auto calibrating Partially Parallel Acquisitions) are the parallel imaging methods utilized in the present day MRI systems to shorten the image gathering time. These techniques help to increase SNR and spatial resolution of the images, when data is acquired at the same time from several coils. This technique helps to obtain high-quality images from collecting samples less than Nyquist rate, making the scan time shorter and the patient's discomfort less while maintaining the image quality. In addition to this, other machine learning and artificial intelligent algorithms refine the image acquisition parameters and compensation for motion, and improve on image reconstruction that gives better quality and more reliable images (Young,2004). These advancement have made MRI diagnosis more accurate and has increase the functional uses of MRI. The impact of improved sequences and methods for MRI imaging has been critical in the improvement of MRI images. The more conventional sequences as spin-echo and gradient-echo have been further developed over the years in order to elaborate a better contrast and a higher resolution. Also, the newer kinds of sequences including fast spin-echo (FSE), inversion recovery (IR) and balanced steady-state free precession (BSSFP) have provided finer and targeted descriptions of tissue and pathological states. Probably the most important breakthrough in MRI is functional MRI and diffusion MRI. Another type of MRI is fMRI, which records the cerebral metabolic activity by mapping the blood-oxygen level dependent signals and this is accomplished via applying of the rapid sequences such as EPI. quickly assist in acquiring images in a temporal duration of milliseconds providing real time imaging of brain functions with temporal and spatial resolutions . This technique has stirred neuroscience since it has offered knowledge on how the brain links and functions that have not been extremely possible to procure. Diffusion Mri such as, Diffusion weighted imaging (DWI) and hence dct diffusion tensor imaging (DTI) depicts the dispersion of water protons in the biological tissues. Which is valuable for imaging of the brain white matter and the detection of acute ischemic stroke. DTI offers white matter tracts that rich detail the connectivity of the brain and the diagnosis of neurological disorders (Attenberger,2015). More recent sequences known as multi-shell diffusion and high-angular resolution diffusion imaging (HARDI) has also enhanced the value of diffusion based sequences. Adoption showed that technological enhancement in MRI expanded in the last few decades enhanced image quality and refinement making MRI important in modern medicine (Blamire,2008). Advancements in all three of these areas have ameliorated the downfalls of the initial MRI systems and have provided better images and overall opening the door to more opportunities for MRI uses. As new technologies emerge today and in the future, MRI has potential to become even more significant in the diagnosis of diseases by enabling the clinician to diagnose, treat and manage diseases in accordance with high quality patient care. These upgrades have not only advanced MRI in a diagnostic capacity but also diversified the uses of MRI in every medical aspect strengthening oncology's role as an integrated component of today's medical imaging (Mansbridge,2019) .

fMRI is a relatively new methodology that allowed researching the brain's functional states by registering changes in blood circulation and oxygen concentrations in the process of its functioning. The development of the TDT was secondary to a sequence of technological enhancements of the MRI particularly in the pre-artificial intelligence (pre-AI) period.The principles of fMRI derive from knowledge from the BOLD contrast mechanisms. The BOLD effect described for the first time by Seiji Ogawa and his collaborators in the early of 1990s, bases its action on the magnetic characteristics of oxygenated and deoxygenated haemoglobin. Neural activation changes blood flow and oxygen level in related area which in turn changes the MR signal. These changes can be observed and then mapped using MRI which then gives an indirect insight into the activity going on in the brains.Before the launching of fMRI, the enhancement of structural imaging was the main concern in the evolution of MRI technology. The pre- Artificial Intelligence or the AI-Preperiod was characterized by improvement of the associated hardware and software that provided for Functional Imaging.Among the most significant achievements related to the pre-AI environment, still, it is possible to highlight the creation of high-field superconducting magnets. Initial MRI machines worked at low fields, well under 1. 0 Tesla and this constraint the SNR and the overall resolutions of the images. The introduction of 1. The 5 Tesla magnet and later the 3 Tesla produced a far greater SNR which allowed for better resolution and greater detail. The improved SNR is very relevant to fMRI since BOLD signal variations triggered by neural activity are comparatively small. At the same time, technology of gradient coil also reached certain development. Precise and stronger magnetic field gradients meant that the faster imaging approaches could be achieved, such as echo-planar imaging (EPI). EPI which was pioneered by Sir Peter Mansfield was adopted as the basis of fMRI due to the features that allowed it to provide information on the immediately preceding brain activity (Hendi,2023). The technique's high temporal resolution assist in capturing the changes in the neural activity such as the sensory, motor and cognitive one. It is also important to note that before the AI advancement, there were also drastic changes in MRI software and computation. First generation of MRI systems had large demands of computational power to process and reconstruct images. As computing power grew, more features could be deal with and more important, bigger datasets could be processed which is needed for high temporal resolution required in fMRI studies. Interpolation methods were enhanced with the help of better algorithms. Processing techniques which transform the basic MR data into images were improved such as Fourier transform methods to yield better image quality as well as less artifacts. Parallel imaging methods for instance SENSE and GRAPPA made it possible to reduce the time for the data acquisition since the data was collected from different receiver coils at the same time. These innovations lowered the scan time and improved the temporal resolution of fMRI making it possible to investigate brief and fast processes in the brain as well as specific cognition (Hu,2004). Organizational structure of fMRI studies also underwent change in the methodological aspects in the pre-AI period. Some of the early investigations that utilized this kind of tactic were the block designs, which are based on cycles of work and rest. It also served the objective of enhancing the contrast between the signal during a task and the signal during rest conditions, a factor that aimed at identification of areas of activation. Event-related designs emerged as the field grew, which enabled researchers to specifically study the brain's activity in response to specific stimuli or event. This design offered more versatility and accuracy in investigations of the time-course of neuronal phenomena (Keenan,,2019).

It marked developments in statistical approaches for the analysis of fMRI results. The nature of the acquired data was composite in that it involved both spatial and temporal aspects, and therefore it demanded the introduction of statistically sound analytic tools to filter signal from noise. The general linear method became one of the most widely used approaches to analyze the fMRI data and using this method researchers were able to model the connection between the conditions and observed BOLD signals. This approach was used to locate areas of the brain that were involved in certain activities, thus improving knowledge of how the brain works.

Table 2. Comparison showing advancements in MRI resolution over time

Time Period	Technology/Technique	Resolution and Image Quality	Key Improvements
1970s	Early MRI Systems	Low resolution, limited image clarity	First human MRI scan with rudimentary images; initial exploration of MRI technology.
1980s	Superconducting Magnets	Improved resolution with increased signal-to-noise ratio	Stronger and stable magnetic fields; introduction of 1.5 Tesla systems
1983	FDA Approval	Standardized clinical use with enhanced image quality	Establishment of MRI in clinical settings
1984	Echo-Planar Imaging (EPI)	Faster imaging with improved temporal resolution	Significant reduction in scan times; better temporal resolution
1990s	Functional MRI (fMRI)	High spatial resolution with dynamic mapping of brain activity	Enabled real-time functional imaging; introduced BOLD contrast
2000s	3 Tesla MRI Scanners	Higher spatial resolution and improved signal-to-noise ratio	Enhanced image detail and diagnostic accuracy
2010s	7 Tesla MRI Scanners	Ultra-high spatial resolution, exceptional detail in imaging	Provided unprecedented image clarity; primarily used in research
2020s	Advanced Imaging Sequences (e.g., dMRI, contrast-enhanced MRI)	Further improved image quality, particularly in complex tissues and structures	Enhanced techniques for visualizing microstructures and functional aspects

INTRODUCTION TO ARTIFICIAL IN MRI

The main methods used in MRI AI are classified as Machine Learning (ML), Deep Learning (DL), Convolutional Neural Networks (CNNs), Recurrent Neural Networks (RNNs) and Generative Adversarial Networks (GANs). These approaches are very effective in handling segmentation, registration and classifying data from MRI. They are also used widely to handle feature extraction and classification. They can detect tumors, lesions or abnormalities with high reliability because they learn the arrangement of features from medical images. At the same time, GANs are used to produce simulated MRI data which helps improve the training process by working with small data, tackling imbalanced classes and boosting the ability of the model to generalize.

AI is also used to reconstruct images automatically by mapping data from the k-space to the final image automatically. Many institutions now use variational autoencoders and transformers to clean images of noise and motion which improves their reliability and quality. AI software in MRI depends on data that has gone through thorough preprocessing for quality output from the training process. Many regularly carried out tasks during preprocessing involve:

1. Normalization: Intensity values can differ a lot between multiple scanners and MRI institutions. Scaling the image's intensity values to fit a certain range (for instance, 0 to 1 or z-score) is normalization and makes all data similar. Multitask learning gets rid of intensity bias, so that deep learning models train faster and perform well on various kinds of datasets.
2. Noise Reduction: Lower-field MRIs and rapid scans tend to have many random noises in the images. Initially, Gaussian and median filters were main tools for reducing noise, but using deep learning-based denoising autoencoders for this purpose is now the norm. Because these models know the difference between noise and important body structures, they can clear up the image while preserving small details needed for accurate diagnosis.
3. Segmentation: The process of singling out areas in the anatomy relevant to the examination being done. Segmentation is when the MRI scan is broken into regions that are important (e.g., gray matter, white matter, lesions). It takes a long time to do manual segmentation and there is a chance of error. These AI models simplify things by automatically finding and labeling areas that are normal or abnormal. This makes it possible to measure the volume, follow diseases and prepare for operations.
4. Data Augmentation: Medical datasets can be quite small because of concerns about patient privacy or the lack of patients.. Tasks like rotating, scaling, flipping and applying elastic deformations can essentially expand the types of data available. Some advanced approaches form fake but realistic pictures using GANs. As a result, AI models tend to generalize better, mainly when datasets are small.
5. Registration: In registration, images from various imaging technologies (such as CT and MRI) or acquired at different times are combined. This makes sure that an area of interest (for example, a tumor) is found at the same point in every image. With AI, registration does not require manual help which helps in studies lasting several tests and diagnoses across different types of images.

They are very important since they decrease the amount of variation, increase the clarity of the data and make the data ready for computer learning. Keeping preprocessing steps the same ensures that MRI tools using AI can be used reliably and help clinicians.

Machine intelligence is steadily entering different areas of medicine, and applications in MRI stand out from the rest. Specifically, there are several artificial intelligence technologies such as machine learning and deep learning that, if integrated with the MRI process, significantly improve image acquisition, processing, and interpretation. In MRI, the first areas of AI application concern the use of these technologies to optimize the imaging processes, increase the diagnostic reliability and, thereby, contribute to better patient outcomes. Discoverer and Machine Learning is astounding many fields through offering systems the means to adapt toward rich data in order to perform in a more efficient manner and also creating the pattern to provide functions that are refined over time without direct programming instructions (Sadeghi,2022). In Medical Imaging, the artificial intelligence especially deep learning algorithms such as Convolutional Neural Networks (CNNs) and Generative Adversarial Networks (GANs) have been identified as extremely potential for imaging enhancement and acquisition improvements. Such models perform well in the recognition of intricate patterns in the imaging data and therefore can contribute toward enhancing the rate and precision of the diagnoses, image construction and interpretation. The implementation of AI in medical imaging present benefits in terms of timings and enhanced precision because measures errors likely to occur when conducting a manual assessment (Jiang,2021). The early approaches of applying AI in MR consisted of the aspects like automatic segmentation of the images, noise removal, reduction of artifacts and other related chores. Establishing work early on involved selection of supervised learning procedures for categorizing anatomic regions and also for detecting abnormalities inside of MRI scans. Such approaches led to the development of the superior kinds of artificial neural networks aimed at dealing with certain imaging issues. As image clarity and diagnostic confidence slowly increased, AI started to look at the edge to become a tool that could augment MRI and make it better.

Machine learning in the context of MRI progressed through a number of stages and made a number of advances, primarily in the sphere of image reconstruction. Baseline MRI methods are well understood to be time consuming and hence involves long hours of scans and distress to patients. The development of newer AI has indexed new algorithms that are about the development of images from a low sample data set and this has long shortened the acquisition time while maintaining high image quality. CNNs, GANs, and compressed sensing methods are now actively used to acquire MRI scans in considerably less time without much compromise in the diagnosis quality (Wang,2016). These innovations are a drastic change from the previous clinical practice in that they bring integrated AI solutions that previously resulted in the trade-off of having faster scans, of better image quality, and better diagnosis.

Table 3. Summary of early AI applications in MRI and their impact

AI Application	Description	Impact	Reference
Image Segmentation	Automating the identification and delineation of anatomical structures.	Improved accuracy and consistency in identifying regions of interest.	Liu, S., et al. "Deep learning in medical ultrasound analysis: A review." Engineering 5.2 (2019): 261-275.
Noise Reduction	Utilizing AI models to filter out noise and enhance image quality.	Enhanced clarity of MRI images, leading to better diagnostic decisions.	Yang, Q., et al. "Deep learning for single-image super-resolution: A brief review." IEEE Transactions on Multimedia 21.12 (2019): 3106-3121.
Artifact Correction	Correcting image distortions caused by patient movement or hardware limitations.	Reduced the need for repeat scans, improving patient experience and workflow efficiency.	Zbontar, J., et al. "fastMRI: An open dataset and benchmarks for accelerated MRI." arXiv preprint arXiv:1811.08839 (2018).
Anomaly Detection	AI-driven systems detecting abnormalities such as tumors or lesions.	Increased detection rates, enabling earlier and more accurate diagnoses.	Litjens, G., et al. "A survey on deep learning in medical image analysis." Medical image analysis 42 (2017): 60-88.
Image Classification	Classifying MRI images into diagnostic categories using machine learning.	Automated and quicker initial assessments, reducing the radiologist's workload.	Esteva, A., et al. "Dermatologist-level classification of skin cancer with deep neural networks." Nature 542.7639 (2017): 115-118.
Accelerated Image Reconstruction	Reconstructing high-quality images from undersampled data for faster MRI scans.	Significantly reduced scan times while maintaining high image fidelity.	Hammernik, K., et al. "Learning a variational network for reconstruction of accelerated MRI data." Magnetic resonance in medicine 79.6 (2018): 3055-3071

CHALLENGES AND LIMITATIONS

The incorporation of AI in MRI processes presents the following technical issues that need to be considered in order to maximise the effectiveness of these technologies as they are applied. By far the most significant is trying to consolidate data into uniformity in its scan across MRI technologies scanners, healthcare centers, and even patients. Conventional MRI systems generate images of a wide range of resolutions, contrast, and image noise by influencing the type of scanner, selected mode, and working parameters. Their effectiveness, however, depends on the ability of AI algorithms to be trained on big standardised datasets. Nevertheless, the variation inherent in data acquisition can act as an obstacle to the creation of standard, always effective AI algorithms. Another technical problem which is crucial is the question of the complexity of AI models In human science. Some of the deep learning techniques which have been applied in image reconstruction and enhancement consume large processing time. MRI data is high-resolution, and the processing of these images in real time involving the application of complex algorithmic models of artificial intelligence requires significant computational power in the form of GPUs and specialised hardware. Such resources may be a necessity, and that may reduce the possibility of implementing the application of AI in MRI in small clinics or facilities . Also, common issues with the AI models are in the model's inability to learn variability and edges in the data stream (Gou,2024). There is a potential that when the AI systems are trained only from the limited or biased datasets, they will not be able to perform well in the real world scenarios where the data distribution is different from the training data. For instance, an AI model trained from a set of images of a particular population may not well interpret images of other population. This issue brings out the reality that training datasets should comprise diverse data, and the validation methods that ought to be in place to see to it that the AI models will work as required in different situations. The employment of AI in MRI workflows provides the following technical considerations that have to be met to optimally harness these technologies. Some of them are public: one is to harmonize the data collected from different MRI, different healthcare institutions, and/or patients. RSTS MRI systems build images with various resolutions, contrasts, and noise levels depending on the type of the scanner, sequence used, and operative environment. This means that AI algorithms must be trained so that they are used to work with big available standard data. There is a problem in data acquisition, as it differs from one site to another; this hinders researchers from establishing general models in AI to perform similarly in different terrains. Yet another of the major technical considerations revolves around the relative dimension of intelligence operational models. Deep learning algorithms, especially those that can be employed in image reconstruction and image enhancement require a lot of computation. MRI is high resolution which means that the images being processed are large and processing these images in real time with high end AI algorithms require a lot of computational power like GPU and purpose built hardware. The requirement of such resources might slow down the use of AI in MRI, particularly in small clinics or facilities with an arrow budget. Furthermore, there is the problem of generalization, that is, the performance of the AI models in relation to variability and boundary conditions. It is argued that AI models that learned on small or biased data sets may perform worse on different data distribution found in real life. For instance, an AI model developed to analyze and interpret images may have been trained on images from the first demographic only and this shortcoming will be seen where it has to perform the same function on images from the second demographic (Frank & Trappe, 1990). It also shows the need both for diverse training sets and a sound validation methodology to check whether models generalise well. Finally, to the issue of the integration of AI into daily clinical practice there are certain difficulties. In the actual implementation, there are always some barriers since the healthcare providers are not ready to accept them due to ignorance, lack of confidences, or threats posed by replacing jobs. Planning and implementation of education of radiologists then clinicians alongside developing AI systems that extend the human learning models would be critical in implementing AI models. Moreover, research should be devoted to improvements of the graphical user interface and compatibility with the well-established MRI systems, as well as the overall routines of the hospitals (Li,2024).

Figure 3. Graphical representation of challenges in AI-MRI integration

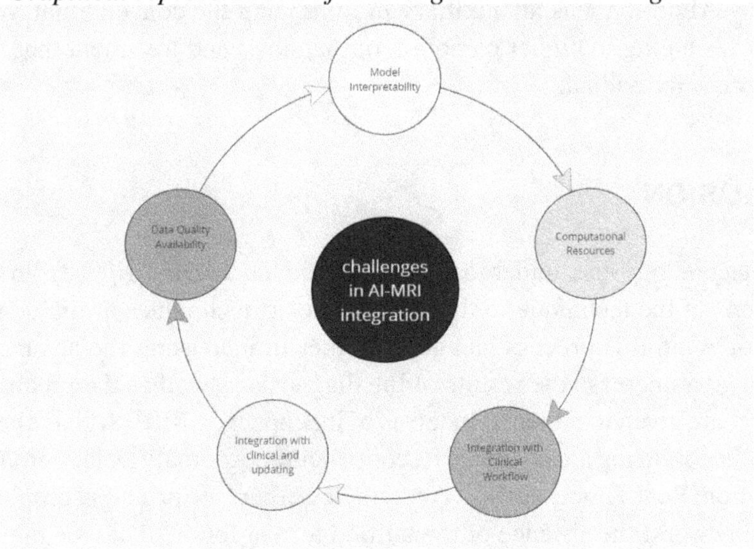

AI MRI diagnosis is still in its modernization stage, however, the future development would help to upgrade the achieved results dramatically. The possibilities of AI and MRI evolution for the future may consist in development of new types of AI that would be able to provide diagnostics in shorter time, with higher accuracy, and tailored to individual needs. They could become a part of MRI systems and perform image processing and analysis in real time something that will obviously ease clinical processes and, in turn, decrease diagnostic times. New technologies and even concepts like quantum computing and other subsequent models of artificial intelligence are likely to have a big impact on this evolution. For example, quantum computing could potentially enhance the amount of computational capacity that is devouted to processing MRI signal data to the extent of making MRI imaging more precise. On the other hand, development of deep learning and neural networks would mean that the AI would not only be able to analyze MRI images with high accuracy but also draw prognosis of the patient, in addition to recommending the optimal treatment regimen depending on a host of parameters.

As for the future, the concept of AI in MRI is to integrate it in all aspects of imaging. With AI integrated MRI it is possible to make MRI systems the core of individualized medicine because the information getting from MRI is patient specific. This would create a change from what is already considered a reactive model of healthcare to a predictive model that is fueled by MRI scans driven by artificial intelligence and designed to not only identify a disease but also to foresee a health problem at its early stage (Khang,2024). As outlined in the context of your paper on the development of MRI these future development point toward the future potentials brought by AI not only as an auxiliary in improving the conventional MRI but as a means of bringing in higher paradigm of diagnosis and treatment that is tailored to the specific individual.

CONCLUSION

MRI technology has undergone constant advancements right from the basic applications of the technique to the state of the art techniques available presently. The use of AI in this process has gone further in increasing the advancement of MRI scans that increase the results of the diagnosis as well as the precision of the results that are given to patients. In terms of its impact on MRI, AI has changed and reshaped the following areas: Image Reconstruction; Anomaly Detection; Workflow Optimization; Real Time Analysis. Nevertheless, there are principal problems exists in this framework: the absence of the unified format for the datasets, the computation problems, and the need to consider the ethical issues like privacy and societal bias of the algorithms. Subsequent research also has to depend on development of valid and generalizable AI models in different healthcare environments and use AI throughout the phases of its development in a transparent and non-bias manner. With development of AI expected to go on, significant benefits in enhancement of MRI is expected in the future to revolutionize medical imaging and diagnostics sector.

REFERENCES

Abuzaid, M. M., Tekin, H. O., Reza, M., Elhag, I. R., & Elshami, W. (2021). Assessment of MRI technologists in acceptance and willingness to integrate artificial intelligence into practice. *Radiography*, *27*, S83–S87. PMID: 34364784

Attenberger, U. I., Morelli, J., Budjan, J., Henzler, T., Sourbron, S., Bock, M., & Schoenberg, S. O. (2015). Fifty years of technological innovation: Potential and limitations of current technologies in abdominal magnetic resonance imaging and computed tomography. *Investigative Radiology*, *50*(9), 584–593. PMID: 26039773

Blamire, A. M. (2008). The technology of MRI—The next 10 years? *The British Journal of Radiology*, *81*(968), 601–617. PMID: 18628329

Calivà, F., Namiri, N. K., Dubreuil, M., Pedoia, V., Ozhinsky, E., & Majumdar, S. (2022). Studying osteoarthritis with artificial intelligence applied to magnetic resonance imaging. *Nature Reviews. Rheumatology*, *18*(2), 112–121. PMID: 34848883

Cau, R., Cherchi, V., Micheletti, G., Porcu, M., Mannelli, L., Bassareo, P., & Saba, L. (2021). Potential role of artificial intelligence in cardiac magnetic resonance imaging: Can it help clinicians in making a diagnosis? *Journal of Thoracic Imaging*, *36*(3), 142–148. PMID: 33769416

de Haën, C. (2001). Conception of the first magnetic resonance imaging contrast agents: A brief history. *Topics in Magnetic Resonance Imaging*, *12*(4), 221–230. PMID: 11687712

Doi, K. (2006). Diagnostic imaging over the last 50 years: Research and development in medical imaging science and technology. *Physics in Medicine and Biology*, *51*(13), R5. PMID: 16790920

Fatahi, M., & Speck, O. (2015). Magnetic resonance imaging (MRI): A review of genetic damage investigations. *Mutation Research/Reviews in Mutation Research*, *764*, 51–63. PMID: 26041266

Fotaki, A., Puyol-Antón, E., Chiribiri, A., Botnar, R., Pushparajah, K., & Prieto, C. (2022). Artificial intelligence in cardiac MRI: Is clinical adoption forthcoming? *Frontiers in Cardiovascular Medicine*, *8*, 818765. PMID: 35083303

Frank, A. M., & Trappe, A. E. (1990). The role of magnetic resonance imaging (MRI) in the diagnosis of spondylodiscitis. *Neurosurgical Review*, *13*, 279–283. PMID: 2280839

Glover, G. H. (2011). Overview of functional magnetic resonance imaging. *Neurosurgery Clinics*, *22*(2), 133–139. PMID: 21435566

Gou, F., Liu, J., Xiao, C., & Wu, J. (2024). Research on artificial-intelligence-assisted medicine: A survey on medical artificial intelligence. *Diagnostics (Basel)*, *14*(14), 1472. PMID: 39061610

Hendi, A. A. (2023). Development of Medical Imaging Techniques: A Review of Technological Advances in the Field of Medical Imaging, Such as Magnetic Resonance Imaging (MRI), Computed Tomography (CT), and Ultrasound Imaging (Ultrasound). *Journal of Positive Psychology and Wellbeing*, *7*(3), 569–578.

Hill, C. E., Biasiolli, L., Robson, M. D., Grau, V., & Pavlides, M. (2021). Emerging artificial intelligence applications in liver magnetic resonance imaging. *World Journal of Gastroenterology*, *27*(40), 6825. PMID: 34790009

Hu, X., & Norris, D. G. (2004). Advances in high-field magnetic resonance imaging. *Annual Review of Biomedical Engineering*, *6*(1), 157–184. PMID: 15255766

Jiang, Y., Edwards, A. V., & Newstead, G. M. (2021). Artificial intelligence applied to breast MRI for improved diagnosis. *Radiology*, *298*(1), 38–46. PMID: 33078996

Joyce, K. A. (2006). From numbers to pictures: The development of magnetic resonance imaging and the visual turn in medicine. *Science as culture*, *15*(01), 1–22.

Joyce, K. A. (2008). *Magnetic appeal: MRI and the myth of transparency*. Cornell University Press.

Katti, G., Ara, S. A., & Shireen, A. (2011). Magnetic resonance imaging (MRI)–A review. *International Journal of Dental Clinics*, *3*(1), 65–70.

Keenan, K. E., Biller, J. R., Delfino, J. G., Boss, M. A., Does, M. D., Evelhoch, J. L., & Sullivan, D. C. (2019). Recommendations towards standards for quantitative MRI (qMRI) and outstanding needs. *Journal of magnetic resonance imaging. Journal of Magnetic Resonance Imaging*, *49*(7), e26. PMID: 30680836

Khang, A. (Ed.). (2024). *Medical Robotics and AI-Assisted Diagnostics for a High-Tech Healthcare Industry*. IGI Global.

Kim, H., Kang, S. W., Kim, J. H., Nagar, H., Sabuncu, M., Margolis, D. J., & Kim, C. K. (2023). The role of AI in prostate MRI quality and interpretation: Opportunities and challenges. *European Journal of Radiology*, *165*, 110887. PMID: 37245342

Li, C., Li, W., Liu, C., Zheng, H., Cai, J., & Wang, S. (2022). Artificial intelligence in multiparametric magnetic resonance imaging: A review. *Medical Physics*, *49*(10), e1024–e1054. PMID: 35980348

Li, X., Zhang, L., Yang, J., & Teng, F. (2024). Role of Artificial Intelligence in Medical Image Analysis: A Review of Current Trends and Future Directions. *Journal of Medical and Biological Engineering*, •••, 1–13.

Lu, J., Feng, F., & Jin, Z. (2013). Cancer diagnosis and treatment guidance: Role of MRI and MRI probes in the era of molecular imaging. *Current Pharmaceutical Biotechnology*, *14*(8), 714–722. PMID: 24372236

Lundervold, A. S., & Lundervold, A. (2019). An overview of deep learning in medical imaging focusing on MRI. *Zeitschrift für Medizinische Physik*, *29*(2), 102–127. PMID: 30553609

Mansbridge, M., Chung, E., & Rhee, H. (2019). The use of MRI and PET imaging studies for prostate cancer management: Brief update, clinical recommendations, and technological limitations. *Medical Science*, *7*(8), 85. PMID: 31387208

McCarthy, M. J. (2011). Introduction to magnetic resonance imaging (MRI). In *Magnetic resonance imaging in foods* (pp. 1–29). Springer US.

Meyer-Base, A., Morra, L., Tahmassebi, A., Lobbes, M., Meyer-Base, U., & Pinker, K. (2021). AI-Enhanced Diagnosis of Challenging Lesions in Breast MRI: A Methodology and Application Primer. *Journal of Magnetic Resonance Imaging*, *54*(3), 686–702. PMID: 32864782

. Rajan, S. S. (1998). MRI: a conceptual overview.

Sadeghi, D., Shoeibi, A., Ghassemi, N., Moridian, P., Khadem, A., Alizadehsani, R., & Acharya, U. R. (2022). An overview of artificial intelligence techniques for diagnosis of Schizophrenia based on magnetic resonance imaging modalities: Methods, challenges, and future works. *Computers in Biology and Medicine*, *146*, 105554. PMID: 35569333

Sadeghi, D., Shoeibi, A., Ghassemi, N., Moridian, P., Khadem, A., Alizadehsani, R., & Acharya, U. R. (2022). An overview of artificial intelligence techniques for diagnosis of Schizophrenia based on magnetic resonance imaging modalities: Methods, challenges, and future works. *Computers in Biology and Medicine*, *146*, 105554. PMID: 35569333

Shahzad, K., & Mati, W. (2020). Advances in magnetic resonance imaging (MRI). In *Advances in Medical and Surgical Engineering* (pp. 121-142). Academic Press.

Smith-Bindman, R., Miglioretti, D. L., & Larson, E. B. (2008). Rising use of diagnostic medical imaging in a large integrated health system. *Health Affairs*, *27*(6), 1491–1502. PMID: 18997204

Wang, S., Zhang, Y., Zhan, T., Phillips, P., Zhang, Y. D., Liu, G., & Wu, X. (2016). Pathological brain detection by artificial intelligence in magnetic resonance imaging scanning (invited review). *Progress in Electromagnetics Research, 156*, 105–133.

Weishaupt, D., Köchli, V. D., Marincek, B., Froehlich, J. M., Nanz, D., & Pruessmann, K. P. (2006). *How does MRI work?: an introduction to the physics and function of magnetic resonance imaging* (Vol. 2). Springer.

Yan, G. P., Robinson, L., & Hogg, P. (2007). Magnetic resonance imaging contrast agents: Overview and perspectives. *Radiography*, *13*, e5–e19.

Young, I. R. (2004). Significant events in the development of MRI. *Journal of Magnetic Resonance Imaging: An Official Journal of the International Society for Magnetic Resonance in Medicine*, *20*(2), 183–186. PMID: 15269941

Chapter 5
Adaptive Devices for Artificial Intelligence of Medical Things

T. Venkat Narayana Rao
https://orcid.org/0000-0002-1996-1819
Sreenidhi Institute of Science and Technology, India

Mohammed Kashif
https://orcid.org/0009-0002-5309-0815
Sreenidhi Institute of Science and Technology, India

T. Thukaram Goud
https://orcid.org/0009-0004-3814-5843
Sreenidhi Institute of Science and Technology, India

P. Sravan Kumar
Sreenidhi Institute of Science and Technology, India

ABSTRACT

Adaptive devices and Artificial intelligence in the realm of medical field have become crucial for enhancing healthcare delivery and patient outcomes. As the virus are evolving with time, it is necessary for our current healthcare system to evolve with it as well. Utilizing artificial intelligence paired with advanced machine learning algorithms incorporated inside a device which can adapt itself based on the instructions from AI might be our best chance to counteract limitations of our current healthcare system. Through Artificial Intelligence of Medical Things (AIoMT) hope to achieve new heights of healthcare systems which significantly. Adaptive devices include advanced health tracking wearables that track vital signs of the patients which can be used as input for the algorithm. However, many several challenges persist,

DOI: 10.4018/979-8-3373-0903-3.ch005

including data security concerns, reliability of algorithm, limitations of hardware and more importantly integrating it with public domain. This chapter would explore many possible and most efficient solutions to the problems regarding AIoMT

1. INTRODUCTION

Adaptive devices and artificial intelligence have emerged as a new key which can unlock new realm of medical technology. In recent years we have seen a rapid growth in artificial intelligence and machine learning, which has allowed surpassed the limitations of traditional diagnostic methods. Given the rapid evolution of AI, it will soon be possible to accurately and efficiently identify diseases. Even though AI is evolving at a rapid pace it might not replace human doctors, but it will definitely help doctors to make proper judgements. The AI machines are more precise and accurate than humans in certain scenarios, which can help doctors to increase the chances of success in surgeries.

During diagnosis or surgery, AI can monitor the condition of patient which will give doctor an opportunity to prioritize his focus on critical part of the surgery. As AI are machines which are capable of doing repetitive tasks which humans find tedious, they can be used to handle enormous amount of such tedious works. AI implemented systems are already being used to handle large number of patients which do not require guidance from a doctor for basic diseases which already have a working diagnosis. AI chatbots have emerged as new consultants for such minor issues, as the technology has advanced it is now cheaper and easier to provide everyone with such services free of cost. The time saved by such AI implemented systems can be used by human doctors to treat more patient which require serious attention. For the patients who are undergoing treatment which requires constant monitoring, the hospital may not be able to facilitate such services can use AI implemented systems to monitor patients.

AI is now able to merge nano technology and health systems to identify early stages of cancer in humans. This significantly increases chances of complete recovery from cancer as diagnosis can be started before the cancer reaches non-treatable stages. As the AI and nano technology continue to evolve it will make treatment affordable and available to everyone.

AI-based radiodiagnosis using chest X-rays has shown great potential in identifying lung conditions such as pneumonia, tuberculosis, COVID-19, and lung cancer with improved accuracy and speed. The integration of AI not only enables efficient analysis of medical images but also supports overburdened healthcare systems, especially in resource-limited settings. Additionally, AI assists in monitoring patients, streamlining repetitive tasks, and handling high patient volumes through systems like AI chatbots. The convergence of AI with nanotechnology also enables early-stage detection of diseases like cancer, making treatment more effective, accessible, and affordable in the evolving landscape of digital healthcare. (Akhter, Singh & Vatsa, et al., 2023)

2. ARTIFICIAL INTELLIGENCE IN HEALTH SYSTEMS

2.1 AI in Present Medical Field

As of now, AI has advanced enough to be integrated into medical field. Infectious diseases which are leading cause to death around the world like, Spanish flu, tuberculosis, Ebola, Severe Acute Respiratory Syndrome, influenza and many more which are harder to identify using traditional methods, in such cases AI integrated systems are being used by doctors to quickly and accurately identify such diseases.

Traditional methods of disease management often suffer from fragmented data and inadequate analyses, leading to ineffective responses, incomplete data collection, insufficient understanding of infection dynamics, and a lack of timely intervention strategies. These issues can hinder effective disease control efforts. One of the key aspects of AI based systems are use of mathematical models like Susceptible-Infectious-Recovered (SIR) model. This model categorizes populations based on their infection status and allows public health officials to simulate various intervention strategies. By adjusting parameters within the model, officials can conduct sensitivity analyses to understand potential outcomes better. This also helps health officials to develop medicines which will be much more effective than traditional ones (Surya, L. et al., 2018).

2.2 Disease Prediction And Prevention Using AI Analytics

AI can also be trained using X-ray images, Electrocardiogram (ECG/EKG), Electroencephalogram (EEG), MRI (Magnetic Resonance Imaging), CT scan, Ultrasound scan and many more to accurately predict the disease such as heart disease, cancer and brain tumor. As the AI is able to predict it early on and also recommend preventions. Doctors can prescribe medicines and treatment early on which can save millions of lives. Since the machines can be designed to take multiple inputs and the give the outputs faster than a human, they are fed a large number of data and the predictions given by the Ai are taken a note off which is further analyzed to be true or not.

2.2.1 Pandemic Control Using AI

As mentioned above, large amount of data is fed to models like SIR to analyze trends of disease, track pandemic progression and advice suitable preventions.

Some of the commonly used models are:

a. Susceptible-Infectious-Recovered (SIR) Model:

It is based on classifying population into three types, first being the people who have been infected.

Second, people who can be infected and third, people who have recovered and gained immunity. Using machine learning algorithms to train AI into such data is found useful in predicting the outbreak of pandemic.

b. SEIR Model (Susceptible-Exposed-Infectious-Recovered):

It is an advanced version of SIR which adds an extra parameter of people who have been exposed yet not infected.

c. Agent-Based Models (ABM):

It is a simulation-based model which is used to simulate individual actions of people in a population to predict how they interact and spread disease.

Using the above models with integration of AI helps us to predict any future outbreak. The data required for models can be continuously fed by current medical records and it is easy for AI to recognize patterns thus, making it easy to prepare ourselves for any future outbreak (Gurev, S. et al., 2023).

2.3 AI Systems

AI systems consist of two types, first one being machine learning, which feeds on the data of patients and also on data from previous medical records to understand all the possible scenarios, and since it also has the record of previous patients it makes the determination of disease more accurate.

The second part of an AI being natural language processing which helps the data organization and management in a well-structured manner. This is also responsible to input as well as give an output to the user in human language which is understandable by doctors (Gadde et al., 2020).

As the data can be processed much faster in computers and is more accurate due to it having more data to refer to, it can be extremely helpful for doctors in determining diseases. AI can make complex structures much simpler and easy to understand for humans so that the doctor can save their time and focus on things of high priority. Since the AI can make things much simpler, the students who are aspiring to become doctors and junior doctors can make use of AI to improve their understanding of medicines, diseases.

Though it is important to be remember that machines as of now tends to make mistake, they cannot be trusted completely thus, it is important to verify the results with an experienced doctor. With our current limitations for technology the AI might be good companion instead of a complete replacement to human doctors.

2.4 Management of Records

Before professional data storing technology was a thing, medical records were being stored manually in a computer. As the previous generations of searching technology was really slow, when a patient is needed to be performed upon immediately it was a challenge to find his previous medical records like his blood type, his previous diagnosis or if he had any chronic disease which significantly affects the type of treatment the patient requires in case of emergencies. The medical record of a patient may also contain consent which gives the doctors to perform any surgery immediately if required. The records take too much time and the patient needs to be operated on quickly in case of emergencies, wrong method of treatment can lead to disastrous results. But such disastrous situation can be prevented using

NLP (Natural Language Processing). In the era of AI, it has become really easy for us to integrate AI into existing medical database management systems. Using this technology searching and summarizing medical records of a patient significantly faster than before (Khanachivskyi, O. et al., 2024).

How does AI in medical records work

a. Optical character recognition (OCR):

The medical records which are available in physical form or in hard disks can be scanned and converted into machine language which can be understood by the algorithm. Since it is digital format, it also makes it faster to search any specifics required by doctor.

b. NLP algorithm:

Systems are designed with specific algorithms which specializes in scanning medical records. This algorithm scans for any special medical condition which can disrupt treatment if treatment is done using traditional methods.

c. Generative AI and medical record indexing:

Generative AIs like UIpath, gpt 4 and many more, can convert the summarized medical record into human readable language. This goes beyond simple keyword extraction from the main medical record, ensuring a nuanced understanding of the content.

AI systems can automatically create a chronological order of all the events and treatments received by the patient, providing a clear timeline of patient's medical history which can be analyzed by doctors, helping them determine the possible cause for patient's current condition (Khanachivskyi, O. et al., 2024).

There are multiple benefits of using AI medical records.

a. AI can accelerate searching and reviewing medical record significantly faster than a human. They also help summarize the records which helps the hospital to be quick and operate on patient if needed.
b. With our current technology, they are highly accurate and designed to be consistent with information so that they do not miss out on any critical information.
c. They are also helpful to hospitals providing them aid in identifying pattern in medical record which strengthens their legal argument.
d. It is cost efficient, as it is one time investment in resources like systems, cooling and storage. Requiring minimal maintenance, it can save both time and cost of the hospital (Khanachivskyi, O. et al., 2024).

2.5 Developing Medicine Using AI

AI algorithms can analyze vast amounts of data to identify potential drug candidates, predicting how molecules will interact, and suggest modifications to enhance efficiency or reduce side effects of a drug. This can speed up the medicine creation process, which traditionally takes years.

AI has been used to identify compounds for diseases like cancer, Alzheimer's, and even COVID-19. Algorithm can analyze individual genetic profiles and other patient data (like lifestyle factors and environment) to develop personalized treatment plans.

By tailoring drugs and therapies to a patient's unique characteristics, AI developed medicine can increase the effectiveness of treatment and reduce adverse effects of the developed medicines (T Venkat Narayana Rao et al.,2020).

Algorithms can also be designed to help researchers discover new uses for existing drugs by simulating the drug molecular model and suggesting any changes in it.

Using machine learning algorithms to analyze vast medical databases, AI can identify drugs that might be effective for diseases other than the ones they were initially approved for, potentially accelerating treatments for conditions with unmet medical needs.

3. AI-ASSISTED TRAINING FOR MEDICAL FIELD

Artificial Intelligence (AI) is revolutionizing medical training by enhancing education, simulation, and decision-making. AI-driven tools, such as virtual patients, machine learning models, and adaptive learning platforms, provide personalized and efficient training experiences for medical students and professionals.

3.1 Virtual Patients

Using modern devices known as Virtual reality headsets, we are able to simulate virtual patient for students to practice upon.

From the previous two decades graphic processing devices has evolved to a point where graphics are photo-realistic and the technology has been compressed into a small wearable headset.

Use of virtual patients offers a multitude of advantages over traditional clinical training. Virtual patients do not need to be physically present with the learner, Virtual patients have a fixed routine of behavior unlike standard patient which can help students who are just at the beginner level. A virtual patient can be updated easily with new information and also provide valuable experience to professionals when there is an outbreak of new disease where patients are hard to reach.

Virtual patients can be easily accessed through internet and also have a large number of medical learning materials. With the revolution in web technologies, it is easy for students to access study materials, virtual patients even in remote places.

As much as there are advantages to a virtual patient created using virtual reality headset, they cannot be equivalent to traditional clinical training but as the technology continues to improve that border becomes thinner and thinner (Combs et al., 2019).

3.2 Simulating Clinical Conditions

Virtual reality headsets have advanced to a point where they are able to provide haptic feedbacks and communicate verbally.

We are able to use AI algorithms to generate a virtual patient using data from a specific category of patients to train a student for particular kind of disease. If a student wants to get hands on experience of a hospital doctor, he is able to by prompting the AI to simulate such conditions.

Depending on the prompt given by user or trainers to train a student under specific conditions, AI can design and render a 3-Dimensional hospital simulation. In this 3-D world, AI generates virtual patients who are capable of interacting with students to simulate intake process of a real hospital.

The intake process may contain recording details of the patient and according to this detail the student is required to choose appropriate treatment for the patient. As the patient is in the digital form, even if the student makes a mistake, it does not cause any harm in real world. There is no shortage of patients and type of patients in virtual world.

With an increase in stress of population over the past decades, suicides have become 2nd leading cause of death in people ages 15-24. But a proper psychiatric interaction can significantly improve the patient's condition (Polanco-Roman, L. et al., 2016).

Virtual patients simulated in clinical conditions portraying the ideology of a typical person exerted by stress can be used as a good practice for students as well as doctors for practice.

This virtual training can significantly improve the quality of clinician-patient interactions, the accuracy of a diagnosis, and the effectiveness of a treatment plan.

After a virtual patient is generated, the student start diagnosing while the AI monitors his actions. After the diagnosis AI analyses the pattern and mistakes done by the students. Based on such data, the AI provides students which correct procedure as well as the areas which needs improvement. Use of such AI based technologies has several advantages over traditional way of teaching clinical skills. The first being accessibility, as the communication technology is at its peak than it has ever been, the data can be transferred really quick which makes it accessible to everyone as the AI can run on remote servers.

It can be reused multiple times and it is capable of handling multiple users thus, making it cost efficient.

As good as its advantages are, there are its shortcomings too.

With our current technological trend, it is expensive to manufacture such devices. The devices might not be available to some population

Even the cost of operating AI on remotes servers are expensive as well as the AI itself are not open-source, meaning the organizations are required to buy them or operate them on subscription-based payment.

As of now, people who are able to take advantage of such sophisticated machines are less, they will emerge larger in future as the technological trend moves towards the AI.

Cons of virtual patients

a. Ethical concerns:

Virtual patients need to accurately diverse populations to prevent bias in medical training. Ethical concerns arise if simulations reinforce stereotypes or exclude certain demographics.

b. Data Privacy & Consent:

Some virtual patients are based on real patient data, raising concerns about informed consent and data anonymization. Institutions must comply with HIPAA, GDPR, and other privacy regulations when using patient-derived data. Any leak of patient's personal medical record can lead to various disastrous issues.

c. Simulation vs. Real-World Skills:

While virtual patients offer valuable practice, over-reliance on simulations might limit exposure to real-life patient interactions and empathy development. Ethical training should balance technical proficiency with human-centered care.

d. Accountability & Decision-Making:

AI-driven virtual patients may influence clinical decision-making. Ensuring trainees understand the limitations of AI-generated diagnoses is critical. Ethical concerns emerge if students rely too heavily on virtual patient simulations without developing independent judgment.

e. Accessibility & Equity:

AI-driven VPs may widen educational disparities if only well-funded institutions can afford them. Ethical deployment should promote equal access to high-quality simulation tools for all medical students (Riva, G. 2024; jagsi, R. 2004).

4. AI IN OPERATING ROOM

Multimodal AI are AI which have been trained on multiple types of data, this makes it easy for such AI to accurately optimise patient selection for surgical intervention.

4.1 Robotic Surgeon

Robotic surgeon, it might sound like a replacement machine to surgeon, but it actually refers to robots used by doctors to assist in surgery. These robots are pinnacle of electric motor technology. The Da Vinci system, the best-selling surgery robot on the market, was approved by the FDA two decades ago. It can operate with a degree of precision down to 1 millimetre (Jee, 2020).

4.1.1 Robotic Surgery Using Robotic Surgeons

Robotic surgery, also known as robot-assisted surgery, is a technique that enables surgeons to perform complex procedures with enhanced precision, flexibility, and control. This method often involves making smaller incisions compared to traditional surgery, which can lead to reduced pain, minimal scarring, and faster recovery times for patients.

A typical robotic surgical system comprises several key components:

a. Surgeon's Console:

A workstation where the surgeon sits and controls the robotic instruments. The console provides a magnified, high-definition, 3D views of the surgical site, allowing for meticulous manoeuvring.

b. Patient-side Cart:

This includes multiple robotic arms that hold surgical instruments and a camera. These arms execute the surgeon's commands with high precision.

c. Vision System:

The system is designed with a high-definition 3D camera. This provides a detailed view of the operative area, thus helping the surgeon perform intricate procedures more effectively.

During the procedure, a surgeon makes small incisions to insert instruments and a camera. Seated at the console, the surgeon manipulates the instruments in real time; the robotic system converts these movements into precise actions inside the patient's body. It should be noted that the robot does not operate independently; it strictly follows the inputs provided by the surgeon.

Robotic surgery has been successfully applied in a range of health care fields, such as:

a. Cardiac Surgery: Performing intricate heart procedures with greater accuracy.
b. Urology: Prostatectomies and other urinary tract surgery.
c. Gynaecology: Patients could have endometriosis or need hysterectomies, among other conditions.
d. Orthopaedics: Joint replacements, spinal surgeries (Morris, B. et al., 2005).

4.1.2 Artificial Intelligence's Role Is Robotic Surgery

AI modeling is allowing surgeons to have advanced intraoperative metrics such as force and tactile measurements, enhanced detection of positive surgical margins, and even allowing for the complete automation of certain steps in surgical procedures (Knudsen, J. E. et al., 2024). Surgical robots rely on data captured through sensors and images to operate, and this data is used by AI to increase their precision and achieve new realm of precision (Hashimoto DA et al., 2018).

Typically, a robotic surgery refers to a surgery in which there is "maser-slave" relation between machine and human. Here human doctors are master which input gestures in a console and the robot performs that operation (Knudsen, J. E. et al., 2024).

However, with the help of integration of AI, this system can be autonomous. During a surgery the robots can be instructed to open skin tissue or drill hole in bones, using the help of AI robot can pinpoint where it needs to perform the operation. High-level of automation is also possible. An AI model which is specifically designed to be optimized based on medical data can be used to perform many tasks during surgery like skin closure after surgery is finished, lymph node dissection and many more. Complete automation of robots is implemented where there is no human input. Such cases can be found where the probability of doctor being available are low like during flights. In robotic surgery native tissue recognition means the ability of surgical systems to spot and tell apart different types of tissues during operations. This skill plays a key role to boost surgical accuracy, keep patients safe, and get better results overall.

A new way to recognize native tissue uses rapid evaporative ionization mass spectrometry (REIMS). This method looks at the spray made during surgical cutting to give real-time molecular details about the tissue. A study in Scientific Reports showed it's possible to combine REIMS with robotic platforms. The research team created a system to remove surgical spray that works with robotic systems allowing steady sample collection during surgery. Their results uncovered specific fat profiles linked to different tissue types making it possible to identify tissues right away during an operation (Mirnezami, R. et al., 2012).

Also, a new sensor using fiber Bragg grating (FBG) arrays has come out to spot tissue mechanical properties during robotic surgery. This sensor built into the instrument, picks out tissues based on how they feel showing it's possible to tell tissues apart better in robot-aided invasive surgeries. These steps forward in spotting native tissue play a key role in boosting what robotic surgery can do. By giving real-time exact naming of tissue types, these tools aim to make surgery more precise cut down the chance of harming healthy tissues by mistake, and in the end, help patients get better results (Sun, S et al., 2022).

4.2 Workflow Recognition

A surgical operation can be divided into steps (e.g., access, execution of surgical objectives, and closure). Steps break down each phase into specific segments that contribute to the overall procedure (e.g., a nerve-sparing step of radical prostatectomy).

Machine learning algorithms are trained using surgical videos which can allow them to compare the data from sensors during an operation to recognize the type of surgery is required. As they have large set of data available, they can predict the possible dangers underlying surgery (Meireles O. R. e al., 2021).

4.3 Surgemes

Surgemes or simply, surgical gestures refer to most basic unit of communication between human tissue and surgical instruments. Understanding these gestures is an important aspect of surgeon skills assessment, surgical training, and autonomous robotic surgery systems. Gesture recognition methods are classified based on input including video, kinematics data, or both. Machine learning models are trained based on surgical videos and kinematic data from previous surgeries to accurately understand these gestures (Ma R et al., 2022).

Operations which take advantage of AI-integrated robotic machines are less likely to fail as some surgeons which are freshers and might make mistake due to interference from their emotions or other ethical reasons but, as the machine operates based on command it is not likely to disobey or make a mistake which might make the surgery unsuccessful.

During the surgery, the AI is used to constantly monitor the patient's condition and alert doctor if it detects any abnormality.

AI is especially effective in postoperative care. As most of the times when the doctor gets tired after surgery and might not be available, AI can be used to monitor patient's condition after the surgery and based on the recovery of the patient provide an optimized discharge plan for the patient which reduces the hospital's burden thus improving their overall efficiency (Gunia, A. e al., 2024).

While autonomous robotic surgery has the potential to revolutionize healthcare, it also comes with several disadvantages and challenges:

a. High Cost of Implementation:

Robotic surgical systems are expensive to acquire, maintain, and upgrade. Hospitals must invest in specialized training for surgeons and staff. The cost of robotic procedures may be higher for patients.

b. Lack of Human Judgment and Adaptability:

Autonomous systems rely on pre-programmed algorithms and may struggle to adapt to unexpected complications. Unlike human surgeons, they lack intuition and experience-based decision-making (Glover, J. et al.,2022)

c. Risk of Malfunction or Technical Failure:

Software bugs, hardware malfunctions, or system errors can lead to serious complications. Power failures or connectivity issues can disrupt surgeries mid-procedure.

d. Ethical and Legal Concerns:

The question of liability in case of surgical errors remains unclear. Ethical dilemmas arise when machines make critical decisions about patient care (Glover, J. et al.,2022).

e. Reduced Surgeon Skill Development:

Over-reliance on automation may hinder the development of hands-on surgical skills. Future surgeons might lack traditional expertise if training shifts entirely to robotic systems.

f. Lack of Emotional Intelligence and Patient Interaction:

Robots cannot offer the reassurance, empathy, and personalized care that human surgeons provide. The absence of human interaction may impact patient trust and satisfaction (Yang, G.-Z. et al., 2017).

While autonomous robotic surgery offers numerous advantages, its drawbacks must be carefully addressed before widespread adoption. A balance between automation and human oversight is essential to ensure safety, efficiency, and ethical medical practices.

5. ARTIFICIAL INTELLIGENCE APPLICATIONS IN MEDICAL IMAGING AND RADIODIAGNOSIS

Artificial intelligence (AI) has emerged as a transformative force in medical imaging and radiodiagnosis, fundamentally changing how medical images are analyzed, interpreted, and utilized in clinical decision-making. The integration of AI technologies, particularly machine learning and deep learning algorithms, enables automated and highly accurate analysis of complex imaging data such as X-rays, computed tomography (CT), magnetic resonance imaging (MRI), and ultrasound. These advancements address longstanding challenges in radiology, including the growing volume of imaging studies, variability in human interpretation, and the need for rapid and precise diagnosis

5.1 Applications of Artificial Intelligence in Radiodiagnosis

a. Automated Image Interpretation: AI algorithms, especially deep learning models, are used to automatically detect and classify abnormalities in medical images such as X-rays, CT scans, MRIs, and ultrasounds. This helps in identifying diseases like pneumonia, tuberculosis, cancers, and fractures with high precision.
b. Early Disease Detection: AI can recognize subtle patterns that may be overlooked by human eyes, enabling earlier diagnosis of conditions such as lung nodules or tumors, which significantly improves patient prognosis.
c. Workflow Optimization: AI tools assist radiologists by prioritizing urgent cases, reducing reporting times, and automating repetitive tasks like measurement and segmentation of anatomical structures.
d. Quantitative Analysis: AI enables precise quantification of lesion size, volume, and progression over time, aiding in treatment planning and monitoring.

e. Decision Support Systems: By integrating patient data and imaging findings, AI systems provide diagnostic suggestions and risk assessments to support clinical decision-making.
f. Remote and Resource-Limited Settings: AI-powered radiodiagnosis tools can provide diagnostic support in areas lacking expert radiologists, improving healthcare accessibility and equity (Akhter, Y. et al., 2023).

5.2 Challenges and Ethical Considerations in AI for Radiodiagnosis

Despite the significant promise of artificial intelligence (AI) in radiodiagnosis, several challenges and ethical issues must be addressed to ensure safe, effective, and equitable deployment.

Challenges:

a. **Data Quality and Availability**: AI models require large, high-quality annotated datasets for training. Limited access to diverse and representative medical imaging data can reduce model accuracy and generalizability across populations.
b. **Interpretability and Transparency**: Many AI algorithms, particularly deep learning models, operate as "black boxes," making it difficult for clinicians to understand how decisions are made, which can hinder trust and adoption.
c. **Integration with Clinical Workflow**: Seamlessly incorporating AI tools into existing radiology systems and workflows poses technical and operational challenges.
d. **Regulatory Approval and Validation:** Ensuring rigorous clinical validation and meeting regulatory standards is essential before AI tools can be widely adopted.
e. **Bias and Fairness:** AI models trained on biased datasets risk perpetuating healthcare disparities by underperforming on underrepresented groups (Rajpurkar, P et al., 2022).

Ethical Considerations:

a. **Patient Privacy and Data Security:** The collection and use of sensitive imaging and health data must comply with privacy regulations (e.g., HIPAA, GDPR) to protect patient confidentiality.
b. **Accountability and Liability:** Clear frameworks are needed to define responsibility in cases of AI-related diagnostic errors.

c. **Informed Consent:** Patients should be informed when AI is involved in their diagnostic process and understand its implications.
d. **Equitable Access:** Efforts should be made to ensure AI benefits are accessible across different healthcare settings, including underserved regions.

Addressing these challenges and ethical considerations is critical to realizing the full potential of AI in radiodiagnosis while maintaining patient safety and public trust (Kelly, C. J. et al., 2019).

5.3 Artificial Intelligence's Role In Radio Diagnosis

AI integration into radiodiagnosis involves embedding advanced computational algorithms into the process of medical image acquisition, interpretation, and reporting. This integration primarily utilizes machine learning (ML) and deep learning (DL) techniques to analyze medical images such as X-rays, computed tomography (CT) scans, magnetic resonance imaging (MRI), and ultrasound images. AI models are trained to recognize patterns, segment anatomical structures, detect abnormalities, and generate diagnostic insights by processing large datasets of labelled medical images.

5.3.1 The Working Mechanism of AI in Radiodiagnosis:

AI systems in radiodiagnosis typically begin with the collection and preprocessing of medical imaging data. Preprocessing includes normalization, noise reduction, resizing, and augmentation to ensure that the input data meets the requirements of the AI models and improves their generalization. The core of AI integration involves developing and training machine learning models, particularly deep neural networks (DNNs) such as convolutional neural networks (CNNs), which are well-suited for image recognition tasks due to their ability to automatically extract hierarchical features from raw pixel data.

During training, these neural networks learn to associate input images with corresponding diagnostic labels through supervised learning. Large datasets annotated by expert radiologists serve as ground truth, enabling the model to learn discriminative features that distinguish between normal and pathological findings. Training involves optimizing the network parameters to minimize the error between predicted outputs and true labels using techniques such as backpropagation and stochastic gradient descent.

Once trained, AI models can be deployed in clinical settings where they analyze new patient images. The input image passes through the network layers, where convolutional filters extract relevant features at different spatial resolutions. The network's final layers typically produce probabilities or classifications indicating the presence or absence of specific abnormalities. Additionally, methods such as heatmaps or saliency maps are generated to visually indicate regions of interest within the image, aiding clinicians in understanding AI predictions (Rajpurkar, P. et al., 2017).

5.3.2 Types of AI Tasks in Radiodiagnosis:

AI integration encompasses several key tasks within the radio diagnostic workflow:

a. Detection and Classification: AI algorithms are designed to detect and classify lesions, nodules, fractures, or other pathological features within medical images. For example, AI models trained on chest X-rays can identify signs of pneumonia, tuberculosis, or lung nodules by recognizing characteristic radiographic patterns.
b. Segmentation: Segmentation involves delineating anatomical structures or abnormal regions within an image. AI models use pixel-level classification to produce precise outlines of organs, tumours, or lesions, which are essential for treatment planning, volumetric analysis, and longitudinal monitoring.
c. Quantification: Beyond detection, AI can measure sizes, volumes, and growth rates of abnormalities by analysing segmented regions, providing quantitative data for clinical assessment.
d. Image Enhancement and Reconstruction: AI is also integrated into the imaging acquisition process itself, where deep learning techniques help improve image quality, reduce noise, and accelerate image reconstruction, especially in modalities like MRI and CT (Lakhani, P. et al., 2017).

5.3.3 Workflow Integration in Clinical Radiology:

AI systems are often embedded into existing radiology workflows through Picture Archiving and Communication Systems (PACS) and Radiology Information Systems (RIS). When a medical image is acquired, it is routed to an AI-powered analysis tool either on local servers or cloud platforms. The AI processes the image and generates outputs—such as diagnostic flags, annotations, or structured reports—which are then made available to radiologists within their standard review environment.

Many AI tools are configured to prioritize cases with suspected abnormalities, helping manage caseloads by flagging urgent studies. Others operate as second readers, providing parallel assessments alongside radiologists' interpretations to improve diagnostic confidence.

5.3.4 Data Requirements and Training Pipelines:

Successful AI integration depends on access to large, diverse, and high-quality datasets. Datasets are typically curated from clinical repositories, often anonymized to protect patient privacy. Data labelling involves expert radiologists manually annotating images, a labour-intensive but critical step to ensure accurate model training.

Training pipelines also incorporate validation and testing phases, where models are evaluated on independent datasets to assess performance metrics such as sensitivity, specificity, accuracy, and area under the receiver operating characteristic curve (AUC-ROC). Continuous model retraining and calibration may occur as new data is acquired, maintaining accuracy and adapting to shifts in imaging protocols or patient populations.

5.3.5 Regulatory and Technical Considerations:

AI tools in radiodiagnosis must comply with regulatory standards before clinical deployment, ensuring safety, efficacy, and reliability. Regulatory bodies require rigorous documentation of development processes, clinical validation studies, and post-market surveillance. Technical integration includes interoperability with existing hospital IT infrastructure, secure data handling, and user interface design that facilitates seamless interaction between AI outputs and radiologists' workflows.

5.3.6 Examples of AI Integration in Radiodiagnosis:

Several AI-powered applications have been integrated into radiology practice worldwide. For instance, automated detection of lung nodules in CT scans is now facilitated by AI systems that highlight suspicious areas for radiologist review. Similarly, AI algorithms analysing mammograms assist in breast cancer screening by classifying lesions and predicting malignancy risk. These implementations demonstrate how AI acts as a complementary tool within radiodiagnosis, streamlining the complex process of image interpretation.

6. NANOTECHNOLOGY IN THE MEDICAL FIELD

Nanotechnology is revolutionizing the medical field by enabling precise diagnostics, targeted drug delivery, regenerative medicine, and advanced imaging techniques. By manipulating materials at the nanoscale (1–100 nanometers), scientists can develop highly effective medical treatments.

6.1 Applications of Nanotechnology in Medicine

a. Targeted Drug Delivery:

Nanoparticles can be engineered to deliver drugs directly to diseased cells, minimizing side effects and improving treatment efficacy. Liposomes and polymeric nanoparticles are commonly used to transport chemotherapy drugs to cancer cells, reducing damage to healthy tissues (Sahoo, S. K. et al., 2003).

b. Cancer Treatment

Gold and silver nanoparticles are used in photothermal therapy, where they absorb light and generate heat to destroy cancer cells. (Brajtburg, J. et al., 1996). Nano-based immunotherapy enhances the body's immune response to fight cancer more effectively (Jain, K. K. et al., 2008)

c. Regenerative Medicine

Nano scaffolds are used in tissue engineering to promote the growth of skin, bone, and nerve cells, aiding in wound healing and organ repair. Stem cell delivery systems use nanocarriers to improve the effectiveness of regenerative treatments (Sahoo, S. K. et al., 2003).

d. Diagnostics and Imaging

Quantum dots and nano sensors enhance the accuracy of MRI, CT scans, and biosensors, improving disease detection at an early stage. (Green, M. M. e al., 2003). Lab-on-a-chip technology integrates nanomaterials for real-time disease monitoring and rapid diagnostics (Sahoo, S. K. et al., 2003).

e. Antibacterial and Antiviral Applications

Silver and copper nanoparticles exhibit strong antimicrobial properties, preventing infections in medical implants and wound dressings. Nano coatings on surgical tools and hospital surfaces reduce the spread of pathogens (Jain, 2008)

6.2 Challenges and Ethical Considerations:

Despite its potential, nanotechnology in medicine faces several challenges:

a. Toxicity Concerns – Some nanoparticles may accumulate in organs, posing long-term health risks (Riehemann, K et al., 2009).
b. Regulatory Hurdles – Strict approval processes are required to ensure the safety and efficacy of nanomedicine (Riehemann, K et al., 2009).
c. Cost and Accessibility – High production costs may limit widespread adoption in developing regions (Ferrari, M. et al., 2005).

6.3 AI Integration In Nano Technology

a. AI-Enhanced Targeted Drug Delivery:

AI optimizes nanoparticle size, shape, and surface chemistry for better drug absorption and minimal side effects.

Machine learning models predict drug release patterns and ensure medications reach the intended target (e.g., cancer cells, neurons, or organs).

Example: AI-designed liposomes and polymeric nanoparticles for precise chemotherapy, reducing toxicity to healthy tissues (Adir, O. et al., 2019).

b. AI-Based Disease Detection and Diagnostics:

Nano sensors and AI-powered biosensors detect diseases in real time by analyzing blood samples or body fluids.

AI assists in early-stage cancer detection by identifying unique molecular signatures in nanoparticle-enhanced imaging.

Example: AI-guided quantum dot nanoparticles for detecting biomarkers of Alzheimer's or Parkinson's disease (Zhu, J. et al., 2023).

c. AI in Nanorobotics for Surgery and Treatment:

AI-controlled nanorobots perform minimally invasive surgeries by precisely navigating within the body.

Nanorobots equipped with AI-based motion control can deliver drugs, remove blockages, or repair damaged tissues.

Example: AI-powered magnetically controlled nanorobots for unclogging arteries in cardiovascular disease treatment (Rajendran, S. et al., 2023).

d. AI-Driven Imaging and Medical Diagnostics:

AI improves nanoparticle-based contrast agents for sharper MRI and CT scans, enhancing medical imaging accuracy.

Deep learning algorithms analyze AI-enhanced nanoscale imaging, helping radiologists detect abnormalities earlier.

Example: Gold and iron oxide nanoparticles combined with AI improve tumor detection in MRIs (Simos, Y. e al., 2021).

e. AI in Personalized Nanomedicine:

AI analyzes genomic and patient data to design customized nanodrugs tailored to an individual's genetic profile.

AI-driven models predict how patients respond to nanomedicine, allowing real-time treatment adjustments.

Example: AI-assisted nano-drug formulations for personalized cancer immunotherapy (Sindhu, R. K. et al., 2021).

AI and nanotechnology are reshaping medicine, enabling personalized treatments, efficient drug delivery, and early disease detection. As research advances, AI-driven nanomedicine will continue to revolutionize healthcare, making treatments more precise, accessible, and life-saving.

7. RESEARCH METHODOLOGY

7.1 Research Design:

a. Experimental Studies – Used for AI-based drug discovery, disease prediction, and medical image analysis.
b. Observational Studies – Analyze real-world clinical data to train and validate AI models.
c. Qualitative Studies – Conduct expert interviews and focus groups to understand AI adoption challenges in healthcare (Esteva, A. et al., 2019).

7.2 Data Collection Methods:

AI models in medicine require high-quality datasets from various sources:

a. Electronic Health Records (EHRs) – Used for AI-based predictive analytics and patient diagnosis.

b. Medical Imaging (MRI, CT, X-rays, Ultrasound) – AI models use deep learning (CNNs) to analyze diseases like cancer.
c. Wearable and IoT Devices – AI analyzes real-time patient data from smartwatches, ECG monitors, and biosensors.
d. Clinical Trial Data – AI assists in drug development by identifying treatment patterns (Nasarian, E. et al., 2023).

7.3 AI Model Development and Implementation

Developing AI solutions in medicine involves multiple steps:

7.3.1 Data Preprocessing:

a. Cleaning and Normalization – Removing missing values and standardizing medical terms.
b. Feature Selection – Identifying relevant biomarkers, symptoms, and risk factors.
c. Data Augmentation – Used in imaging AI to improve model robustness.

7.3.2 Model Selection:

Common AI techniques in medical research include:

a. Machine Learning (ML) – Decision Trees, Random Forests, and SVMs for disease prediction and diagnostics.
b. Deep Learning (DL) – CNNs and RNNs for medical image analysis and NLP-based EHR processing.
c. Natural Language Processing (NLP) – Extracting insights from clinical notes and research papers.

7.3.3 Model Training and Validation:

a. Supervised Learning – Trains AI using labeled datasets (e.g., cancer detection models).
b. Unsupervised Learning – Finds patterns in unlabeled medical data.
c. Reinforcement Learning – Used in robotic surgery and personalized treatment planning (Khanachivskyi, O. et al., 2024).

7.4 Model Evaluation and Performance Metrics:

AI models in medicine must be rigorously validated using:

a. Accuracy, Precision, Recall, F1-Score – Evaluate classification performance.
b. ROC-AUC Curve – Measures diagnostic ability in disease prediction models.
c. Cross-Validation – Ensures model generalizability across different datasets (Topol, E. J. e al., 2019).

7.5 Ethical Considerations & Regulatory Compliance:

a. Patient Privacy – Compliance with HIPAA, GDPR, and FDA regulations.
b. Explainability – Using interpretable AI (XAI) to justify medical decisions (Jiang, F. et al., 2017).

7.6 Deployment & Real-World Validation:

AI models must be tested in clinical settings before full implementation:

a. Pilot Studies & Clinical Trials – Testing AI tools in hospitals and research labs.
b. Integration with Hospital Systems – AI is embedded in electronic health record systems, diagnostic tools, and robotic surgeries.
c. Real-Time Monitoring & Feedback – Continuous improvement of AI accuracy based on clinical feedback (Cohen, R. Y. et al 2021).

AI research in medicine requires structured data collection, model development, rigorous evaluation, ethical compliance, and real-world validation. This methodology ensures AI-driven medical innovations are safe, effective, and trustworthy for clinical applications.

8. FUTURE DIRECTIONS

Artificial Intelligence (AI) is transforming the healthcare industry by improving diagnostics, treatment planning, patient monitoring, and administrative efficiency. With the integration of machine learning (ML), deep learning (DL), natural language processing (NLP), and robotics, AI is set to revolutionize healthcare further in the coming years. This paper explores the future directions of AI in healthcare, focusing on advanced medical diagnostics, personalized medicine, AI-driven robotics, predictive analytics, and ethical considerations (Juang, W.-C et al., 2022).

8.1 AI-Powered Diagnostics and Early Disease Detection

One of the most promising uses of AI in healthcare is its ability to improve disease detection and diagnostics. AI-driven imaging systems are already enhancing the accuracy of radiology, dermatology, and pathology. In the future, AI will play a crucial role in detecting diseases at their earliest stages, often before symptoms become apparent. For instance, deep learning algorithms trained on large datasets of X-rays, MRIs, and CT scans can identify patterns that indicate the presence of cancer, cardiovascular diseases, or neurological disorders with high precision. AI-powered diagnostics will reduce human error, increase efficiency, and ensure faster decision-making, leading to better patient outcomes.

Also, AI will be integrated with wearable devices and biosensors to continuously monitor vital signs and detect early markers of diseases. Patients with chronic conditions such as diabetes, hypertension, and heart disease will benefit from AI systems that analyze data in real time and provide instant alerts to doctors if abnormalities are detected. This proactive approach will help in preventive medicine, allowing healthcare professionals to intervene before a patient's condition worsens (Zhang, Y. et al., 2016).

8.2 Personalized Medicine and AI-Driven Drug Discovery

AI is reshaping the field of personalized medicine by tailoring treatments based on an individual's genetic profile, lifestyle, and medical history. The future of healthcare will witness AI-driven precision medicine that customizes drug therapies and treatment plans to meet each patient's unique needs. AI models trained on genomic data will help predict how patients will respond to certain medications, minimizing adverse effects and optimizing treatment effectiveness.

Additionally, AI is expected to accelerate drug discovery and development by analyzing biological and chemical interactions at an unprecedented scale. Traditional drug discovery is expensive process, taking 10-15 years to bring a new drug to market. AI algorithms can analyze millions of compounds, simulate drug interactions, and identify potential drug candidates much faster. Pharmaceutical companies like Pfizer, AstraZeneca, and Google DeepMind are already leveraging AI to develop novel treatments for diseases such as cancer, Alzheimer's, and rare genetic disorders. In the coming years, AI-powered drug repurposing will gain momentum, where existing drugs are analyzed for their potential to treat new diseases. This approach will significantly reduce R&D costs while ensuring faster availability of treatments for emerging health threats, such as pandemics.

8.3 AI-Driven Robotics and Automation in Healthcare

The future of AI in healthcare will see a rise in AI-driven robotics for both surgical and non-surgical applications. Surgical robots, such as the da Vinci Surgical System, will continue to advance, allowing for more precise, minimally invasive procedures. AI-powered robotic surgeons will assist in complex surgeries, reducing complications and improving patient recovery times. In addition to surgical robots, AI-driven care robots will support healthcare professionals by assisting in patient care, rehabilitation, and elderly care. These robots will help address staff shortages by performing routine tasks, such as medication delivery, patient monitoring, and lifting patients. AI-powered robotic exoskeletons will also become more sophisticated, helping paralyzed patients regain mobility and supporting stroke rehabilitation therapies. Beyond hospitals, AI chatbots and virtual health assistants will provide patients with instant medical advice, symptom checking, and appointment scheduling. These virtual assistants will use NLP to engage in natural conversations with patients, reducing the burden on healthcare providers while ensuring continuous patient support.

8.4 Predictive Analytics using AI in Healthcare

AI's ability to analyze vast amounts of healthcare data will be instrumental in predicting disease outbreaks and preventing health crises. Predictive analytics will leverage AI to analyze electronic health records (EHRs), environmental factors, and genetic data to identify individuals at high risk of developing chronic diseases. By recognizing early warning signs, AI will enable healthcare providers to implement preventive measures, lifestyle modifications, and early interventions, reducing hospitalizations and healthcare costs. Moreover, AI will be crucial in predicting and managing global health threats, such as pandemics. By analyzing real-time data from multiple sources, including social media, government reports, and travel patterns, AI will detect early signs of infectious disease outbreaks and help public health officials implement containment measures before they escalate into global crises.

8.5 AI in Mental Health and Cognitive Care

The mental health sector will benefit a lot from AI-driven interventions. AI-powered chatbots and virtual therapists will provide round-the-clock mental health support for patients suffering from depression, anxiety, PTSD, and other mental health conditions. These AI tools will use sentiment analysis and voice recognition to assess a patient's emotional state and offer appropriate coping strategies or alert human therapists if intervention is needed.

Furthermore, AI is expected to play a major role in early detection of neurodegenerative diseases such as Alzheimer's and Parkinson's disease. AI algorithms analyzing speech patterns, facial expressions, and movement data can detect early cognitive decline, allowing for timely intervention and better disease management. AI-driven cognitive training programs will also be developed to help patients maintain brain health and slow disease progression.

8.6 Ethical Considerations and AI Governance in Healthcare

Despite its transformative potential, AI in healthcare raises significant ethical, legal, and regulatory challenges. The widespread adoption of AI must be accompanied by strict data privacy and security protocols to protect patient information. AI models must be transparent, explainable, and unbiased to ensure ethical decision-making in medical practice.

Bias in AI models remains a major concern, as algorithms trained on non-diverse datasets may produce inaccurate or unfair outcomes, especially for underrepresented populations. Future research will focus on developing unbiased AI models that ensure fairness across different demographics. Governments and regulatory bodies, such as the FDA and WHO, will establish global AI healthcare policies to regulate AI-based medical applications and ensure patient safety.

8.7 AI Integration with Smart Hospitals and IoT

The future of AI in healthcare will witness the rise of smart hospitals, where AI, IoT (Internet of Things), and blockchain technology work together to enhance patient care. AI-powered hospital management systems will optimize bed management, patient flow, and resource allocation to improve hospital efficiency. Additionally, AI will integrate with IoT-enabled smart devices to provide continuous patient monitoring. Smartwatches, biosensors, and remote monitoring devices will collect real-time health data, allowing AI to detect health deterioration and trigger alerts for medical intervention. This technology will be particularly beneficial for elderly care, post-surgery monitoring, and managing chronic diseases like diabetes and heart disease (T Venkat Narayana Rao, et al., 2016).

AI is set to revolutionize healthcare by improving diagnostics, enabling personalized treatments, enhancing robotic-assisted surgeries, and driving predictive analytics. The future of AI in medicine will be shaped by advancements in machine learning, robotics, and real-time data processing, making healthcare more efficient, accessible, and patient-centric. However, as AI becomes deeply embedded in medical decision-making, ethical concerns, data privacy, and regulatory frameworks must evolve to ensure responsible and equitable AI adoption. With continuous innovation and collaboration between healthcare providers, AI researchers, and policymakers, AI-driven healthcare solutions will enhance patient outcomes, reduce medical errors, and usher in a new era of intelligent and personalized medicine. The next decade will likely see AI becoming an integral part of clinical workflows, telemedicine, robotic surgeries, and mental health interventions, making healthcare smarter, safer, and more effective than ever before.

9. CASE STUDIES

9.1 Case Study-1: AI in Early Detection of Diabetic Retinopathy

Diabetic Retinopathy (DR) is a leading cause of blindness among diabetic patients worldwide. Early detection and timely intervention are crucial to prevent vision loss. (Gong, Q. Y. et al., 2022). However, due to a shortage of trained ophthalmologists, particularly in low-resource settings, many patients are diagnosed at an advanced stage. Artificial Intelligence (AI) has emerged as a game-changing solution by automating DR screening, improving accuracy, and making diagnosis more accessible.

9.1.1 Background

Google's DeepMind and Verily, in collaboration with the Indian Ministry of Health and Aravind Eye Hospital, developed an AI-based screening system for DR. The system utilized deep learning algorithms trained on thousands of retinal images to detect early signs of diabetic eye disease (Clement, 2024).

9.1.2 Implementation of AI in DR Diagnosis

The AI model was trained using a dataset of 128,000 retinal images, labeled by experienced ophthalmologists. The system analyzed new retinal scans and classified them into different severity levels, ranging from no retinopathy to severe retinopathy.

The AI model was integrated into primary care centers and diabetic clinics, enabling non-specialist healthcare workers to conduct preliminary screenings. Patients identified as high-risk were then referred to specialists for confirmation and treatment.

9.1.3 Impact and Outcomes

a. Higher Accuracy and Speed – Studies showed that the AI model achieved an accuracy of 94-96%, comparable to human ophthalmologists. It detected subtle retinal changes that could be missed by general physicians.
b. Increased Accessibility – AI screenings allowed rural and underserved populations to access diabetic eye exams without needing a specialist on-site.
c. Faster Diagnosis and Treatment – The AI system significantly reduced diagnosis time from days to minutes, enabling early treatment and reducing complications.
d. Scalability – The AI model was expanded to hospitals and clinics in India, Thailand, and the U.K., screening thousands of patients daily.

9.1.4 Challenges and Ethical Considerations

While AI improved DR detection, challenges remained:

a. Data Bias – AI models trained on specific populations needed further refinement to perform well across diverse ethnicities.
b. Regulatory Approvals – Healthcare AI tools required strict FDA and WHO approvals before large-scale adoption.
c. Doctor-AI Collaboration – Ophthalmologists needed to be trained to interpret AI recommendations accurately and make final clinical decisions.

The use of AI in diabetic retinopathy screening demonstrated its potential to revolutionize early disease detection, reduce diagnostic workloads, and improve patient care suffering from such diseases. AI can bridge healthcare gaps, especially in developing regions with limited medical expertise. As AI continues to evolve, its integration with telemedicine and mobile screening units will further enhance preventive healthcare and global accessibility (Google n.d.).

9.2 Case Study-2: AI-Based Radiodiagnosis for Tuberculosis Detection Using Chest X-rays

Background:

Tuberculosis (TB) remains a major public health concern in low- and middle-income countries. Chest X-rays (CXR) are a standard screening tool, but the shortage of skilled radiologists often delays diagnosis and treatment.

AI Implementation:

An AI-powered tool developed by Qure.ai, known as qXR, was deployed in rural clinics across India to automatically interpret chest X-rays for TB detection. The deep learning model was trained on thousands of labelled CXR images to identify radiological patterns consistent with TB.

Process:

a. Patients were screened using standard digital X-ray machines.
b. The AI model analysed each scan in under one minute and flagged those with probable TB signs.
c. High-risk cases were then prioritized for further testing (e.g., GeneXpert) and treatment.
d. The AI system provided probability scores and visual heatmaps to assist physicians.

Outcomes:

a. Diagnostic accuracy comparable to expert radiologists (sensitivity >90%, specificity ~85%).
b. Turnaround time reduced drastically from hours or days to minutes.
c. Increased screening capacity in remote areas with no on-site radiologists.
d. Facilitated early treatment, reducing community spread and improving patient outcomes.

Challenges & Lessons:

a. Required validation across diverse populations.
b. Needed integration with local health IT systems and workflows.
c. Interpretability tools (like heatmaps) helped build trust with healthcare professionals.

AI in radiodiagnosis, especially for diseases like TB, offers transformative potential by enhancing diagnostic reach and speed, particularly in underserved areas. Tools like qXR exemplify how AI can bridge gaps in healthcare access and expertise. (Pasa, F et al., 2019).

10. CONCLUSION

Artificial Intelligence (AI) is redefining the future of healthcare through its integration into diagnostics, treatment, patient monitoring, and medical education. From enhancing radiodiagnosis accuracy to enabling real-time patient data analysis, AI empowers healthcare professionals to make faster and more informed decisions. The use of AI in adaptive devices such as smart prosthetics, AI-powered wheelchairs, and virtual patient simulations is significantly improving the quality of life for patients and the effectiveness of clinical training. Furthermore, AI-driven systems streamline medical record management, aid in early disease detection, and accelerate drug development through data-driven insights. The synergy of AI with technologies like nanotechnology and robotics has introduced minimally invasive surgeries and personalized medicine that are more efficient and accessible. However, challenges such as data privacy, algorithmic bias, and the need for human oversight must be addressed to ensure ethical AI adoption. Overall, the continued evolution of AI in healthcare holds the promise of smarter, safer, and more equitable medical systems, where both patients and providers benefit from technology-driven innovation.

REFERENCES:

Adir, O., Poley, M., Chen, G., Froim, S., Krinsky, N., Shklover, J., & Schroeder, A. (2019). Integrating artificial intelligence and nanotechnology for precision cancer medicine. *Advanced Materials*, *32*(13), 1901989. PMID: 31286573

Akhter, Y., Singh, R., & Vatsa, M. (2023). AI-based radiodiagnosis using chest X-rays: A review. *Frontiers in Big Data*, *6*, 1120989. PMID: 37091458

Akhter, Y., Singh, R., & Vatsa, M. (2023). AI-based radiodiagnosis using chest X-rays: A review. *Frontiers in Big Data*, *6*, 1120989. PMID: 37091458

Brajtburg, J., & Bolard, J. (1996). Lipid-based formulas of amphotericin B. *Drugs*, *51*(6), 1025–1044.

Clement, C. (2024, February 29). Real-world examples and applications of AI in healthcare. OpenLoop Health.

Cohen, R. Y., & Kovacheva, V. P. (2021). A methodology for a scalable, collaborative, and resource-efficient platform to facilitate healthcare AI research. arXiv preprint arXiv:2112.06883.

Combs, C. D., & Combs, P. F. (2019). Emerging roles of virtual patients in the age of AI. *AMA Journal of Ethics*, *21*(2), E153–E159. PMID: 30794125

Esteva, A., Robicquet, A., Ramsundar, B., Kuleshov, V., DePristo, M., Chou, K., Cui, C., Corrado, G., Thrun, S., & Dean, J. (2019). A guide to deep learning in healthcare. *Nature Medicine*, *25*(1), 24–29. PMID: 30617335

Ferrari, M. (2005). Cancer nanotechnology: Opportunities and challenges. *Nature Reviews. Cancer*, *5*(3), 161–171. PMID: 15738981

Gadde, S. S., & Kalli, V. D. R. (2020). Applications of artificial intelligence in medical devices and healthcare. [IJCST]. *International Journal of Computer Science Trends and Technology*, *8*(2), 182–188.

Glover, J., & Young, A. (2022). Autonomous surgical robotic systems and the liability dilemma. *Frontiers in Surgery*, *9*, 1015367. PMID: 36277285

Gong, Q. Y., Hu, G. Y., Yu, S. Q., Qian, T. W., & Xu, X. (2022). Comprehensive assessment of growth factors, inflammatory mediators, and cytokines in vitreous from patients with proliferative diabetic retinopathy. *International Journal of Ophthalmology*, *15*(11), 1736–1742. PMID: 36404978

Green, M. M., & Wittcoff, H. A. (2003). Chapter 9: Polymers: The Fourth Dimension of Chemistry. In Organic Chemistry Principles and Industrial Practice (pp. 275–312).

Gunia, A., Varma, P., Zhang, J., Fehervari, M., & Ashrafian, H. (2024). Artificial Intelligence in Surgery: The Future Is Now. *European Surgical Research, 65*(1), 22–39.

Gurev, S. (2023, September 15). EVEScape: Predicting Virus Evolution with AI. *Time.*

Hashimoto, D. A., Rosman, G., Rus, D., & Meireles, O. R. (2018). Artificial intelligence in surgery: Promises and perils. *Annals of Surgery, 268*(1), 70. DOI: 10.1097/SLA.0000000000002693 PMID: 29389679

jagsi, R., & Lehmann, L. S. (2004). The ethics of medical education. BMJ, 329(7461), 332–334.

Jain, K. K. (2008). Nanomedicine: Application of nanobiotechnology in medical practice. *Medical Principles and Practice : International Journal of the Kuwait University, Health Science Centre, 17*(2), 89–101. PMID: 18287791

Jee, C. (2020, February 11). Robot-assisted high-precision surgery has passed its first test in humans. *MIT Technology Review.*

Jiang, F., Jiang, Y., Zhi, H., Dong, Y., Li, H., Ma, S., Wang, Y., Dong, Q., Shen, H., & Wang, Y. (2017). Artificial intelligence in healthcare: Past, present and future. *Stroke and Vascular Neurology, 2*(4), 230–243. PMID: 29507784

Juang, W.-C., Hsu, M.-H., Cai, Z.-X., & Chen, C.-M. (2022). Developing an AI-assisted clinical decision support system to enhance in-patient holistic health care. *PLoS One, 17*(10), e0276501. PMID: 36315554

Kelly, C. J., Karthikesalingam, A., Suleyman, M., Corrado, G., & King, D. (2019). Key challenges for delivering clinical impact with artificial intelligence. *BMC Medicine, 17*(1), 195. PMID: 31665002

Khanachivskyi, O. (2024, October 17). Transforming healthcare: The role of AI in medical records summarization.

Kirchner, E. A., Fernandez, J. G., Kampmann, P., Schröer, M., Metzen, J. H., & Kirchner, F. (2015). Intuitive interaction with robots - Technical approaches and challenges. In Drechsler, R., & Kühne, U. (Eds.), *Formal modeling and verification of cyber-physical systems* (pp. 225–240).

Knudsen, J. E., Ghaffar, U., Ma, R., & Hung, A. J. (2024). Clinical applications of artificial intelligence in robotic surgery. *Journal of Robotic Surgery, 18*(1), 102. PMID: 38427094

Kumar, A., & Gaharwar, M. (2020). Artificial intelligence based wireless smart wheelchair. *Journal of Applied Research and Technology, 18*(6), 262–267.

Lakhani, P., & Sundaram, B. (2017). Deep learning at chest radiography: Automated classification of pulmonary tuberculosis by using convolutional neural networks. *Radiology, 284*(2), 574–582. PMID: 28436741

Ma, R., Ramaswamy, A., & Xu, J.. (2022). Surgical gestures as a method to quantify surgical performance and predict patient outcomes. *NPJ Digital Medicine, 5*(1), 187. DOI: 10.1038/s41746-022-00738-y PMID: 36550203

Meireles, O. R., Rosman, G., Altieri, M. S., Carin, L., Hager, G., Madani, A., Padoy, N., Pugh, C. M., Sylla, P., Ward, T. M., & Hashimoto, D. A., & SAGES Video Annotation for AI Working Groups. (2021). SAGES consensus recommendations on an annotation framework for surgical video. *Surgical Endoscopy, 35*(9), 4918–4929. PMID: 34231065

Mirnezami, R., Nicholson, J., & Darzi, A. (•••). Preparing for precision medicine. *The New England Journal of Medicine, 366*, 489–491. PMID: 22256780

Morris, B. (2005). Robotic surgery: Applications, limitations, and impact on surgical education. *MedGenMed : Medscape General Medicine, 7*(3), 72. PMID: 16369298

Nasarian, E., Alizadehsani, R., Acharya, U. R., & Tsui, K. L. (2023). Designing interpretable ML systems to enhance trust in healthcare: A systematic review to propose a responsible clinician-AI collaboration framework. arXiv preprint arXiv:2311.11055.

Pasa, F., Golkov, V., Pfeiffer, F., Cremers, D., & Pfeiffer, D. (2019). Efficient deep network architectures for fast chest X-ray tuberculosis screening and visualization. *Scientific Reports, 9*(1), 6268. PMID: 31000728

Polanco-Roman, L., Gomez, J., Miranda, R., & Jeglic, E. (2016). Stress-related symptoms and suicidal ideation: The roles of rumination and depressive symptoms vary by gender. *Cognitive Therapy and Research, 40*(5), 606–616. PMID: 27695146

Rajendran, S., Sundararajan, P., Awasthi, A., & Rajendran, S. (2023). Nanorobotics in medicine: A systematic review of advances, challenges, and future prospects. arXiv preprint arXiv:2309.10881.

Rajpurkar, P., Chen, E., Banerjee, O., & Topol, E. J. (2022). AI in health and medicine. *Nature Medicine, 28*(1), 31–38. PMID: 35058619

Riehemann, K., Schneider, S. W., Luger, T. A., Godin, B., Ferrari, M., & Fuchs, H. (2009). Nanomedicine—Challenge and perspectives. *Angewandte Chemie International Edition*, *48*(5), 872–897. PMID: 19142939

Riva, G., & Wiederhold, B. K. (2024). Ethical challenges of virtual reality technology interventions for the vulnerabilities of patients with chronic pain: Exploration of technician responsibility. *Journal of Medical Internet Research*, *26*, e40056.

Sahoo, S. K., & Labhasetwar, V. (2003). Nanotech approaches to delivery and imaging drug delivery. *Drug Discovery Today*, *8*(24), 1112–1120. PMID: 14678737

Simos, Y. V., Spyrou, K., Patila, M., Karouta, N., Stamatis, H., Gournis, D., & Tsougos, I. (2021). Trends of nanotechnology in type 2 diabetes mellitus treatment. *Asian Journal of Pharmaceutical Sciences*, *16*(1), 62–76. PMID: 33613730

Sindhu, R. K., Kaur, H., Kumar, M., Sofat, M., Yapar, E. A., Esenturk, I., & Zengin, G. (2021). The ameliorating approach of nanorobotics in the novel drug delivery systems: A mechanistic review. *Journal of Drug Targeting*, *29*(8), 822–833. PMID: 33641551

Singh, A. K., & Gaharwar, M. (2018). Artificial intelligence-based wireless smart wheelchair. [IJETER]. *International Journal of Emerging Technologies in Engineering Research*, *6*(3), 162–167.

Singh, A. K., & Gaharwar, M. (2020). Artificial intelligence based wireless smart wheelchair. *Journal of Applied Research and Technology*, *18*(6), 262–267.

Sun, S., Dutson, E. P., & Geoghegan, R. (2022, July). A novel sensor for tissue mechanical property detection during robotic surgery. *Proceedings of the Annual International Conference of the IEEE Engineering in Medicine and Biology Society*, 2022, 4834–4838.

Surya, L. (2018). How government can use AI and ML to identify spreading infectious diseases. [IJCRT]. *International Journal of Creative Research Thoughts*, *6*(1), 899–902.

Topol, E. J. (2019). High-performance medicine: The convergence of human and artificial intelligence. *Nature Medicine*, *25*(1), 44–56. PMID: 30617339

Venkat Narayana Rao, T., & Reddy, G. R. (2016). Prediction of soil quality using machine learning techniques. *International Journal of Scientific & Technology Research*, *8*(11), 1309–1313.

Venkat Narayana Rao, T., Unnisa, A., & Sreni, K. (2020). Medicine recommendation system based on patient reviews, International Journal of Science and Technology. *Res*, *9*, 3308–3312.

World Health Organization. (2024, April 16). Spinal cord injury. World Health Organization.

Yang, G.-Z., Cambias, J., Cleary, K., Daimler, E., Drake, J., Dupont, P. E., & Taylor, R. H. (2017). Medical robotics—Regulatory, ethical, and legal considerations for increasing levels of autonomy. *Annual Review of Control, Robotics, and Autonomous Systems*, *1*(1), 1–28. PMID: 33157870

Zhang, Y., & Zhang, D. (2016). Deep learning-based classification of hyperspectral data. *IEEE Journal of Selected Topics in Applied Earth Observations and Remote Sensing*, *9*(2), 868–879.

Zhu, J., Li, Y., & Shi, J. (2023). Application of artificial intelligence in the exploration and optimization of biomedical nanomaterials. *Nano Biomedicine and Engineering*, *15*(1), 1–14.

Chapter 6
AI in Wearable Imaging Devices

Adebayo Paul Olujide
https://orcid.org/0000-0002-4088-0634
University of Ilorin, Nigeria

Aremu Issa Babatunde
https://orcid.org/0009-0006-1701-8591
University of Ilorin, Nigeria

Ayinde Junaid Babatunde
https://orcid.org/0000-0002-8440-0268
Evercare Hospital Lekki, Nigeria

ABSTRACT

AI and wearable imaging devices are technologies changing real-time diagnostics, especially remote patient monitoring. This chapter explores AI's role in wearable imaging by highlighting its potential to enhance healthcare through greater accuracy, efficiency, and accessibility. It begins by examining wearable imaging applications in radiology and emphasizing their role in early disease detection. It delves into AI-driven advancement by improving image quality and diagnostic precision of ultrasound and MRI. Vital applications discussed include heart health monitoring, brain disorder assessment, and sports injury evaluation. AI's ability to analyze data, identify patterns, and predict health risks is also discussed. Additionally, the chapter covers device miniaturization, portability, and battery efficiency. Real-world examples illustrate AI's impact while challenges such as privacy, ethics, and regulatory concerns are addressed. Finally, the chapter looks ahead to AI's integration with telemedicine and emerging device innovations.

DOI: 10.4018/979-8-3373-0903-3.ch006

A. INTRODUCTION TO WEARABLE IMAGING IN RADIOLOGY

Wearable imaging devices are changing how we look at health care. In the past, if patients needed X-rays, MRIs, or ultrasounds, they had to go to a hospital or clinic, make an appointment, and wait (Kassay & De Silva, 2022; Monteagudo, 2016; Smith & Adhami, 1999). It took time and could be a hassle. But now, technology is stepping in. With new tools and intelligent machines, we can monitor health in real time without long waits. These wearable devices let people watch their health from home or wherever they are (Thacharodi et al., 2024). For example, imagine wearing a device that tracks the heart's activities daily. If something unusual happens, the device quickly alerts you or your doctor (Rákay & Galajdová, 2020). This live data can help catch problems early, which is important, especially for those with a higher risk of health issues.

One of the most incredible things about these devices is that they do not just take one picture of the health; they can keep track of it over more extended periods. Instead of gathering information in a big one-time test, you get constant updates. This ongoing monitoring can help find trends that a single scan might miss. Now, let us discuss why these devices are even better with AI or artificial intelligence. While the wearables can do a lot on their own, when paired with AI, they become super intelligent. AI is capable of analyzing captured medical images and identifying issues identify quickly.

For example, a wearable ultrasound device with AI could take high-quality images of your body and analyze them immediately for any signs of trouble. This enables doctors to decide faster, helping patients even when they are remotely located.

Artificial intelligence significantly enhances the quality of images. Medical imaging sometimes reflects noise or lack of clarity. Yet, AI has the potential to rectify such issues virtually in seconds. AI processes the images and makes them instantly usable. Moreover, AI has the capacity to scan health data longitudinally to identify potential threats even before they have turned into serious diseases. This transformation from a reactive approach to a preventive one has the potential to revolutionize healthcare practices.

A deeper examination of the intersection of wearable technology and AI indicates the technologies can significantly transform the healthcare system. AI-enabled devices could deliver this by presenting explainable health information on medical imaging. These technologies would decrease the load on medical centers, decrease expenses, and enhance patient care.

In the subsequent sections, we will cover the operating principles of such devices, their current applications, and the future challenges that can be anticipated. Such a convergence of high-tech has the capability to realize an active healthcare system that is personalized to the needs of the individual. This is an inspiring time for the medical fraternity as we advance towards a more customized way of healthcare delivery.

B. TECHNOLOGICAL FOUNDATIONS OF AI-ENHANCED WEARABLE IMAGING DEVICES

Wearable imaging technology combined with artificial intelligence is revolutionizing the tech landscape. The devices have combined high-degree AI features with wearable technology for enhanced health monitoring, data analysis, and human-machine interaction. Table 1 presents an overview of wearable imaging and AI. This section will examine the imaging function of the devices and how AI enhances the precision and user-friendliness of the resulting images.

Table 1. Wearable Imaging and AI: A Smart Synergy in Modern Diagnostics

Overview of Wearable Imaging Devices	**AI Technologies in Imaging**
Function: Wearable imaging devices capture visual data through integrated cameras and sensors, enabling real-time image processing and analysis.	*Function*: Artificial Intelligence enhances image recognition and analysis through machine learning algorithms, allowing for better data interpretation.
Applications in Healthcare	**Implications for Privacy and Ethics**
Function: AI-enhanced imaging devices have transformative applications in healthcare, from remote diagnostics to patient monitoring.	*Functions*: The integration of imaging and AI raises significant concerns regarding privacy, data security, and ethical use of technology.

The wearable device powered by AI is sophisticated because of its hardware and software features. These components enable instantaneous recording and processing of visual information. They are helpful in multiple sectors like healthcare, fitness, sports medicine, etc. Let us now consider the prime elements of wearable imaging devices.

i. *Image Sensor*: Cameras and sensors are key for wearable imaging tools. Most of these gadgets use CMOS sensors. They take great pictures and use very little power. Some even add thermal and infrared sensors. This lets users see things not visible to the naked eye (Goossens et al., 2017; Santos et al., 2020).
ii. *Miniaturization and Comfort*: It refers to reducing the size of devices while enhancing user experience. Thanks to advances in making things smaller, today's devices can fit powerful chips and sensors into light, comfy designs. This means people can wear them all day long without feeling discomfort.

iii. *AI Algorithms:* Artificial intelligence is super crucial for processing images. Deep learning algorithms help improve image quality, recognize objects, and give helpful insights. So, with these features, users can figure out what plants are or even learn about health issues using their wearables.

iv. *Real-Time Data Processing*: Wearable devices need to process data right away. That is why they use strong processors, usually ARM-based. These processors help with tasks like analyzing and encoding video quickly. This allows users to get immediate feedback while using the device.

v. *Cloud and Edge Computing*: Many wearables store and analyze lots of data in the cloud. They use cloud computing for innovative features, like personalized suggestions based on user info. Lately, some devices have also been processed locally. This makes things faster and works better when the internet connection is not strong.

vi. *Battery Life and Energy Efficiency*: For a wearable to be practical, it must last a long time on a single charge. This means using parts that do not drain the battery quickly. Intelligent design and energy-efficient algorithms strengthen battery life so users do not have to recharge often.

vii. *User Interface and Experience*: AI makes using wearables easier. Features like voice commands help users navigate without much hassle. Plus, adaptive displays show relevant information at the right time. This makes the whole experience better and more user-friendly.

viii. *Connectivity and Integration*: Good wearables can talk to other devices through Bluetooth, Wi-Fi, and even 5G. This smooth communication helps with sharing data and images quickly, which adds to the overall usefulness of the system.

ix. *Privacy and Security:* Keeping user information safe is important. Devices take steps like advanced encryption and getting user consent to handle data securely. This way, personal information stays protected (Z. Li et al., 2022; Vizitiu et al., 2021).

AI in Wearable Devices

AI is revolutionizing wearable devices. It helps these gadgets process any data that comes from their sensors. This makes them way better than older devices. AI plays a significant role in keeping track of health and spotting diseases early (Jin, 2019; Shajari et al., 2023). Devices use smart AI models, like deep neural networks and CNNs. These models examine the data from sensors. They find patterns and look at information over time. Because of this, wearables can be more precise and work faster (Brutzman et al., 2024).

Imaging Technology in Wearables

Wearable imaging tools are compact yet powerful, providing clear, real-time images of the body using technologies like ultrasound, MRI, and NIRS. Their portability allows doctors and patients to access crucial imaging data outside traditional clinical settings. With AI integration, these devices are becoming more innovative, user-friendly, and increasingly effective in health monitoring—marking just the beginning of their potential.

a. *Ultrasound in Wearables*: Doctors usually use ultrasound imaging, but now it is small enough to be embedded in wearables. These devices can continuously monitor heart health, blood vessels, and muscles (Mierzwa et al., 2016; Yang et al., 2019). For example, an ultrasound patch can show blood flow in real time. This can help detect issues like deep vein thrombosis at an early point.
b. MRI in Wearables: Researchers are investigating the possibility of shrinking MRI technology for wearable applications due to developments in low-field MRI systems (Tricoli et al., 2017). This could increase access to non-invasive brain imaging and promote personalized healthcare (Block et al., 2016). The potential for real-time brain monitoring with wearable MRI technology could improve sports training, rehabilitation, and mental health. Even if issues like image quality and energy usage still exist, ongoing advancements highlight the potential for more tailored and accessible care.
c. Near-Infrared Spectroscopy (NIRS): NIRS is an important technology for wearable devices. It helps check tissue makeup and blood flow without needing any cuts. Near-infrared light (700-900 nm) can measure oxygenated and deoxygenated hemoglobin levels. NIRS makes advanced health checks easy to use in daily life. It connects high-tech testing with regular health monitoring. This tech offers smarter and more personalized healthcare solutions.

Types of AI Algorithms Used in Wearable Imaging

Wearable imaging technologies have advanced significantly. It now incorporates artificial intelligence algorithms to process, analyze, and interpret data with exceptional precision—figure 1 presents AI algorithm types used in wearable imaging and their unique characteristics and contributions.

1. Supervised Learning Algorithms

Supervised learning algorithms form the foundation of wearable imaging, using labeled data to train models. They are necessary for analyzing real-time sensing data by wearable sensors. It provides clinical-grade data for personalized health (Xiao et al., 2024). However, supervised Learning performance is often limited by the availability of labeled data, which would require much time and funds (Ek et al., 2024).

2. Unsupervised Learning Algorithms

Unsupervised learning models greatly value analyzing data obtained from wearable imaging devices. Their value is reinforced by their ability to detect outliers or uncover hidden patterns, such as skin imaging that could indicate melanoma (Adegun & Viriri, 2020; Y. Li & Shen, 2018; Prathiba et al., 2019). One of the prominent algorithms for unsupervised learning is clustering algorithms. In this family of algorithms, K-Means and Hierarchical Clustering are commonly used. This has been applied to segment wearable imaging data into the appropriate groups. The segmentation assists in highlighting areas for further medical investigation.

3. Reinforcement Learning (RL) Algorithms

Reinforcement learning algorithms are most appropriate for adaptive decision-making, and it is most appropriate for wearables that interact with users continuously (H. Zhang et al., 2022; J. Zheng et al., 2020). RL systems learn optimal actions by receiving feedback through rewards or punishments. In wearable imaging, RL can control devices to adjust imaging parameters dynamically for improved images. An RL-based smart wristband can control the camera's exposure settings. This enables the capture of vein structures precisely under different lighting conditions.

4. Deep Learning Algorithms

Deep learning (DL) models, i.e., Convolutional Neural Networks (CNNs), are a significant innovation in wearable imaging, meaning visual data processing (X. Zhang, 2021). DL models excel in the extraction of features and the hierarchy generation of representations. They thus are suitable for application in disease diagnosis and biometrics. An influential example is a wearable retinal camera that employs CNN technology to diagnose diabetic retinopathy (Zhu et al., 2023).

5. Transfer Learning

Transfer learning is a method in machine learning in which a model developed for a task is modified or adjusted for another similar task (Chavez et al., 2023). It is beneficial when there are limited computational resources or labeled data. A wearable ultrasound imaging powered by an AI model can be an edge device for effective performance.

6. Generative Adversarial Networks (GANs)

GANs are also potent in wearable imaging to generate synthetic data and improve image quality(Suzuki et al., 2020). By opposing two neural networks against one another—a generator and a discriminator—GANs can complete missing image details or enhance resolution. In telemedicine wearable imaging, GANs can enhance low-resolution thermal images to allow clinicians to provide more precise remote diagnoses (L. Zhang et al., 2022).

7. Ensemble Learning Algorithms

Ensemble learning integrates several models to render them more accurate and resilient (Y. Guo et al., 2020). Random Forests, Gradient Boosting, or stacking are frequently used in wearable imaging to integrate information from many sources. A wearable system for diagnosing skin lesions can aggregate results from several algorithms to aid in deciding if a lesion is malignant or benign.

8. Edge AI Algorithms

Edge AI is a model intended for on-device calculation, with privacy and real-time capability(Sharma & Sarkar, 2022). The algorithms are tuned to the limited computational capacity of the wearable device, using lightweight architectures like MobileNet or quantized neural networks (Nandi et al., 2022). An example is a wearable gait analyzer using Edge AI to process local foot pressure imaging data, alerting users to balance issues without requiring a cloud connection.

9. Hybrid AI Systems

Hybrid systems utilize different AI methods in conjunction with one another to increase their performance. As shown, integrating deep Learning with reinforcement learning, for instance, can make wearable imaging devices learn very quickly across diverse environments without compromising accuracy(Xu et al., 2020; G. Zheng et al., 2023). Similarly, a hybrid AI-based wearable blood glucose sensor could utilize deep Learning to analyze imaging data and reinforcement learning to improve its non-invasive sensing ability.

Figure 1. Type of AI Algorithms and some of their examples

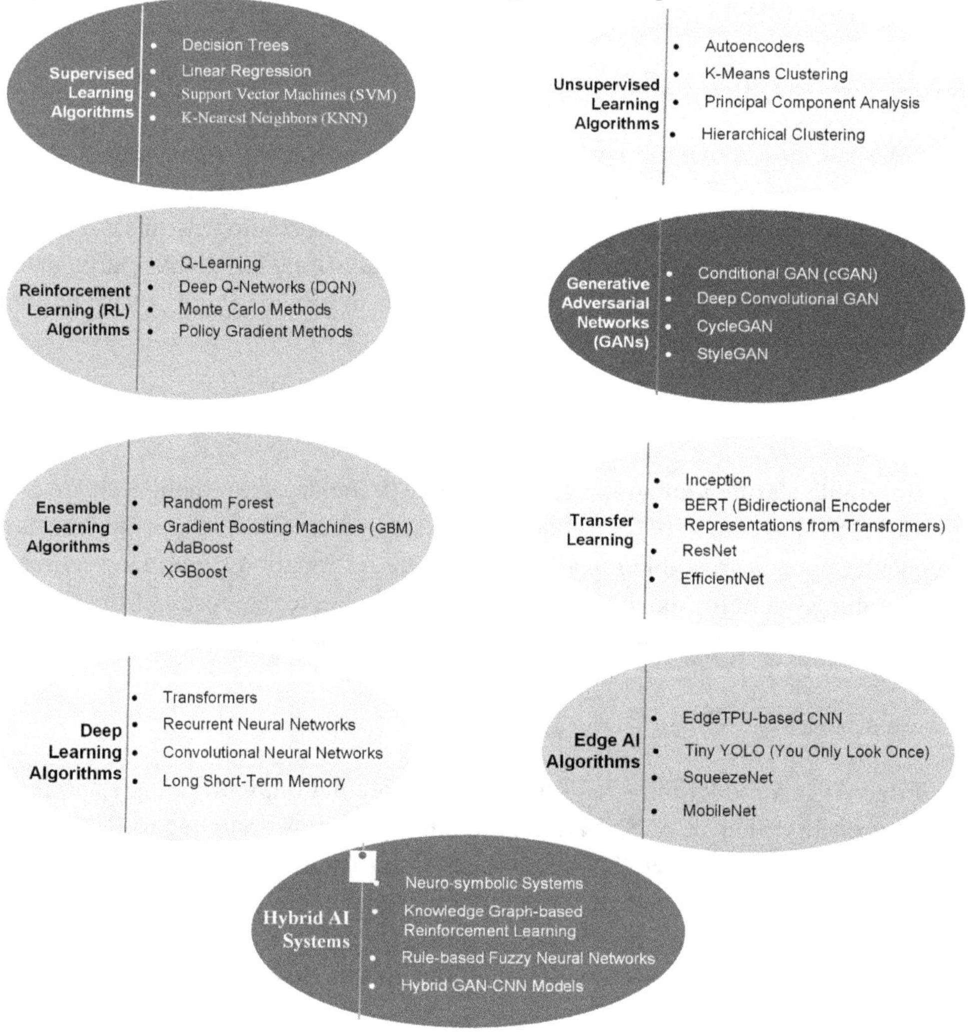

Role of AI in Data Preprocessing, Image Quality Enhancement, and Noise Reduction

Artificial intelligence has now become an integral part of contemporary imaging technologies. It provides a means of addressing difficulties involved in preprocessing raw information. It adds to the enhancement of image quality and reduces noise (Saw & Ng, 2022). Such functions are inevitable when accurate and authentic results are obtained, particularly for medical diagnosis, remote sensing, and wearable imaging (Smeraldo et al., 2023). The following section describes the groundbreaking work of AI in these disciplines.

1. Data Preprocessing: From Raw to Clean

Artificial Intelligence assists in data preprocessing. It is a fundamental process of getting the raw data ready for analysis. Activities such as error correction and identifying valuable features are part of this process. AI algorithms, including machine learning, identify patterns within the dataset. Such tools assist in reducing and normalizing the data (Adebayo et al., 2024). In medical imaging, AI can automatically highlight organs or tumors in scans so researchers can focus on them (Strolin et al., 2023). A wearable MRI device might use AI to match images from different scans, even if the patient moves a bit. This step is crucial. It is an essential stage, as preprocessing minimizes manual intervention, reduces error rates, and improves the reproducibility of results. Thereby enable more precise downstream analysis.

2. Image Quality Enhancement: Clarity Unleashed

AI is excellent for making low-quality images better. It uses methods like super-resolution, contrast boost, and filling in image gaps. These techniques rely on intelligent algorithms called CNN and GAN (Fatima, 2020; Kumar & Jain, 2022; Rane et al., 2023). These methods help bring out details that are useful for diagnosis or analysis. For example, a GAN can improve blurry X-ray pictures from portable imaging devices. This could be achieved through restoring critical details that might have been lost due to limited hardware capabilities. Unlike traditional methods, AI can learn complex transformations and adapt to varying imaging conditions. It then produces tailored enhancements that align with the specific needs of a given application.

3. Noise Reduction: Precision Through Purity

Noise is a common imaging issue arising from sensor limitations, environmental interference, or low-light conditions. AI-based noise reduction techniques go beyond conventional filtering methods by leveraging deep Learning to distinguish between meaningful data and irrelevant artifacts(Cui et al., 2023; Lee, 2021). Neural networks trained on large datasets can effectively suppress noise without sacrificing important details in the image. However, a deep learning model applied to ultrasound imaging can filter out speckle noise, revealing clearer tissue structures and improving diagnostic accuracy(Hyun et al., 2022; Lee et al., 2022). Human-Like Insight: Imagine hearing a whispered conversation in a noisy room. Traditional filters would lower all sounds, including the voice you are trying to hear. AI, in contrast, can "learn" what the voice sounds like and isolate it, leaving the noise behind.

4. Synergy Between AI and Domain Knowledge

The effectiveness of AI in these roles is amplified when combined with domain expertise. For example, in medical imaging, expert-labeled datasets often guide AI models (Azizi et al., 2022; Lang et al., 2024). The techniques ensure that enhancements or reductions align with clinical significance. This collaboration bridges the gap between raw computational power and practical application. In wearable thermal imaging, domain knowledge might inform an AI model about typical heat signatures of inflammation, helping it preprocess and enhance images for remote diagnosis.

5. Real-Time Applications in Wearable Imaging

In wearable devices, the importance of AI is magnified due to constraints like limited computational resources and the need for real-time processing. Edge AI algorithms (Figure 1) are designed to preprocess, enhance, and denoise data directly on the device, ensuring timely and actionable insights (MENDİ, 2023; Shuvo, 2022). A wearable camera for visually impaired users can preprocess images, enhance low-light visuals, and remove noise in real-time (Z. Chen et al., 2021; Vivek, 2022). This capability enables smoother navigation. AI's role in these areas is supportive and transformative, redefining how data is prepared, enhanced, and purified for analysis. AI enhances the reliability and impact of imaging technologies across numerous fields by ensuring that every pixel or data point contributes meaningfully.

Figure 2. Wearable scanners

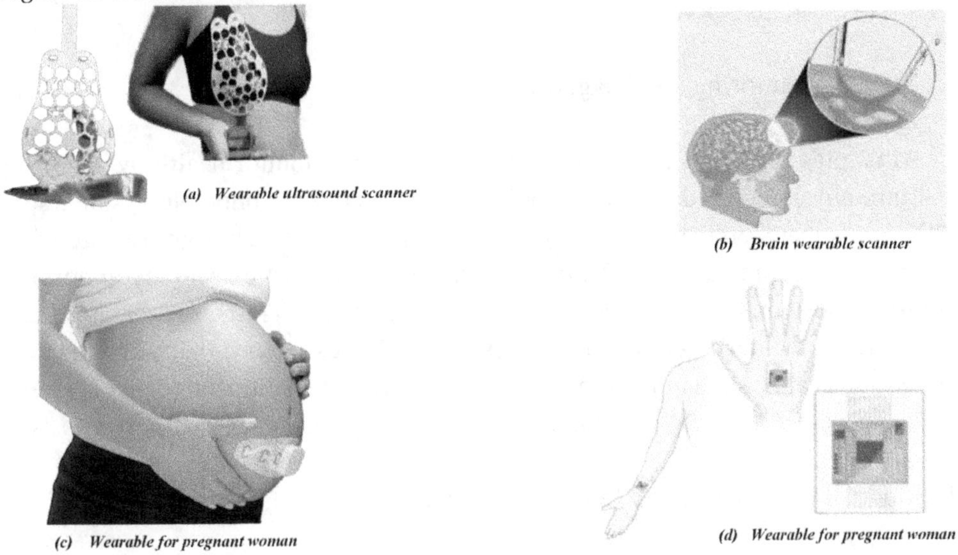

(a) Wearable ultrasound scanner

(b) Brain wearable scanner

(c) Wearable for pregnant woman

(d) Wearable for pregnant woman

Consider a wearable device for fetal pregnancy monitoring (see Figure 2 (c)). It uses wearable ultrasound to track the baby's heart rate and movements in real-time. Smart software cleans up the data by filtering out noise from mom's movement and boosting weaker signals. At the same time, it looks at the images for signs of issues like growth problems. It then provides clinicians with actionable insights remotely. This integration of imaging and AI transforms prenatal care, making it more proactive and accessible.

Nevertheless, the technologies that underpin AI-driven wearable imaging gadgets are complex imaging modalities and advanced AI approaches. Combined, they meet the challenge of miniaturized diagnostics while widening the swath of real-time healthcare. Technological advances will present a new way to perceive and deliver medical imaging, leading to more intelligent applications and actionable insights in healthcare.

C. APPLICATION AREAS OF AI IN WEARABLE IMAGING

AI technology is now being integrated with an emerging field of wearable imaging technology that is about to open up new dimensions in the healthcare industry. These technologies are known for their uniqueness of continuous non-invasive monitoring and precise diagnostics in several medical domains. These innovations transform personalized medicine from cardiovascular health to musculoskeletal disease. Here, we discuss some central areas of work in AI for wearable imaging, emphasizing their transformative potential.

1. Health Monitoring and Diagnostics

AI is integrated into wearable imaging devices to monitor health by analyzing real-time physiological data. For example, a smartwatch with a photoplethysmography (PPG) sensor and embedded AI can detect arrhythmias or early signs of cardiovascular disease (Liao et al., 2022). AI also enhances diagnostic accuracy in portable ultrasound systems, enabling doctors to assess organ health remotely (Dicle, 2023). Combined with internet connectivity, these technologies extend quality healthcare to remote areas. One such innovation—a wearable AI-driven ultrasound patch—helps physicians detect blood-flow abnormalities for early vascular disease diagnosis.

2. Sports Performance and Injury Prevention

Wearable imaging devices paired with AI analyze athletes' biomechanics and muscle activity to optimize training and prevent injuries (Sharanyanivasini et al., 2023). Machine-learning algorithms process motion-capture data to detect joint or muscle stress patterns before injuries occur. AI-driven motion sensors monitor gait and flag abnormalities that may lead to stress fractures. These advances in sports medicine help reduce unexpected injuries and serious health risks.

3. Rehabilitation and Physical Therapy

Wearable imaging devices driven by AI are crucial for monitoring patients throughout rehabilitation since they allow for constant progress monitoring. Exoskeletons and motion cameras record motion data. AI algorithms modify treatment regimens and offer real-time feedback to enhance recovery. This guarantees individualized and flexible care. For instance, wearable gloves with AI incorporated monitor finger movements and recommend remedial activities to assist stroke victims in regaining fine motor abilities (K. Guo et al., 2023; Luca et al., 2020).

4. Mental Health and Neurological Disorders

Wearable imaging devices with AI are priceless in identifying and treating neurological and mental health disorders (Hassantabar et al., 2022; Orfanidis et al., 2022). Sophisticated imaging devices interpret brain activity patterns or eye movement to spot signs of stress, anxiety, or neurodegenerative disorders such as Parkinson's. In today's cutting-edge devices, AI algorithms can analyze functional near-infrared spectroscopy (fNIRS) signals from wearable headbands to identify the onset of cognitive impairment.

5. Remote Patient Monitoring in Telemedicine

AI increases the usefulness of wearable imaging in telemedicine by facilitating close remote examination. AI-enabled devices can take good-quality diagnostic images and analyze them locally, which lessens the necessity for in-person consultation (Omotajo & Lang, 2022). The application is specifically vital in remote or underserved areas. The fruitful innovation, a wearable imaging device combined with AI, may examine skin lesions and diagnose them as benign or malignant. This tool allows dermatologists to give precise remote consultations.

6. Fitness and Lifestyle Monitoring

AI in wearable imaging devices helps users monitor their fitness goals and lifestyle trends. AI can recommend personalized fitness regimes, diet plans, or stress-reduction methods by merging imaging information with health data, building a complete wellness experience. Wearable AI-enabled smart glasses with imaging that assesses body alignment during yoga are a case in point. It provides real-time feedback for better alignment and balance.

7. Elderly Care and Fall Detection

Wearable imaging devices with AI are also crucial in the care of the elderly, specifically in fall prevention and detection. The systems use predictive analytics and real-time imaging data to evaluate the possibility of falls. The contributing factors may be instability or muscle weakness, and the systems notify caregivers promptly. Wearable cameras with artificial intelligence are being implemented to monitor movement patterns, providing alerts before incidents occur.

8. Industrial Safety and Ergonomics

Wearable imaging technologies with artificial intelligence can add safety in industrial environments by tracking workers' movement and position (Balaji & Srinivasan, 2023; Muanme et al., 2023). The systems detect dangerous behavior, send alerts to reduce workplace injuries, and enhance ergonomics by suggesting reducing stains.

9. Augmented Reality (AR) in Wearable Imaging

Wearable imaging technology, powered by AI, transforms medicine by expanding its application into cardiovascular, neurological, and musculoskeletal areas. It is now being utilized to address more complex diseases like diabetes and cancer. These advancements enable real-time monitoring and early disease detection. This development improves patient outcomes through proactive interventions.

Other Relevant Applications of AI in Wearable Imaging

Artificial intelligence-driven wearable imaging technology is poised to drive the growth of the healthcare system. It would be utilized in cardiovascular, neurological, and musculoskeletal fields. It is being employed to address more advanced diseases like diabetes and cancer. Such technologies enable early disease detection and real-time monitoring. Real-time monitoring enhances patient outcomes by providing proactive interventions.

Diabetes Management

The artificial intelligence-powered wearable imaging devices enhance diabetes management by enabling real-time, non-invasive monitoring. Using techniques like near-infrared and Raman spectroscopy, they estimate glucose levels painlessly and detect complications early by simultaneously monitoring blood flow and skin temperature (Dremin et al., 2021; Heise et al., 2021; Loyola-Leyva et al., 2024). Early detection prevents late complications like neuropathy and retinopathy.

Cancer Detection

Effective cancer therapy depends on early tumor diagnosis, and wearables combining optical imaging and AI constitute a significant advancement in this area. In order to prevent needless biopsies and speed up diagnosis by sophisticated pattern recognition, these gadgets examine skin lesions to identify subtle indications of melanoma or other malignancies. Beyond dermatology, researchers are creating wearables powered by AI that can detect breast cancer without radiation as a practical substitute for conventional mammography.

D. AI-DRIVEN DATA ANALYSIS AND INTERPRETATION IN WEARABLE IMAGING

This section examines how machine learning (ML) drives real-time data processing in clinical settings and the challenges it must overcome. Wearable imaging devices generate massive volumes of data, underscoring the urgent need for effective medical data analysis.

Use of AI to Identify Patterns, Detect Anomalies, and Predict Potential Health Risks

AI enhances wearable imaging by uncovering subtle patterns invisible to the naked eye. Deep learning algorithms can extract image features, track changes over time, and accurately classify health conditions (Begum & Vidyullatha, 2022). In anomaly detection, AI-powered wearables spot deviations early—such as using retinal imaging and segmentation algorithms to detect microvascular changes that predict diabetic retinopathy before clinical symptoms appear (Lin et al., 2022). Beyond detection, AI excels in predictive analytics by combining historical and real-time data to assess an individual's disease risk. This preventive approach reduces hospitalizations and improves outcomes. Yet, making AI predictions interpretable and clinically actionable remains challenging, demanding close collaboration among clinicians, data scientists, and researchers.

Challenges in Real-Time Data Processing and Decision-Making for Clinical Relevance

AI holds the potential to transform wearable imaging and real-time clinical decision-making; however, several obstacles still need to be overcome. Running large AI models locally is hampered by limited on-device processing power and battery limitations, necessitating reliance on cloud or edge computing—which also introduces latency and privacy problems (Azizi et al., 2022; Singh et al., 2020; Tuncel et al., 2022). Additionally, it is crucial to balance sensitivity and specificity; too sensitive models might result in false positives and anxiety, while too little sensitivity could cause important health signals to be missed.

For instance, to prevent serious repercussions, a skin cancer detector must accurately differentiate between benign moles and melanoma. Explainable AI (XAI) solutions are essential for promoting clinician trust; however, integrating AI outputs into clinical workflows has been rendered more difficult by deep learning's “black-box” nature (Tjoa & Guan, 2021). Ultimately, overcoming these challenges and reaching broad clinical acceptance will depend on developments in interpretability, federated learning, and model optimization (Y. Chen & Wu, 2023; Malcangi, 2021; Zahid et al., 2022).

E. ADVANCEMENTS IN MINIATURIZATION AND DEVICE MOBILITY

In this section, we examine the key technological advancements in miniaturization, the balance between image quality and resource efficiency, and highlight the promising future of wearable imaging in remote and out-of-hospital care. Wearable imaging devices are becoming increasingly portable and compact, allowing seamless integration into everyday healthcare and expanding their availability and utility across diverse medical settings.

Technological Innovations in Device Size and Portability

Over the years, advancements in miniaturization have significantly impacted wearable imaging technologies. The improvement focuses on making high-performance imaging systems smaller, lighter, and more convenient. Unlike traditional medical imaging devices, such as MRI or CT scanners (Figure 3) (Attenberger et al., 2020; Bhuva et al., 2020), they tend to be large and confined to hospital settings. In contrast, emerging wearable imaging technologies utilize microelectronics, flexible sensor technology, and artificial intelligence-based processing to extend diagnostic capabilities to patients.

Figure 3. Device Size and Portability

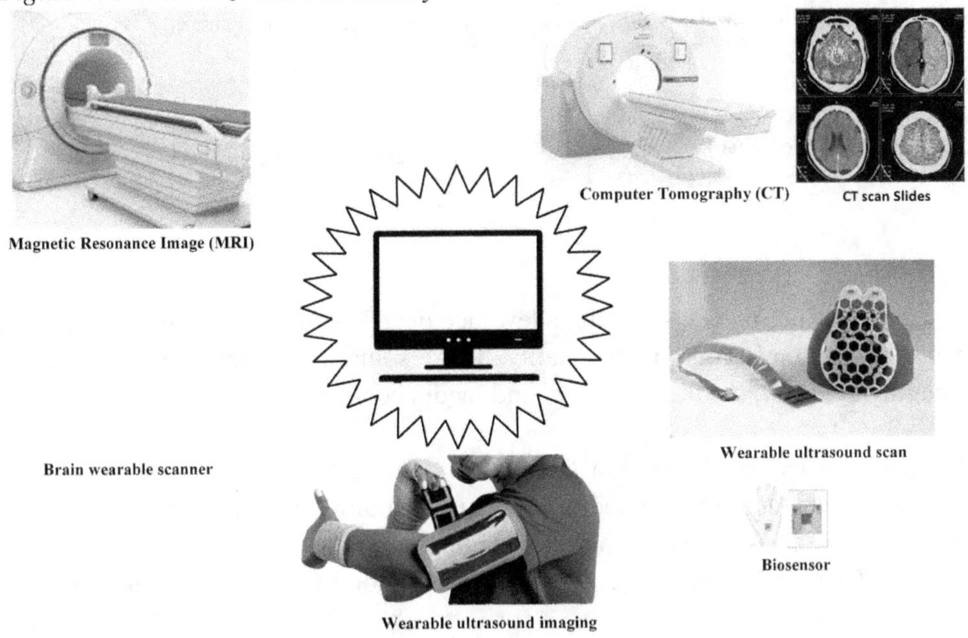

Advancements in nanofabrication and bio-integrated electronics have been instrumental in this revolution (Aljabali et al., 2021; Chow et al., 2005). For example, scientists have created ultra-thin, skin-conformal ultrasound patches that continuously track deep tissue structures without hindering movement (Liu et al., 2022). Likewise, advances in compact optics and micro-LEDs have enabled miniaturized retinal imaging devices, bringing eye disease screening to remote locations.

Aside from minimizing physical size, these innovations also make devices more straightforward. The trend for wireless, battery-conserving designs reduces the necessity for awkward cables and external power supplies, increasing mobility and comfort. As these technologies continue to develop, wearable imaging devices will become essential to clinical and personal health monitoring. This closes the gap between professional diagnostics and day-to-day wellness monitoring. The technology will assist in check-mate human activities.

AI-Powered Super-Resolution Techniques

AI-based super-resolution algorithms utilize the strength of DL to increase the resolution of an image or video beyond its original quality level. The algorithms are instrumental in refining satellite imaging, security, medical imaging, and media content.

Figure 4. AI-Powered Super-Resolution Techniques

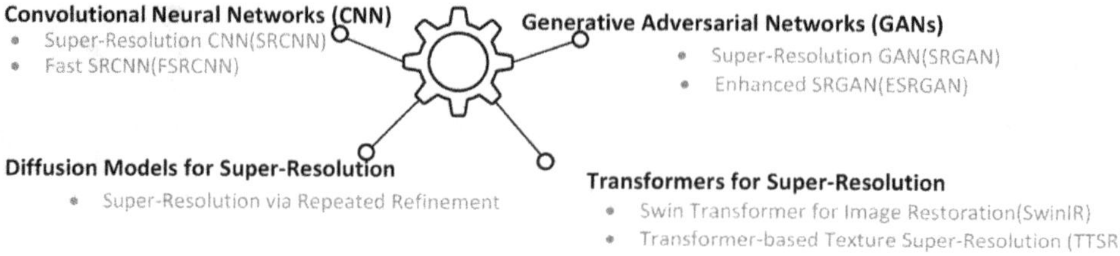

Super-resolution CNN solutions leverage deep Learning to enhance image and video resolution beyond native quality. These solutions are important in satellite imaging, security, medical imaging, and media content.

i. SRCNN (Super-Resolution CNN) was among the earliest super-resolution techniques that utilized deep Learning. It employs a simple three-layer CNN to restore low-resolution images to high-resolution images.
ii. FSRCNN (Fast SRCNN): An improved version of SRCNN enhances performance and speed.
iii. SRGAN (Super-Resolution GAN): Employing a generator-discriminator architecture in which the generator increases the image's resolution, and the discriminator checks its realism. This method generates high-quality textures and realistic details. This approach produces high-quality textures and realistic information.
iv. ESRGAN (Enhanced SRGAN): An improved version of SRGAN that reduces artifacts and generates sharper images.
v. SwinIR (Swin Transformer for Image Restoration) uses self-attention mechanisms to capture long-range dependencies and improve super-resolution results.
vi. TTSR (Transformer-based Texture Super-Resolution): this model leverages transformers to refine image textures.
vii. SR3 (Super-Resolution via Repeated Refinement): A diffusion probabilistic that can reconstruct high-resolution images progressively from noise.

Future Possibilities for Wearable Imaging in Out-of-Hospital Settings and Remote Patient Monitoring

Wearable imaging is reshaping healthcare beyond the clinic, enabling personalized, proactive monitoring as devices become smaller. Early disease detection and intervention become routine: patients with cardiovascular conditions might use wearable ultrasounds to track blood flow and heart function continuously, while AI-powered retinal wearables offer at-home diabetic eye screening to catch complications sooner.

In remote and underserved areas, AI-driven imaging patches can record and transmit diagnostic images from rural clinics to specialists worldwide—no advanced infrastructure needed—helping to close healthcare gaps. As wearable imaging converges with AI and 5G connectivity, future devices won't just capture images; they'll analyze them in real-time, transforming care from reactive treatment to ongoing, data-driven health management.

F. CASE STUDIES OF AI IN WEARABLE IMAGING DEVICES

i. AI-Enabled Smart Contact Lenses for Diabetic Retinopathy Monitoring

Recent innovations in miniaturized imaging and AI-based analysis have created smart contact lenses with embedded microscopic sensors and imaging. The contact lenses are designed to monitor retinal changes in diabetic patients continuously(Deng et al., 2022; Kim et al., 2020), with early detection of diabetic retinopathy using AI-augmented image processing. Incorporating deep learning models facilitates real-time analysis, decreasing the necessity for frequent in-clinic appointments.

Future Direction of Research: An exciting direction is to complement these lenses with Federated Learning to enable secure, decentralized AI training across diverse patients. Additional development of edge AI functionality can also enhance real-time image processing and energy efficiency to make these lenses more feasible for everyday use.

ii. AI-Driven Wearable Ultrasound for Monitoring Cardiovascular Health

Wearable ultrasound patches based on artificial intelligence are revolutionizing cardiovascular monitoring with the potential for continuous, real-time imaging of blood vessels and cardiac function (Hu et al., 2023; Steinberg et al., 2022). The wearables employ advanced deep-learning algorithms to identify arterial plaque accumulation, abnormal heart rhythms, and hypertension at early stages, facilitating early medical interventions (Forghani et al., 2022). In contrast to conventional echocardiograms, AI-driven wearables eliminate the necessity for experienced operators, increasing access to cardiac diagnostic equipment.

Future Research Direction: Exploring self-adaptive artificial intelligence models with flexible responses to individual patient variation can significantly enhance diagnostic accuracy. In addition, using generative AI for image enhancement can increase signal quality in poor-quality ultrasound images. Thus, this enables more reliable assessment across diverse demographic populations.

iii. AI-Enhanced Smart Helmets for Detection of Traumatic Brain Injury (TBI)

Intelligent headgear equipped with wearable imaging and artificial intelligence diagnostic systems is transforming the real-time detection of traumatic brain injury(Asani et al., 2023; Fabrizio & Termine, 2023), especially in contact sports and the military. The helmets acquire cranial imaging information, identify microhemorrhages, and determine concussion severity through deep learning image segmentation. The AI-enhanced system notifies medical experts in real time, enabling prompt intervention.

Future Research Direction: The creation of AI models for predictive analytics can allow these helmets to foresee the risk of injury before it occurs, using biomechanical data coupled with imaging data. AI's ability to separate low-level concussions from catastrophic TBIs developed further can guide decision-making among athletes and military members.

iv. Wearable Infrared Imaging System with AI to Detect Skin Cancer

Integrating infrared imaging in wearable devices like smartwatches and skin patches provides non-invasive early detection of melanoma and other skin cancers(Chhatlani et al., 2022; Elouerghi et al., 2022). The machine learning algorithms trained on thermal and multispectral image datasets interpret slight temperature variations relevant to tumor tissues (Xing et al., 2023). Continuous tracking through this methodology minimizes periodic dermatological monitoring while maximizing cancer detection in its early phase.

Future Research Direction: Developing AI models distinguishing between benign and malignant lesions with higher specificity remains an essential challenge. In addition, incorporating personalized AI models that learn from an individual's skin type and history could improve the accuracy of diagnostics and reduce false positives. Each case study underscores the transformative impact of artificial intelligence on wearable imaging technologies, presenting innovative possibilities for early detection and continuous monitoring. Subsequent investigations should enhance AI frameworks concerning personalization, energy efficiency, and privacy-preserving methodologies, guaranteeing that these advancements are clinically efficacious and widely accessible.

G. CHALLENGES AND CONSIDERATIONS

i. *Data privacy and Security:*

There are privacy and security concerns because wearable imaging equipment gathers many private health information. Adherence to laws such as HIPAA and GDPR is crucial. Patient data can be protected through federated learning, decentralized storage, and robust encryption.

ii. *Precision and Dependability*

For precise diagnosis, wearables with AI rely on high-quality, validated training data. Continuous data validation and safeguarding of real-world monitoring data are essential for avoiding misdiagnosis and fostering confidence.

iii. *System Integration*

The majority of healthcare infrastructures do not seamlessly integrate AI wearables. To incorporate imaging data into hospital networks and electronic health records, defined data formats and interoperability standards must be adopted.

iv. Energy Efficiency and Battery Life

Wearable imaging systems require continuous power for real-time monitoring and AI processing. It is observed that frequent charging or short battery life can limit their usage. Thus, developing low-power AI chips and low-power consumption algorithms is adequate to extend usage time and enhance usability.

v. *Ethical and Regulatory Issues*

Using AI in wearables for healthcare delivery systems also introduces ethical concerns. The issue includes bias in algorithms and decision-making. In addition, the regulatory approval processes of any decision can be delayed. However, transparent ethical principles and agile regulatory frameworks are needed to address these concerns while fostering innovation.

vi. *Cost and Accessibility*

The AI-powered wearables are expensive, especially for low and medium-income countries. The exorbitant price and its maintenance costs discourage its widespread adoption. However, the stakeholders, policymakers, and governments should subsidy AI-powered wearable costs. This is required to facilitate its adoption in the healthcare systems of developed and developing nations.

vii. *Real-Time Processing and Latency*

Real-time processing and latency have been a concern in healthcare with AI-powered wearables. The high latency is due to a lower network generation version. Hence, researchers and policymakers are encouraged to adopt advanced techniques such as transfer learning for better prediction.

Data Privacy and Security Issues in Wearable Imaging

The process by which AI-powered wearable imaging captures data raises security concerns. The wearables frequently capture relevant healthcare information. Hence, the transmission channel of data raises susceptibility to data breaches, unauthorized access, and exploitation. What will protect patient confidentiality are secure encryption methods, trustworthy authentication protocols, and decentralized storage.

One of the primary interests of researchers is the development of artificial intelligence techniques that preserve privacy, such as Federated learning and differential privacy, which allow data analysis without exposing individual data records to disclosure. Further, integrating biometric authentication with blockchain-based access control systems can enhance security without sacrificing user convenience.

Cybersecurity experts, artificial intelligence researchers, and clinicians need to collaborate on creating security protocols that balance data protection and usability. It is also imperative that policymakers and regulatory bodies implement strict compliance requirements to balance the governance of wearable imaging data with current laws, including HIPAA in the US and GDPR in the EU.

Ethical and Regulatory Concerns Around AI's Role in Continuous Monitoring

AI-driven wearable imaging technologies also bring significant ethical questions, such as consent, data ownership, and bias in AI-driven decision-making. As much as continual health monitoring is valuable—disease detection early on, remote patient monitoring—it can also be intrusive. The users must control what is being monitored, by whom, and for what.

Among the challenges facing scientists is ensuring AI models are explainable and interpretable. If, for example, a wearable imaging device detects something wrong with a person's health, patients and practitioners must understand the AI's reasoning to arrive at this conclusion and not merely a "black box" prediction. Explainable AI (XAI) methods will play a central part in bridging the gap.

On the regulatory front, establishing global standards for AI-enabled wearables is a challenging but necessary task. Collaboration between medical ethicists, AI governance specialists, and attorneys is needed to develop policies that prevent discrimination and bias, particularly in AI model training datasets. Harmonize approval pathways for AI-enabled wearable medical devices regulatory bodies such as the FDA (United States), EMA (Europe), and WHO.

Technical Limitations: Device Durability, Battery Life, and Connectivity

The operation of wearable AI-enabled imaging devices is often hardware-constrained. The devices must be comfortable and light yet offer high-resolution imaging. However, compact form factors usually cost processing capacity, battery duration, and robustness.

A critical priority for researchers is the development of energy-efficient AI algorithms that reduce computational requirements without compromising accuracy. Advances in neuromorphic computing and edge AI can reduce energy consumption, allowing for prolonged battery life and enabling real-time processing of the device itself rather than relying on cloud servers.

Further, the availability of stable connectivity is a significant challenge, especially in remote or underprivileged areas with poor network infrastructure. AI-based compression techniques that facilitate efficient transmission of imaging data through low-bandwidth networks can somewhat alleviate these difficulties. Electrical engineers, material scientists, and biomedical engineers must collaborate to enhance wearable hardware. In contrast, telecommunications engineers must strive to advance IoT connectivity to ensure uninterrupted data transmission.

H. FUTURE DIRECTIONS FOR AI IN WEARABLE IMAGING DEVICES

The future of wearable imaging devices that use artificial intelligence has many possibilities for improving healthcare and patient outcomes. As technology keeps evolving, several significant trends and new ideas are set to transform the application of these devices. The innovation will make them more central to providing personalized, effective, and easily accessible care.

Integration with AI-Driven Healthcare Tools and Telemedicine

Integrating wearable imaging devices with artificial intelligence with telemedicine software advances digital medicine. These real-time diagnostic tools facilitate the easy transfer of medical images to distant health professionals. AI analysis of such images provides quick and precise evaluation. This aspect helps clinicians diagnose medical conditions and suggest interventions without face-to-face consultation.

A critical area of research in this discipline includes improving the interoperability of wearable imaging devices with existing electronic health record (EHR) systems. Standardized protocols will enable seamless data exchange between different healthcare infrastructures. In addition, integrating artificial intelligence-based decision support systems can enhance remote monitoring through early identification of anomalies, thus reducing the burden on healthcare facilities.

Future research should address the potential of federated Learning for wearable devices in telemedicine. By allowing decentralized artificial intelligence model training, patient data can be processed locally and kept private, a highly applicable feature for large-scale applications in regulation-sensitive environments.

Enhancing Personalization and Predictive Analytics

AI-powered wearable imaging devices have the potential to revolutionize personalized medicine. It is tailoring healthcare interventions based on the user profile. The wearables can detect health risks before symptomatic manifestation through constant monitoring and advanced machine learning algorithms. This offers preventive and proactive care interventions.

For instance, AI-powered imaging wearables in cardiology can gauge vessel changes and calculate the likelihood of cardiac incidents by prompting early intervention. Similarly, in dermatology, AI-enabled skin imaging devices can warn about melanoma early with invisible changes to the naked eye.

An up-and-coming line of research is the development of reinforcement learning algorithms tailored to specific physiological profiles. Instead of generalized data sets, artificial intelligence systems can evolve through continuous Learning processes, increasing their predictive power over time. Moreover, the prospects for integrating AI imaging with multimodal biometric data—heart rate variability, blood oxygen levels, and movement patterns—offer exceedingly great accuracy for personalized health coaching.

Advancements in AI Algorithms, Device Wearability, and Clinical Applications

The future trajectory of artificial intelligence in wearable imaging devices hinges on three interconnected elements: machine learning algorithms, improvements in device ergonomics, and the extension of clinical uses. Deep learning models, including self-supervised Learning and transformer-based architectures, can potentially facilitate more sophisticated image analysis with reduced reliance on labeled datasets. These advancements would be particularly valuable in low-resource environments where the availability of expert-annotated datasets is a critical limitation.

From a hardware standpoint, future generations of wearable imaging devices must emphasize comfort and robustness while maintaining high image resolution and computation power. Incorporating light, pliable materials, and energy-saving artificial intelligence chips will be critical to allowing extended use and an unobtrusive user experience.

Clinically, AI-powered wearables that deliver imaging technologies have the potential to revolutionize diagnosis in specialties such as neurology, ophthalmology, and orthopedics. For example, AI-powered retinal imaging using wearables could make diabetic retinopathy diagnosis possible at an early stage. In contrast, handheld ultrasound devices could make prenatal care more available in poor communities. More research is required on creating regulatory frameworks under which AI-powered wearables undergo rigorous clinical testing and validation parameters to enable widespread adoption in the mainstream healthcare setting.

REFERENCES

Adebayo, P. O., Jimoh, R. G., & Yahya, W. B. (2024). Hybridization of data-driven threshold algorithm with fuzzy particle swarm optimization technique for gene selection in microarray data. *Scientific African, 23*. Advance online publication. DOI: 10.1016/j.sciaf.2023.e02012

Adegun, A. A., & Viriri, S. (2020). Deep learning-based system for automatic melanoma detection. *IEEE Access : Practical Innovations, Open Solutions, 8*, 7160–7172. DOI: 10.1109/ACCESS.2019.2962812

Aljabali, A. A. A., Qar, J., Al Zoubi, M. S., Al-Batanyeh, K. M., Al Trad, B., Alkaraki, A. K., Al Khateeb, W., Hussein, E. I., Alrababaa, A., Muhaidat, R., & El-Oqlah, A. (2021). A new frontier in switchable bioelectronics and bionanotechnology interfaces. *Functional Materials Processing for Switchable Device Modulation*, 25–42. https://doi.org/DOI: 10.1016/B978-0-12-823972-8.00010-1

Asani, F., Patel, B., Srikanthan, S., & Agu, E. (2023). BioscoreNet: Traumatic Brain Injury (TBI) detection using a multimodal self-attention fusion neural network and a passive bioscore monitoring framework from smartphone sensor data. *Smart Health (Amsterdam, Netherlands), 27*. Advance online publication. DOI: 10.1016/j.smhl.2022.100352

Attenberger, U. I., Biber, S., & Wichtmann, B. D. (2020). Technological Advances of Magnetic Resonance Imaging in Today's Health Care Environment. *Investigative Radiology, 55*(9), 531–542. DOI: 10.1097/RLI.0000000000000678 PMID: 32487969

Azizi, S., Culp, L., Freyberg, J., Mustafa, B., Baur, S., Kornblith, S., Chen, T., MacWilliams, P., Mahdavi, S. S., Wulczyn, E., Babenko, B., Wilson, M., Loh, A., Chen, P.-H. C., Liu, Y., Bavishi, P., McKinney, S. M., Winkens, J., Roy, A. G., & Natarajan, V. (2022). *Robust and Efficient Medical Imaging with Self-Supervision*. http://arxiv.org/abs/2205.09723

Balaji, T. S., & Srinivasan, S. (2023). Detection of safety wearable's of the industry workers using deep neural network. *Materials Today: Proceedings, 80*, 3064–3068. DOI: 10.1016/j.matpr.2021.06.464

Begum, S. H., & Vidyullatha, P. (2022). A Study of Deep Learning Models in Diagnosis and Prediction of Chronic Diseases. *2022 3rd International Conference on Issues and Challenges in Intelligent Computing Techniques, ICICT 2022*. https://doi.org/DOI: 10.1109/ICICT55121.2022.10064613

Bhuva, A. N., Moralee, R., Moon, J. C., & Manisty, C. H. (2020). Making MRI available for patients with cardiac implantable electronic devices: Growing need and barriers to change. *European Radiology, 30*(3), 1378–1384. DOI: 10.1007/s00330-019-06449-5 PMID: 31776746

Block, V. A. J., Pitsch, E., Tahir, P., Cree, B. A. C., Allen, D. D., & Gelfand, J. M. (2016). Remote physical activity monitoring in neurological disease: A systematic review. *PLoS One, 11*(4). Advance online publication. DOI: 10.1371/journal.pone.0154335 PMID: 27124611

Brutzman, K., Burns, Q., Cammisa, V., Peracchio, J., Phillips, C., Sarpong, K., & Liu, L. (2024). Integrating AI and ChatGPT in Wearable Devices for Enhanced Abnormal Activity Reporting: A Mixture of Experts Approach. *2024 4th IEEE International Conference on Software Engineering and Artificial Intelligence, SEAI 2024*, 231–235. https://doi.org/DOI: 10.1109/SEAI62072.2024.10674191

Chavez, C., Gangadharan, K., & Zhang, Q. (2023). Knowledge Transferring in Deep Learning of Wearable Dynamics. *Digest of Technical Papers - IEEE International Conference on Consumer Electronics, 2023-Janua*. https://doi.org/DOI: 10.1109/ICCE56470.2023.10043543

Chen, Y., & Wu, M. (2023). Artificial Intelligence-enabled contactless sensing for medical diagnosis. *Medical Review (Berlin, Germany), 3*(3), 195–197. DOI: 10.1515/mr-2023-0022

Chen, Z., Liu, X., Kojima, M., Huang, Q., & Arai, T. (2021). A wearable navigation device for visually impaired people based on the real-time semantic visual slam system. *Sensors (Basel), 21*(4), 1–14. DOI: 10.3390/s21041536 PMID: 33672146

Chhatlani, J., Mahajan, T., Rijhwani, R., Bansode, A., & Bhatia, G. (2022). Derma-Genics - Early Detection of Melanoma using YOLOv5 Deep Convolutional Neural Networks. *2022 IEEE Delhi Section Conference. DELCON, 2022*. Advance online publication. DOI: 10.1109/DELCON54057.2022.9753227

Chow, D. C., Johannes, M. S., Lee, W. K., Clark, R. L., Zauscher, S., & Chilkoti, A. (2005). Nanofabrication with biomolecules. *Materials Today, 8*(12, SUPPL. 1), 30–39. DOI: 10.1016/S1369-7021(05)71287-6

Cui, Y., Li, L., Tao, Z., Chen, M., & Wei, T. (2023). Filtering Out High Noise Data for Distributed Deep Neural Networks. *IEEE Transactions on Automation Science and Engineering, 20*(1), 101–111. DOI: 10.1109/TASE.2022.3208027

Deng, M., Song, G., Zhong, K., Wang, Z., Xia, X., & Tian, Y. (2022). Wearable fluorescent contact lenses for monitoring glucose via a smartphone. *Sensors and Actuators. B, Chemical, 352*. Advance online publication. DOI: 10.1016/j.snb.2021.131067

Dicle, O. (2023). Artificial intelligence in diagnostic ultrasonography. *Diagnostic and Interventional Radiology, 29*(1), 40–45. DOI: 10.4274/dir.2022.211260 PMID: 36959754

Dremin, V., Marcinkevics, Z., Zherebtsov, E., Popov, A., Grabovskis, A., Kronberga, H., Geldnere, K., Doronin, A., Meglinski, I., & Bykov, A. (2021). Skin Complications of Diabetes Mellitus Revealed by Polarized Hyperspectral Imaging and Machine Learning. *IEEE Transactions on Medical Imaging, 40*(4), 1207–1216. DOI: 10.1109/TMI.2021.3049591 PMID: 33406038

Ek, S., Presotto, R., Civitarese, G., Portet, F., Lalanda, P., & Bettini, C. (2024). *Comparing Self-Supervised Learning Techniques for Wearable Human Activity Recognition*. http://arxiv.org/abs/2404.15331

Elouerghi, A., Bellarbi, L., Khomsi, Z., Jbari, A., Errachid, A., & Yaakoubi, N. (2022). A Flexible Wearable Thermography System Based on Bioheat Microsensors Network for Early Breast Cancer Detection: IoT Technology. *Journal of Electrical and Computer Engineering, 2022*. Advance online publication. DOI: 10.1155/2022/5921691

Fabrizio, C., & Termine, A. (2023). Artificial Intelligence Applications for Traumatic Brain Injury Research and Clinical Management. *Contemporary Clinical Neuroscience*, (Part F276), 391–402. DOI: 10.1007/978-3-031-24930-3_18

Fatima, N. (2020). AI in Photography: Scrutinizing Implementation of Super-Resolution Techniques in Photo-Editors. *International Conference Image and Vision Computing New Zealand, 2020-Novem*. https://doi.org/DOI: 10.1109/IVCNZ51579.2020.9290737

Forghani, N., Maghooli, K., Dabanloo, N. J., Farahani, A. V., & Forouzanfar, M. (2022). DeepPAD: Detection of Peripheral Arterial Disease Using Deep Learning. *IEEE Sensors Journal, 22*(16), 16254–16262. DOI: 10.1109/JSEN.2022.3188810

Goossens, S., Navickaite, G., Monasterio, C., Gupta, S., Piqueras, J. J., Pérez, R., Burwell, G., Nikitskiy, I., Lasanta, T., Galán, T., Puma, E., Centeno, A., Pesquera, A., Zurutuza, A., Konstantatos, G., & Koppens, F. (2017). Broadband image sensor array based on graphene-CMOS integration. *Nature Photonics, 11*(6), 366–371. DOI: 10.1038/nphoton.2017.75

Guo, K., Orban, M., Lu, J., Al-Quraishi, M. S., Yang, H., & Elsamanty, M. (2023). Empowering Hand Rehabilitation with AI-Powered Gesture Recognition: A Study of an sEMG-Based System. *Bioengineering (Basel, Switzerland), 10*(5). Advance online publication. DOI: 10.3390/bioengineering10050557 PMID: 37237627

Guo, Y., Wang, X., Xiao, P., & Xu, X. (2020). An ensemble learning framework for convolutional neural network based on multiple classifiers. *Soft Computing*, *24*(5), 3727–3735. DOI: 10.1007/s00500-019-04141-w

Hassantabar, S., Zhang, J., Yin, H., & Jha, N. K. (2022). MHDeep: Mental Health Disorder Detection System Based on Wearable Sensors and Artificial Neural Networks. *ACM Transactions on Embedded Computing Systems*, *21*(6). Advance online publication. DOI: 10.1145/3527170

Heise, H. M., Delbeck, S., & Marbach, R. (2021). Noninvasive monitoring of glucose using near-infrared reflection spectroscopy of skin—Constraints and effective novel strategy in multivariate calibration. *Biosensors (Basel)*, *11*(3). Advance online publication. DOI: 10.3390/bios11030064 PMID: 33673679

Hu, H., Huang, H., Li, M., Gao, X., Yin, L., Qi, R., Wu, R. S., Chen, X., Ma, Y., Shi, K., Li, C., Maus, T. M., Huang, B., Lu, C., Lin, M., Zhou, S., Lou, Z., Gu, Y., Chen, Y., & Xu, S. (2023). A wearable cardiac ultrasound imager. *Nature*, *613*(7945), 667–675. DOI: 10.1038/s41586-022-05498-z PMID: 36697864

Hyun, D., Brickson, L., Zhuang, L., Simson, W. A., Pinton, G., & Dahl, J. (2022). Applications of ultrasound image reconstruction using deep learning. *The Journal of the Acoustical Society of America*, *152*(4, Supplement), A113–A113. DOI: 10.1121/10.0015721

Jin, C. Y. (2019). A review of AI Technologies for Wearable Devices. *IOP Conference Series. Materials Science and Engineering*, *688*(4). Advance online publication. DOI: 10.1088/1757-899X/688/4/044072

Kassay, A., & De Silva, A. (2022). Necessity of Diagnostic Imaging and its Lacking Availability. *University of Western Ontario Medical Journal*, *90*(1). Advance online publication. DOI: 10.5206/uwomj.v90i1.13506

Kim, S.-K., Koo, J., Lee, G.-H., Jeon, C., Mok, J. W., Mun, B. H., Lee, K. J., Kamrani, E., Joo, C.-K., & Shin, S. (2020). Wireless smart contact lens for diabetic diagnosis and therapy. *Science Advances*, *6*(17), eaba3252. PMID: 32426469

Kumar, L., & Jain, M. (2022). A Novel Image Super-Resolution Reconstruction Framework Using the AI Technique of Dual Generator Generative Adversarial Network (GAN). *Journal of Universal Computer Science*, *28*(9), 967–983. DOI: 10.3897/jucs.94134

Lang, O., Yaya-Stupp, D., Traynis, I., Cole-Lewis, H., Bennett, C. R., Lyles, C. R., Lau, C., Irani, M., Semturs, C., Webster, D. R., Corrado, G. S., Hassidim, A., Matias, Y., Liu, Y., Hammel, N., & Babenko, B. (2024). Using generative AI to investigate medical imagery models and datasets. *EBioMedicine*, *102*. Advance online publication. DOI: 10.1016/j.ebiom.2024.105075 PMID: 38565004

Lee, H. (2021). Noise reduction system by using cnn deep learning model. *Indonesian Journal of Electrical Engineering and Informatics*, *9*(1), 84–90. DOI: 10.11591/ijeei.v9i1.2494

Lee, H., Lee, M. H., Youn, S., Lee, K., Lew, H. M., & Hwang, J. Y. (2022). Speckle Reduction via Deep Content-Aware Image Prior for Precise Breast Tumor Segmentation in an Ultrasound Image. *IEEE Transactions on Ultrasonics, Ferroelectrics, and Frequency Control*, *69*(9), 2638–2650. DOI: 10.1109/TUFFC.2022.3193640 PMID: 35877808

Li, Y., & Shen, L. (2018). Skin lesion analysis towards melanoma detection using deep learning network. *Sensors (Switzerland)*, *18*(2). Advance online publication. DOI: 10.3390/s18020556 PMID: 29439500

Li, Z., Wang, B., Li, J., Hua, Y., & Zhang, S. (2022). Local differential privacy protection for wearable device data. *PLoS ONE*, *17*(8 August). https://doi.org/DOI: 10.1371/journal.pone.0272766

Liao, M. T., Yu, C. C., Lin, L. Y., Pan, K. H., Tsai, T. H., Wu, Y. C., & Liu, Y. Bin. (2022). Impact of recording length and other arrhythmias on atrial fibrillation detection from wrist photoplethysmogram using smartwatches. *Scientific Reports*, *12*(1). Advance online publication. DOI: 10.1038/s41598-022-09181-1 PMID: 35354873

Lin, P.-K., Chiu, Y.-H., Huang, C.-J., Wang, C.-Y., Pan, M.-L., Wang, D.-W., Mark Liao, H.-Y., Chen, Y.-S., Kuan, C.-H., Lin, S.-Y., & Chen, L.-F. (2022). PADAr: Physician-oriented artificial intelligence-facilitating diagnosis aid for retinal diseases. *Journal of Medical Imaging (Bellingham, Wash.)*, *9*(04). Advance online publication. DOI: 10.1117/1.jmi.9.4.044501 PMID: 35903415

Liu, Y., Menon, R., Putcha, A., Huang, K., Bonilla, L., Vora, R., Li, J., Zhang, L., Wang, Y., Fletcher, L., Lassiter, A., Huang, C., Buse, J. B., Cheng, K., & Bai, W. (2022). Skin-Interfaced Deep-Tissue Sensing Patch via Microneedle Waveguides. *Advanced Materials Technologies*, *7*(9). Advance online publication. DOI: 10.1002/admt.202200468

Loyola-Leyva, A., Hernández-Vidales, K., Loyola-Rodríguez, J. P., & González, F. J. (2024). Noninvasive Glucose Measurements Through Transcutaneous Raman Spectroscopy: A Review. *Journal of Diabetes Science and Technology*, *18*(2), 460–469. DOI: 10.1177/19322968221109612 PMID: 35815609

Luca, C., Andritoi, D., Corciova, C., & Fuior, R. (2020). Intelligent Glove for Rehabilitation of Hand Movement in Stroke Survivor. *EPE 2020 - Proceedings of the 2020 11th International Conference and Exposition on Electrical And Power Engineering*, 546–549. https://doi.org/DOI: 10.1109/EPE50722.2020.9305619

Malcangi, M. (2021). AI-Based Methods and Technologies to Develop Wearable Devices for Prosthetics and Predictions of Degenerative Diseases. *Methods in Molecular Biology (Clifton, N.J.)*, *2190*, 337–354. DOI: 10.1007/978-1-0716-0826-5_17 PMID: 32804375

MENDİ, A. F. (2023). Edge ai technology in the defense industry via reinforcement learning in simulation environments. *Gümüşhane Üniversitesi Fen Bilimleri Enstitüsü Dergisi*. https://doi.org/DOI: 10.17714/gumusfenbil.1266035

Mierzwa, A. P., Huang, S. P., Nguyen, K. T., Culjat, M. O., & Singh, R. S. (2016). Wearable ultrasound array for point-of-care imaging and patient monitoring. *Studies in Health Technology and Informatics*, *220*, 241–244. DOI: 10.3233/978-1-61499-625-5-241 PMID: 27046585

Monteagudo, J. L. R. (2016). Medical imaging needs in a rural health center from a clinical point of view. *Defining the Medical Imaging Requirements for a Rural Health Center*, 7–39. https://doi.org/DOI: 10.1007/978-981-10-1613-4_2

Muanme, W., Pararach, S., & Kaeprapha, P. (2023). An Artificial Intelligence Camera System to Check Worker Personal Protective Equipment Before Entering Risk Areas. *Lecture Notes in Electrical Engineering, 1045 LNEE*, 747–755. https://doi.org/DOI: 10.1007/978-981-99-2287-1_102

Nandi, P., Anupama, K. R., Bajaj, A., Shukla, S., Musale, T., & Kachadiya, S. (2022). Performance evaluation of Machine Learning algorithms on System on Chips in Wearables for Healthcare Monitoring. *Procedia Computer Science*, *218*, 2755–2766. DOI: 10.1016/j.procs.2023.01.247

Omotajo, D., & Lang, E. (2022). *149 Impact of AI in diagnostic imaging: establishing its role in contributing to or mitigating harms from overdiagnosis*. A35.1-A35. https://doi.org/DOI: 10.1136/bmjebm-2022-podabstracts.71

Orfanidis, C., Darwich, A. S., Cheong, R., & Fafoutis, X. (2022). Monitoring neurological disorders with AI-enabled wearable systems. *DigiBiom 2022 - Proceedings of the 2022 Emerging Devices for Digital Biomarkers*, 24–28. https://doi.org/DOI: 10.1145/3539494.3542755

Prathiba, M., Jose, D., & Saranya, R., & Nandhinidevi. (2019). Automated Melanoma Recognition in Dermoscopy Images via Very Deep Residual Networks. *IOP Conference Series. Materials Science and Engineering*, *561*(1). Advance online publication. DOI: 10.1088/1757-899X/561/1/012107

Rákay, R., & Galajdová, A. (2020). Concept for Physiological Function Monitoring With Wearable Sensors. *Technical Sciences and Technologies*, *4*(22), 190–197. DOI: 10.25140/2411-5363-2020-4(22)-190-197

Rane, M., Kulkarni, M., Dalvi, A., Kulkarni, A., Singh, A., Bhave, A., & Arawat, V. (2023). AI Algorithm for Image Enhancement. *2023 3rd International Conference on Advances in Electrical, Computing, Communication and Sustainable Technologies, ICAECT 2023*. https://doi.org/DOI: 10.1109/ICAECT57570.2023.10117819

Saw, S. N., & Ng, K. H. (2022). Current challenges of implementing artificial intelligence in medical imaging. *Physica Medica*, *100*, 12–17. DOI: 10.1016/j.ejmp.2022.06.003 PMID: 35714523

Shajari, S., Kuruvinashetti, K., Komeili, A., & Sundararaj, U. (2023). The Emergence of AI-Based Wearable Sensors for Digital Health Technology: A Review. *Sensors (Basel)*, *23*(23). Advance online publication. DOI: 10.3390/s23239498 PMID: 38067871

Sharanyanivasini, J. S., Nirmalprithivraj, M., Tharanipriya, S., Pradeepkumar, G., Arun Prasath, M. M., & Saravanakumar, R. (2023). Sports Applications of Biomechanics Wearable Sensors using IoT. *Proceedings of the 2023 2nd International Conference on Electronics and Renewable Systems, ICEARS 2023*, 613–618. https://doi.org/DOI: 10.1109/ICEARS56392.2023.10085068

Sharma, D., & Sarkar, S. (2022). Enabling Inference and Training of Deep Learning Models for AI Applications on IoT Edge Devices. *Internet of Things : Engineering Cyber Physical Human Systems*, •••, 267–283. DOI: 10.1007/978-3-030-87059-1_10

Shuvo, M. M. H. (2022). Edge AI: Leveraging the Full Potential of Deep Learning. *Studies in Computational Intelligence*, *1061*, 27–46. DOI: 10.1007/978-3-031-14748-7_2

Singh, R. P., Hom, G. L., Abramoff, M. D., Campbell, J. P., & Chiang, M. F. (2020). Current challenges and barriers to real-world artificial intelligence adoption for the healthcare system, provider, and the patient. *Translational Vision Science & Technology*, *9*(2), 1–6. DOI: 10.1167/tvst.9.2.45 PMID: 32879755

Smeraldo, S., Busboom, A., Bendisch, S., Hriskov, H., Morgenstern, T., & Prandini, M. (2023). A data-driven approach to fault diagnostics for industrial process plants based on feature extraction and inferential statistics. *2023 International Conference on Control, Automation and Diagnosis, ICCAD 2023*. https://doi.org/DOI: 10.1109/ICCAD57653.2023.10152324

Smith, B. J., & Adhami, R. R. (1999). Medical imaging. *IEEE Potentials*, *17*(5), 9–12. DOI: 10.1109/45.730965

Steinberg, S., Huang, A., Ono, Y., & Rajan, S. (2022). Continuous Artery Monitoring Using a Flexible and Wearable Single-Element Ultrasonic Sensor. *IEEE Instrumentation & Measurement Magazine*, *25*(1), 6–11. DOI: 10.1109/MIM.2022.9693453

Strolin, S., Santoro, M., Paolani, G., Ammendolia, I., Arcelli, A., Benini, A., Bisello, S., Cardano, R., Cavallini, L., Deraco, E., Donati, C. M., Galietta, E., Galuppi, A., Guido, A., Ferioli, M., Laghi, V., Medici, F., Ntreta, M., Razganiayeva, N., & Strigari, L. (2023). How smart is artificial intelligence in organs delineation? Testing a CE and FDA-approved Deep-Learning tool using multiple expert contours delineated on planning CT images. *Frontiers in Oncology*, *13*. Advance online publication. DOI: 10.3389/fonc.2023.1089807 PMID: 36937399

Suzuki, N., Watanabe, Y., & Nakazawa, A. (2020). GAN-based Style Transformation to Improve Gesture-recognition Accuracy. *Proceedings of the ACM on Interactive, Mobile, Wearable and Ubiquitous Technologies*, *4*(4). Advance online publication. DOI: 10.1145/3432199

Thacharodi, A., Singh, P., Meenatchi, R., Tawfeeq Ahmed, Z. H., Kumar, R. R. S., Neha, V., Kavish, S., Maqbool, M., & Hassan, S. (2024). Revolutionizing healthcare and medicine: The impact of modern technologies for a healthier future—A comprehensive review. *Health Care Science*. Advance online publication. DOI: 10.1002/hcs2.115 PMID: 39479277

Tjoa, E., & Guan, C. (2021). A Survey on Explainable Artificial Intelligence (XAI): Toward Medical XAI. *IEEE Transactions on Neural Networks and Learning Systems*, *32*(11), 4793–4813. DOI: 10.1109/TNNLS.2020.3027314 PMID: 33079674

Tricoli, A., Nasiri, N., & De, S. (2017). Wearable and Miniaturized Sensor Technologies for Personalized and Preventive Medicine. *Advanced Functional Materials, 27*(15). Advance online publication. DOI: 10.1002/adfm.201605271

Tuncel, Y., Krishnakumar, A., Chithra, A. L., Kim, Y., & Ogras, U. (2022). A Domain-Specific System-On-Chip Design for Energy Efficient Wearable Edge AI Applications. *Proceedings of the International Symposium on Low Power Electronics and Design*. https://doi.org/DOI: 10.1145/3531437.3539711

Vivek, K. P. V. (2022). A Smart Wearable Guiding Device for The Visually Impaired People. *International Journal for Research in Applied Science and Engineering Technology, 10*(6), 1568–1572. DOI: 10.22214/ijraset.2022.44153

Vizitiu, A., Nita, C. I., Toev, R. M., Suditu, T., Suciu, C., & Itu, L. M. (2021). Framework for privacy-preserving wearable health data analysis: Proof-of-concept study for atrial fibrillation detection. *Applied Sciences (Switzerland), 11*(19). Advance online publication. DOI: 10.3390/app11199049

Xiao, X., Yin, J., Xu, J., Tat, T., & Chen, J. (2024). Advances in Machine Learning for Wearable Sensors. *ACS Nano, 18*(34), 22734–22751. DOI: 10.1021/acsnano.4c05851 PMID: 39145724

Xing, J., Guo, J., Cui, S., Li, W., & Chang, X. (2023). Graphical multispectral radiation temperature inversion algorithm based on deep learning. *Optics Letters, 48*(8), 2166. DOI: 10.1364/ol.487425 PMID: 37058668

Xu, M., Qian, F., Zhu, M., Huang, F., Pushp, S., & Liu, X. (2020). DeepWear: Adaptive local offloading for on-wearable deep learning. *IEEE Transactions on Mobile Computing, 19*(2), 314–330. DOI: 10.1109/TMC.2019.2893250

Yang, X., Chen, Z., Hettiarachchi, N., ... (2019). A wearable ultrasound system for sensing muscular morphological deformations. *IEEE Transactions on ..., Query date: 2024-01-31 11:57:47*. https://ieeexplore.ieee.org/abstract/document/8760415/

Zahid, N., Sodhro, A. H., Kamboh, U. R., Alkhayyat, A., & Wang, L. (2022). AI-driven adaptive reliable and sustainable approach for internet of things enabled healthcare system. *Mathematical Biosciences and Engineering, 19*(4), 3953–3971. DOI: 10.3934/mbe.2022182 PMID: 35341282

Zhang, H., Li, S., Zhao, Q., Rao, A. K., Guo, Y., & Zanotto, D. (2022). Reinforcement Learning-Based Adaptive Biofeedback Engine for Overground Walking Speed Training. *Proceedings of the IEEE RAS and EMBS International Conference on Biomedical Robotics and Biomechatronics, 2022-Augus*. https://doi.org/DOI: 10.1109/BioRob52689.2022.9925339

Zhang, L., Dai, H., & Sang, Y. (2022). Med-SRNet: GAN-Based Medical Image Super-Resolution via High-Resolution Representation Learning. *Computational Intelligence and Neuroscience, 2022*. Advance online publication. DOI: 10.1155/2022/1744969 PMID: 35747717

Zhang, X. (2021). Application of human motion recognition utilizing deep learning and smart wearable device in sports. *International Journal of System Assurance Engineering and Management, 12*(4), 835–843. DOI: 10.1007/s13198-021-01118-7

Zheng, G., Lai, S., Braverman, V., Jacobs, M. A., & Parekh, V. S. (2023). A framework for dynamically training and adapting deep reinforcement learning models to different, low-compute, and continuously changing radiology deployment environments. *ArXiv, abs/2306.0*. https://api.semanticscholar.org/CorpusID:259108791

Zheng, J., Cao, H., Chen, D., Ansari, R., Chu, K. C., & Huang, M. C. (2020). Designing Deep Reinforcement Learning Systems for Musculoskeletal Modeling and Locomotion Analysis Using Wearable Sensor Feedback. *IEEE Sensors Journal, 20*(16), 9274–9282. DOI: 10.1109/JSEN.2020.2986768

Zhu, W., Qiu, P., Lepore, N., Dumitrascu, O. M., & Wang, Y. (2023). *NNMobile-Net: Rethinking CNN Design for Deep Learning-Based Retinopathy Research*. http://arxiv.org/abs/2306.01289

Chapter 7
Integrating Large Language Models for Advanced Imaging Applications

Samyukta Rongala
https://orcid.org/0009-0002-0254-2420
University of Missouri, Saint Louis, USA

Teja Krishna Kota
https://orcid.org/0009-0006-8979-4311
New England College, USA

ABSTRACT

This chapter explores the transformative potential of large language models (LLMs) in conjunction with image technology, highlighting their ability to redefine limitations in language production and comprehension. By examining their integration into various fields, including medical imaging, autonomous systems, and multimedia content analysis, the chapter underscores the potential for revolutionizing these domains. The discussion also considers the role of LLMs and artificial intelligence in regulatory technology (RegTech) solutions, aimed at streamlining policy processes and mitigating risks. A detailed overview of current studies evaluates the effectiveness of AI and machine learning (ML) combinations. The chapter presents a methodology wherein an AI-based model, utilizing LLMs, analyzes data from diverse processes and datasets. This approach reveals the advantages of AI applications in corporate finance, particularly in enabling financial specialists to derive meaningful insights from extensive datasets.

DOI: 10.4018/979-8-3373-0903-3.ch007

I. INTRODUCTION

Increased oversight in the wake of the 2008 financial crisis, lightning-fast technical developments, and the imperative to improve market dynamics have all contributed to the current trend of increasingly stringent regulatory standards for the financial industry. It is demonstrated as standard regulations procedures as usual arduous, expense, and employee intensivly as to handle the extent and difficulty in the rule duties that are already in place. RegTech, which stands for regulatory technology, has emerged as a acting force with the setting. RegTech offers cutting-edge technical solutions that can speed up regulatory processes, boost transparency, and reduce risk. Artificial Intelligence (AI), Machine Learning (ML), blockchain, and big data analytics are the technologies that are changing the way financial companies handle risk and compliance.

Consequently, there is a growing need for creative manipulation that can meet the demands as simultaneously enhancing activity effectively and strategic execution. Reaction to economic shocks, technological developments, shifts in leadership, and new policies, the regulatory framework under which the banking industry functions is intricate and ever-evolving (Jha et al., 2023) Authorities are claose to the business and becomes more complex as integrated. The implementation of tight limitations has been done in order to protect customers, maintain constant marketing, and pull stop to economial improper activity. In the current regulatory environment, economial organization are subject to a wide variety of rules and regulations that govern risk management, data protection, Know Your Customer (KYC) rules, and Anti-Money Laundering (AML) measures (Cao and Zhai, 2023).

There are significant challenges that financial institutions must overcome in order to maintain compliance within this intricate system. An effective compliance infrastructure is necessary to monitor, report, and resolve regulatory requirements due to the amount and complexity of regulations (Chen et al., 2023). standard rules and regulations, alternation typically implemented manually, require a significant amount of resources, and are compartmentalised, which leads to inefficiencies and increased operating expenditures. If these procedures are slow to adapt to new regulations, it could be difficult for institutions to remain compliant on time. Compliance inspections that are performed manually may result in errors and discrepancies, which can then lead to violations of regulations and significant fines (Dong et al., 2023). The demand for competent compliance personnel is also on the rise in response to increasingly complicated regulatory requirements, which puts additional pressure on available resources and budgets (Rizinski et al., 2024). By failing to satisfy the requirements of a regulatory environment that is always evolving, the traditional method of compliance is putting institutions in a position where they are exposed to new challenges and (Rane, 2023).

Using the certain attributes, K-nearest neighbours (KNN) grouping, which was developed by Fix and Hodges in 1989, is frequently utilised in order to locate photos within the database that are comparable to one another. On the other hand, such a single-modal method has two significant obstacles to overcome. To begin, it places an excessive amount of detail on the visuals. The image embedding model usually finds goods with images that are similar, but they don't always come from the same category. Take, for example, the query for dental foss that is shown in Figure 1. The owner retains all rights. The I2I only MIEM and the I2I dental floss Cotton Swab for Charging Batteries Cotton Swab for Charging. Floss for the teeth Floss for the teeth Floss for the teeth Floss for the teeth Pepsi Bottle Necklace is a product that is available. Only I2I together with MIEM and I2I Pepsi (Dowling & Lucey, 2023).

The comparison of search results using a variety of criteria. For example, the left column shows pictures of user queries, and the right column shows the top 4 things that were found. The image of each item is accompanied by the product name that corresponds to that item. Particularly noteworthy is the fact that the utilisation of Image-to-image (I2I) only places an emphasis on visual elements, ignoring semantic information. Combining MIEM with I2I with the constraints as effectively mitigated. goods with similar packaging (like battery chargers and cotton swabs) are often taken back. Subsequently, it disregards expressive data containedin the image. The introduction of sounds as identifying the model as to the item may result in improper generation when various item added are present in the data image. It is possible to reduce the impact of problematic situations like these. In addition, the process of image embedding presents difficulties for engineers.

Because of the vast number of products in Shopee's e-commerce platform1 and the requirement for numerous replications (Kokina & Blanchette, 2019), creating an embedding for each image necessitates a significant index volume. In addition, the process of dealing with many images for each product necessitates mapping and deduplication, which further increases the complexity of engineering. Technologies that have the potential to alleviate these obstacles have been developed (Met et al., 2020). The concept-aware modality fusion technique was utilised by (Cheng et al., 2023). in order to integrate information from a single image with texts; however, it is not capable of accommodating numerous images (Deveranjan, 2018). Also, the fact that it uses KnnSoftmax (Thekkethil et al., 2021) for training makes execution more difficult during training.

METER (Thekkethil et al., 2021) and X-VLM (Villar & Khan, 2021) are two earlier papers that looked at data image-to-rating the information using a aggegration attention transformer with matched rate with a couple of data images and information. Nevertheless, these approaches listed as some drawbacks when it comes to combining information from many modalities during the recall phase. The Multi-modal Item Embedding Model (MIEM) is proposed as a means of addressing these difficulties that are comprehensive in nature. In this paper, construct and establish the experience of MIEM is proposed on the real time platform. MIEM uses a Merge Attention Transformer Module to combine information from photos and texts in order to provide an embedding for a specific product. The inputs consist of numerous images and product titles. MIEM then uses this information to process the information.

Injecting explicit semantic information into the embedding through product titles solves the problem of the image embedding model fixating on picture details too much. MIEM has being used by the real time enviorment to fuel the picture identification operation. A stunning 8.70% rise in clicks per user and a 5.45% lift in the orders per user statistic have been achieved as a result of the implementation of MIEM in comparison to the solution that was previously selected.

Figure 1. Co-occurrence analysis of Regulatory

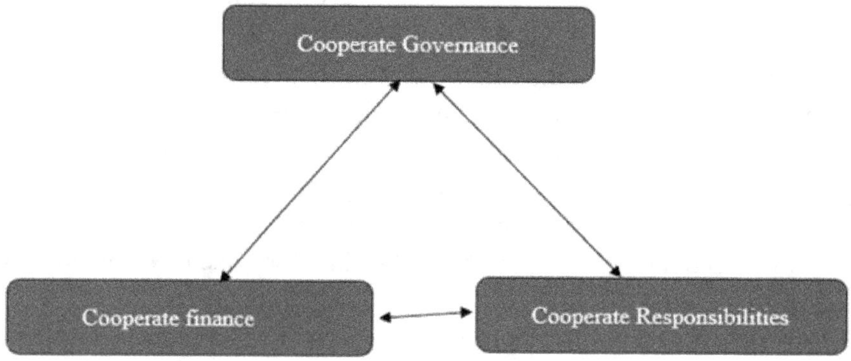

A. Introducing SupTech, RegTech, and FinTech:

The financial industry is thought to be highly regulated because it is so important to customers, countries, and the whole world. Because of this, it is believed that the financial industry has been at a high level of concentration for many years. Large companies, like banks, insurance organization, and money managment, have long provided economial activity because they can follow strict rules. There is a high probability that when industries become overly consolidated, competition is eliminated and progress is halted. After overcoming these obstacles, the banking business has developed into one of the most active fields in the contemporary economy since it emerged. This shift was mostly brought about by the advent of new technology, which was the principal agent of change. Many innovations in the banking industry had their start around the middle of the twentieth century . Certain shifts as the ability to denote the new criteria such as financial technology being introduced (Cao and Zhai, 2023).

When there were global financial problems in 2008, the word "fintech" was made up to describe them. As the name suggests, "FinTech" is a group of technologies used in finance to make operations run more smoothly and automatically (Chen et al., 2023). As a result of the collapse of several economial transaction in that year, the economial organization was shaken, and transaction were weakened. Recent rules and regulations are made it easier for regulators to have more power in the financial sector, which is tough for players. Over $300 billion in penalties was assessed against transaction gobally for noncompliance with the recent rules (Cao and Zhai, 2023). In contrast, the things listed above created an environment that was good for the growth of FinTech. The development of business models that avoid the traditional structures of banks and make use of computers to better meet the requirements of clients was promoted for start-ups in the financial technology industry (Rane, 2023).

Figure 2. Regulatory procedure in finance sector

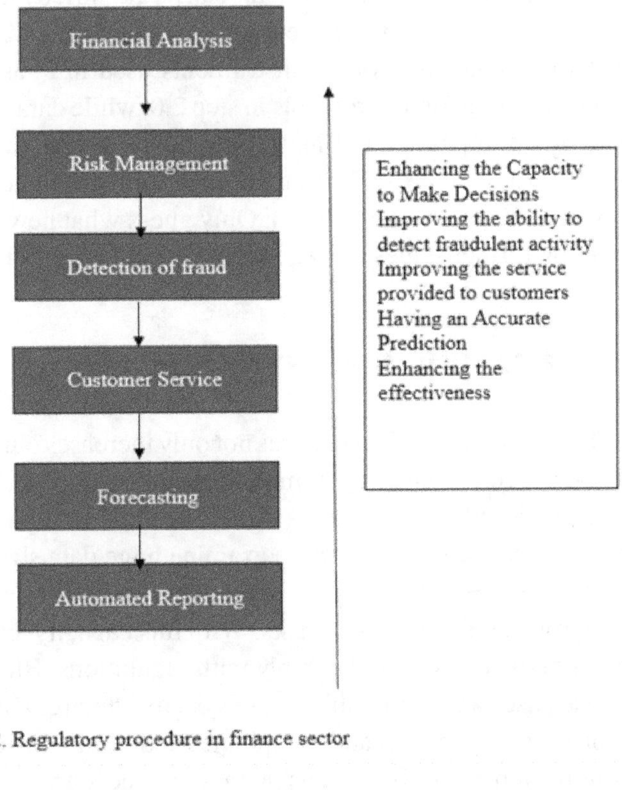

Figure 2. Regulatory procedure in finance sector

In spite of this, there was still a significant problem that needed to be solved. Licensed financial institutions nevertheless had trouble complying with regulations. The post-crisis rules and standards and managing the diifculty and challenges were a significant and costly obstacle for the established enterprises in the financial industry. RegTech was clearly in high demand at this point.

The use of technology to handle financial industry regulations is called RegTech. (Dong et al., 2023): Due to their obvious benefits, these tools are becoming more and more popular. RegTech solutions are useful for things like effcient price with rules and standard tasks, better knowledge of rules needed, feasible in managing the risk and secure the information in the financial industry. There was a $4.5 billion investment pool in RegTech startups in 2018, a nearly fivefold increase from the previous year (Villar & Khan, 2021). As the focus moves from "know your customer" to "know your data," the ecosystem is expected to attain its peak performance in Phase 3.0, according to the participants. Because data serves as the connecting factor between FinTech and RegTech, the laws that govern the economial organization is required to update so that they are founded on information. A completely updated set of regulations that encompass all from digital identification to data owner will be necessary in order to do this (Thekkethil et al., 2021).

On top of that, RegTech systems can be classified into four various stages according to the features they come equipped with. Manual data collection based on cycle time was a capability of the instruments used in Phase 1.0. Compliance software established consistent protocols in step 2.0, while data science supported automated back office in phase 3.0. Finally, in phase 4.0, both artificial intelligence and machine learning approaches that are able to foresee and identified difficulty before they occur (Smeets et al., 2021). Only guess what new possibilities will be brought about by further stages of RegTech, since it has probably not yet reached its limits.

II. LITERATRUE SURVEY

The automation of procedures not only increases output but also reduces the likelihood of errors caused by humans (Smeets et al., 2021) and (Asatiani & Penttinen, 2016), which ultimately results in more accurate compliance evaluations. AI and ML make it feasible for RegTech to examine huge data size as in real time, make them to detect the sets of strategies, anomalies, and potential dangers. The end outcome is improved information on risks. With this capacity, companies can quickly detect fraud, mitigate risks, and comply with regulations. Blockchain technology offers a decentralised and immutable ledger system, which enables transparent and auditable records of transactions and compliance activities (Doguc, 2021). This brings about an improvement in both transparency and accountability. Increased transparency and accountability in stakeholder, regulator, and consumer interactions is a direct outcome of RegTech solutions' scalability, which allows institutions to swiftly respond to changing market conditions and updated laws. A location in which rules and regulations are always being updated is one in which adaptability such as this is absolutely necessary.

(Wang et al., 2022) assert that Robotic Process Automation (RPA) is a developing technology that has a significant potential to impact auditing procedures. File organisation, auditing data preparation, and data integration from several sources are just a few examples of the many simple, repetitive, manual, and rule-based tasks that make up an auditor's duty set. People make a lot of mistakes on these jobs, which takes a lot of time and hard work to finish. Robotic process automation (RPA) is designed to work with data that computers can interpret, which means auditing processes are more accurate and efficient. In addition, the characteristics of RPA have the potential to significantly enhance auditing procedures. At first, robotic process automation (RPA) has the potential to make data transmission between programs easier, which is a task that auditors have traditionally carried out by manually copying and pasting. Secondly, in conjunction with the capability to correlate and evaluate significant amounts of data across a number of different platforms. Third, the development of complex and logic-based business judgements, despite the fact that it can be used to rule-based tasks.

Further, RPA can simplify the grouping the informaiton as procedure, traditional way to standardise the data, and may have synergistic effects, which would lead to increased efficiency. According to (Amini et al., 2021), the terms RPA and AI are repeateadly used interchangeably because both have had a significant impact on and will continue to influence accounting practices. Occasionally, particular segments of the industry are affected by the widespread expansion of artificial intelligence. As talked about in academic articles, the literature review will look at how new technologies have changed the auditing industry and how it works. His literature review focusses on three emerging technologies: AI, robotic process automation, and blockchain. Expert systems, machine learning, and natural language processing will be the focal points of this examination of the role of AI in auditing, which will also look at its background and present uses. In this evaluation, take and look at the tech, its features, and how it works in an auditing setting. Additionally, these parts consist of an analysis of the numerous implications, benefits, and issues that are associated with the technology. As the examination comes to a close, the implications will become more extensive with regard hazards.

Blockchain technology has many potential benefits, according to (Wyrobak, 2020), but it also has certain negative aspects, like any other technology. Immutability, updates to smart contracts, and issues around privacy are all things that are included in these hurdles. In spite of the fact that immutability is frequently considered to be a feature of blockchains, it may cause problems with the terms of smart contracts. Data that is stored in blockchain can't be deleted or changed. This is a problem for smart contracts because the terms of the contracts might not be correct. Data modification is excessively complex, which could cause problems if smart contract rules need to be changed. According to (Goodell et al., 2021), a blockchain system where every transaction is visible on the ledger could cause problems because some contracts could be secret and the data could include sensitive information. Moreover, blockchains have a major challenge when it comes to scalability, which includes latency (the time it takes for a transaction to be confirmed), size, and storage as necessary parts of the system. The growing number of nodes over time shows that the growing amount of data may cause problems.

Moreover, (Aziz et al. 2022) investigates the factors that should be taken into account while deploying blockchains within organisations. A solution used by one company might not work for another, even if it has many benefits, especially if it is not the best or most practical way to improve a process. To reiterate what was stated earlier, blockchain implementations offer a multitude of benefits, one of which is the validation of transactions involving several parties; yet, difficulties still exist. Due to the fact that they require consensus in order to function at their full capacity, blockchains are vulnerable to hacker security problems. It is expected that companies will not completely replace their current IT systems with blockchain technology down the road. Blockchains are seen as a valuable asset that can enhance current systems. However, there is a misconception that RPA is an outdated technology. They do, however, have different purposes, so they can work together instead of against each other.

The use of artificial intelligence in auditing can be traced back to the 1980s. Several expert systems that increased the efficiency of decision-making were included in the research that was carried out by (Kim, 2021), which acknowledged the use of computer-based applications in the auditing process. Constructs the argument that, as was mentioned before, certain accounting responsibilities are characterised as being repetitive and manual activities. Due to the fact that accounting information is gathered and organised during these operations, the auditing profession is extremely reliant on accounting data. According to (Gan et al., 2020), the field of accounting is particularly well-suited for a wide range of applications involving artificial intelligence. Reducing human error in specific tasks, like primary entry bookings, AI improves procedures and makes accounting information more dependable. While auditors are responsible for ensuring that these entries are accurate and reliable, they are confronted with a more substantial basis, which improves the efficiency of the confirmation process, particularly with regard to reliability. There are a number of activities that are required for auditing, including the selection of samples and the making of decisions.

Generally speaking, all rule-based auditing jobs, particularly those that need the maximum amount of time, have the potential to experience significant benefits from the implementation of AI. In addition, the research conducted by (Cheng et al., 2023) investigated a number of components that may be utilised to enhance auditing operations. At first, it can be used to analyse textual material in order to detect and anticipate fraud. In the process of identifying fraudulent actions in financial accounts and detecting abnormalities, it has been established that NPL models can improve the effectiveness of the process.

By using machine learning, Deloitte can improve its place in the advisory services market by making document analysis faster and more accurate. Deloitte put together different versions of the Kira platform along with its own models and called them "Argus" in the accounting business. Their accomplishments were recognised with the "Audit Innovation of the Year" award (Devlin et al., 2018) from the International Accounting Bulletin. PwC has been making investments in artificial intelligence and machine learning for a number of years. This allows the robot to discover irregularities and transactions that are considered to be dubious. PwC's innovation has offered a competitive edge, which has resulted in an increase in corporate value. The GL.ai robot performs auditory duties in the same manner as an experienced professional. 2018 according to PWC. Machine learning technologies have been included into EY's services in order to improve the effectiveness of the auditing profession. The goal was to create a fraud detection software that would use their FIDS (Fraud Investigation and Dispute Service) to find suspicious invoices with a 97% success rate. Moreover, Naoto Ichihara, an Assurance Partner at EY, investigated the viability of artificial intelligence in the auditing industry. Consequently, this led to the establishment of EU Helix GL, which makes use of machine learning in order to identify anomalies in large datasets as well as unstructured data.

Business Emotion Analysis Tool (BEAT) is a product of Deloitte that helps in managing and evaluating voice communications. Break down the BEAT tool into its three main components. At first, it listens in on voice conversations between customers. Second, it is able to make use of natural language processing in order to identify potential used to determine the regulatory parameters for the contract that is being executed. Approximately thirty-three communications have the potential to have undesirable outcomes, and the system will outline these outcomes along with the relevant information. The technology enables the employees of Deloitte to perform an analysis of unstructured data with increased precision and efficiency. In addition, EY has incorporated natural language processing technology into a variety of aspects of its auditing procedures. One example of such an implementation is the capability to remove information from a variety of contracts in response to new legislation or other changes (Devlin et al., 2018).

Language-based voice-based chatbots like Siri, Alexa, and Google Home Assistant have made voice-based chatbots very popular, and people are now studying automated talking agents. Conversations with people that are coherent and interesting on a wide range of subjects should be a long-term objective for conversation systems (Dosovitskiy et al., 2020). The problem is that these systems necessitate either a large amount of engineering work or a large amount of training data collected and annotated, or both. The following is a survey of previous methods that have been utilised for the purpose of training conversational agents to collect and annotate data (Dou et al., 2022). Extensions that may be possible in the future.

Task Completion Agents must be specifically to design to incorporate dynamFor well-structured tasks like travel reservations (Drabas & Lee, 2017) have continuously increased in sophistication and versatility (Goebel et al., 2023).

End-to-end learning for automated conversational agents has become more common recently. This is partly because neural architectures have gotten better and there is more general-purpose training data available. Additionally, the concept of conversation has been presented as a means of eliciting user interests for the purpose of performing item suggestion. An end-to-end reinforcement learning framework was presented in (Gormley & Tong, 2015) for a personalised conversational sales bot, while (Ibrahimi et al., 2022) both of these examples are examples of previous research.

The (Savarese & Hoi, 2023) provides a summary of the accessible corpora up to the year 2017, which includes online human-human interactions, Twitter, and dialogue from films. Recently, a number of teams have created frameworks that incorporate external information in answer creation and actively acquire concepts through talks (Li et al., 2022). This is done with the intention of improving the process of knowledge retrieval.

Although significant advancements have been made, the fundamental knowledge is still encoded, for example in a neural network. If the domain is big, can be expanded, or is changed often, like product information, this is not possible. The same goes for sources that don't have a rich search function. It is a system that has been described that has learnt. This is the closest effort that has been made to accomplish this. It is only reasonable that such logs would not be accessible due to privacy concerns. Therefore, in order to train such agents, a conversation collecting tool retrieved external knowledge from a search engine, together with the queries and actions that were linked with it. Crowd workers and real users assess Alexa Prize Conversational AI challenge talks (Selvaraju et al., 2021). An unintended consequence of the challenge is the availability of certain public datasets.

Although there was no set agenda for the conversations, the "Wizards" were told to stick to a generic script and ask predetermined questions regarding movie tastes, which was different from their previous attempts. The data set that was produced as a consequence might be useful (Liu et al., 2021a). The data collection that was produced, despite its beneficial nature, was restricted to a relatively small number of individuals who took part in the laboratory investigation. Because of the open-ended character of the study, it is difficult to scale up to generate a sufficiently large and robust data collection, which is necessary for the training of efficient automated search agents.

This pattern is echoed in (Loshchilov & Hutter, 2019), in which the authors publish a collection of sixty-four high-quality talks about shopping that cover a variety of objectives. It is also a reflection of the difficulties that arise with increasing data collecting in this sector, which is a significant element that are working to overcome. Recently, LLMs gave workers advice on what to say, supposedly to make it easier to record these complicated conversations, but they only recorded about half of the talks (Oord et al., 2018)

(Paszke et al., 2019) conducted a survey in which fifty persons from five different local enterprises in and around Tochigi Prefecture, Japan, participated in order to measure consumer perception. Based on the outcomes of the study, it was determined that the purchasers showed an interest in acquiring used products. Furthermore, the pricing was found to be appropriate, as the consumers will not suffer any sentiments of shame or social guilt while purchasing such used things. This article also analysed the characteristics that contribute to client loyalty in those firms and made the comment that this particular store ought not to be deemed improper for antique products and artefact shops.

As a result of the availability of excess products that may be sold on the market, the development of the secondhand sector and the competitiveness for new things have both been dropping. Due to the fact that there is no regular availability of previously owned items, there will be an increase in rivalry among buyers of secondhand goods to purchase new items, which will also contribute to an increase in the cost of materials. Furthermore, if the supply of new items is reduced as a result of the sale of old goods, this will not tend to be a one-for-one situation. In the event that the cost of recycled products is more than the expense of getting new merchandise, this will be an obvious advantage made available by recycled merchandise in comparison to new merchandise. The goal of this study was to evaluate some of the most significant trends in the market for used products, as well as their causes and the consequences they have on retail in the digital age (Qian et al., 2019).

This study employed the Naive Bayes Classifier, Logistic Regression, and Support Vector Machines as its classifiers to examine and determine the review's veracity. Researchers created a model to identify bogus reviews using linguistic properties including unigrams, bigrams, and review length.

They utilised harvesting techniques to construct a dataset for the classification of false reviews in four distinct cities and established a feature structure for the detection of fakes. To classifying bogus reviews, the dataset was utilised. Moreover, (Radford et al., 2021) provided a system for recognising the false feedback measured in the consumer electronics business as well as for classifying the fake reviews that are found in the consumer electronics domain. This system encompasses both the identification and classification of the fake reviews. A method that can detect phoney evaluations for consumer devices has also been presented. Additionally, to classify reviews, they have developed a fictitious system that is based on the structure that was provided for the purpose of conducting the classification. This system was created to categorise reviews. Through the application of statistical methods, they were able to attain an F-score level of 82% on the categorisation function. Additionally, the Ada Boost classifier was shown to be effective in the Friedman test, which provides further evidence that it is beneficial.

(Song et al., 2002) addresses the problem of ranking systems that are regularly affected by profile injection attacks or anomalous scores created by collective suggestion techniques. These types of assaults can have a significant impact on ranking systems. These are the kinds of attacks that have the potential to do harm to ranking systems. Injecting detrimental profiles that tend to reduce an item's popularity or injecting malicious profiles that strongly rate a specific item are the most common obstacles that attackers confront.

Furthermore, a quintile regression model was integrated to examine the important factors related to online shoppers' preferences; this allowed to uncover how promotional efforts affected product sales. Considerations such as the intruder's potential to take advantage of the circumstance, the unique qualities of the sought-after valuable product, and the industry's intrinsic motivation are considered when assessing these repercussions. This research served as the catalyst for the development of a novel iterative rating attack, which was subsequently validated through the trials to determine whether it was effective. Additionally, they carried out research and prepared a list of the economic impact of a variety of elements that influence product sales and downloads. This was done in addition to the statement.

All the components that are taken into consideration in the new neural network models that have been developed by (Sun et al., 2020) include the typical bag-of-words, the context of the words, and the emotions of the user. Specifically, these models employ three distinct sets of features to endeavour to comprehend the text: Grammes of n-grams, phrase embedding, and the combination of words and phrases different lexicon-based emotion cues can be found in a variety of contexts.

An approach that is known as high-dimensional categorisation was employed in order to categorise the incorrect input into four unique groups of its own. By contrasting the proposed technique with the other ways that have been explored, it has been proved that categorisation is a successful method.

A new framework for using machine learning techniques to figure out the ratings of web reviews was suggested by (Wang et al., 2018). They found that a number of different text preprocessing techniques, such as the detection of negation words, the correction of word elongation, and the lemmatisation of parts of speech in conjunction with terms frequency and N-gram words, have the potential to improve accuracy. This was established through their research. They also illustrated how well the general mood of lexicons like SenticNet 4 and SentiWordNet 3.0 can be used to construct the features. This was done in addition to the previous.

An innovative method for the finding of de-blocking was presented during the presentation. This method would dynamically collect object demos from a deep learning system. Prior to the beginning of the deblocking process, hierarchical properties were investigated with the help of a convolutional neural network (CNN) that was implemented. Utilising the moving window, CNN then found the most useful features.

Attaining online automatic product classification is currently the principal goal of the pursuit of electronic commerce development. Looking at the features of product pictures, created a quick supervised image classifier using the class-specific Pyramid Histogram of Words (PHOW) description and Image-to-Class distance (PHOW/I2C). The local attributes are represented as soft-voting PHOW descriptors during the training phase, which involves intense sampling of the characteristics. When reach this point, the training phase will start. Next, distributional means and variances of each visual word are used in each class to generate the class-specific descriptors. After the preceding step has been finished, this is the next step that is carried out.

The expansion of used goods has been discovered to decrease the necessity for new ones, as evidenced by the works. However, it has been discovered that the warranty duration has an impact on sales and the behaviour of consumers when purchasing used items. Currently, there is a substantial level of demand for used items that are available on the market. Furthermore, it analyses the difficulties that purchasers face when making purchases based on manufactured evaluations, as well as the strategies that were employed to identify these reviews through the implementation of machine learning models. Moreover, it also investigates the approaches that were taken to detect these reviews.

Nevertheless, most projects have the unintended consequence of causing errors and outcomes that cannot be identified (Wang et al., 2019). The use of machine learning tactics to the investigation of feelings and sentiments was another subject that was covered in the publications that were mentioned before. Therefore, no study has yet attempted to combine the methods of analysing product photos with those of identifying emotions in product reviews. Since these works do not compare the same things with those supplied by other dealers and do not take into consideration elements such as product quality, appearance, wear and tear, or quality, the model that was built took into account all of these aspects. Considerations like product quality, aesthetics, and durability have been omitted from these works. Additionally, this work does not compare the same product with different dealers; accordingly, all of these elements have been taken into consideration in the model that has been offered since it was introduced.

III. RESEARCH METHODOLOGY

In the proposed approach, the LLM's based AI model is deployed as it helps to construct the data warehouse as the modeling process takes certain stages as mentioned below,

A. LLM's Based AI Model:

The data's are modelled based on the process of data warehouse with kimbell's approach as, Initial step helps to identify the business process as analyse the students entry, their registering for the new course, analyse the student grade obtained, student payment and their graduation count of students. Then data can be grained and declared based on the data measure as it is integrated with the data granularity. The data measurement is based on the student information with every year, information of the student who is registering, distribution of grade of the student, graduation data and payment done by the student. The data dimension is identified based on role associated with the student.

B. Modified LLM Process:

Figure 3. Data Warehouse Architecture using LLM Process

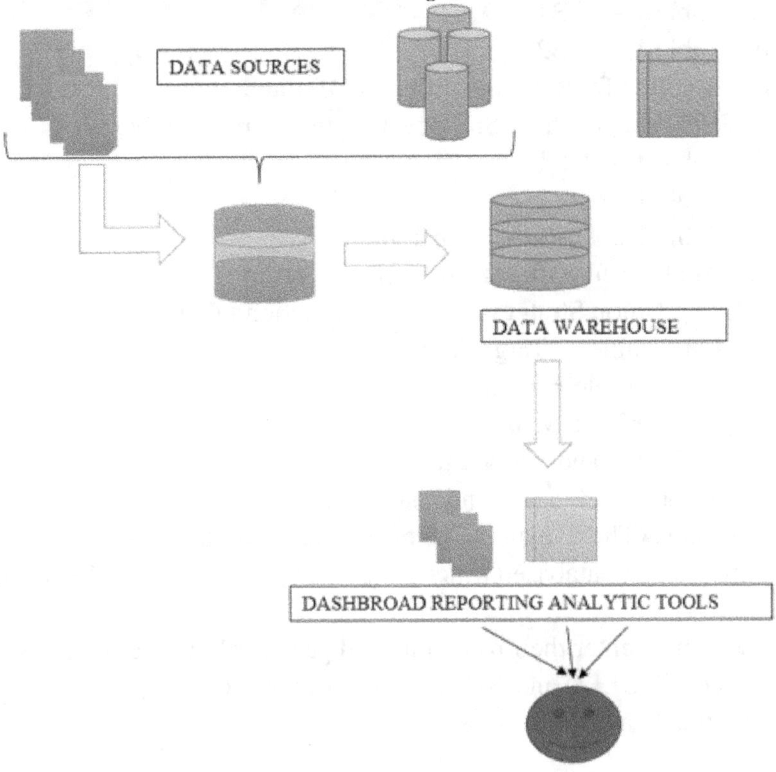

In the LLM process, the server, mainframe, source production is taken as the input as it get the initial process of extraction as takes the unstructured data and perform extraction on the data stage and generalize the data as structured one. Then it performs data cleaning as it cleans the unwanted data into useful one. Then data conforms and deliver make the data to be analysed and processed. Finally it is sent back to the use application by the end user as it operates several processes such as, scheduling the data, handling the data exception, data recovery, and data restart, checking the data quality and reliability with certain user support.

Algorithm 1: Modified LLM Process for Data Integration

Input: Server; Mainframe; Data Source
Output: Data Integration

1. Identify the data source to perform data extraction
2. The data tables are structured and their explanation
    - Using a merging strategy, create the master table
        a. Table 1 → DB1
        b. Table 1 → DB2
        c. Merger (Table 1 from different DB1 and 2)
    - Using Merge Union Strategy, Create the master table
        a. Table 1 → DB1
        b. Table 1 → DB2
        c. Table 1 not influence on Table 2
        d. Apply Merge strategy with Union Action
    - Using Union Strategy, create a transaction table
        a. Large table → Target Table
        b. Target Table = {Pilot Table}
3. Heterogeneoour Data Source
4. DB = DB {Merge and Union Strategy}
5. Perform Data identification and analyze the data source
    A. Hostname (The domain name or IP address of the database server)
    B. Name of the database (which may include certain identifiers such as the schema)
    C. Users must enter their username and password in order to access the data source.IFNULL() and NULL Values Expression
6. Creating the data dimension tables.

The process of data integration is performed and represented in Algorithm 1.

C. Data Cleaning and Conforming:

In the cleaning process, the data errors are detected and removed as inconsistent data's are identified as it results in enhancing the data quality.

- Analysis the data
- Refining the data
- Verify the data

Based on the data rule and value, re-analyze the data based on LLM process to perform data confirmation, data join and association. Then the data helps to create conform data dimension as it takes data hierarchy and dimension

D. Data Delivery and Loading:

In this data table, only user analysis data's are present and for each data table, the key is generated. Here the start schema being used as it helps to de normalize the data and then deliver the data as the targeted data table.

- Slow Changing Dimension (SCD)
- Loading the Fact Table

E. DATA Process Testing:

The main objective of LLM process is to test the data by identifying and collecting the data errors as it occurs before the process of data analytical and reporting. Various data testing are performed i.e. validate the data completion, testing the Meta data and LLM test incrementing. All loaded data are measured as it helps to validate the objective if data completion. The table defined are verified while performing the Meta data testing. Data document can be mapped based on checking the data type, length of the data, checking the data index between the source and destination table. Then the unwanted data duplication can be determined based on the incremented LLM testing.

IV. INTEGRATING MULTI MODAL WITH LLM

The Structure of the MIEM According to Figure 3, MIEM utilises a dual-tower architecture that is composed of two separate components. These towers are the query tower and the item tower. The query tower receives the customer's uploaded query image as input and produces the corresponding query embedding as output. The item tower, in contrast, takes text and numerous product photos as input and outputs the item embedding. Notably, the image encoder is shared between the query and the item towers, which results in a reduction in the amount of parameters that are necessary and brings about an improvement in the recall score.

A. Design of MIEM:

In the following, find the specifics of the model's design:

1. Image Encoder: The Swin Transformer (Wang et al., 2020) is utilised in the construction of the image encoder. This is a brand-new vision transformer model that uses hierarchical feature representations and costs the same amount of computing power no matter how big the input picture is.

Compared to the previous Vision Transformer (Dosovitskiy et al., 2020), Swin Transformer has done better at ImageNet classification, COCO object recognition, and semantic segmentation challenges. In MIEM, the Swin Transformer basis is utilised in order to achieve a delicate equilibrium between speed and accuracy.

2. Title Encoder: In accordance with (Wang et al., 1993), construct the title encoder by utilising the multilingual BERT basis.
3. The Fusion Module: the fusion module consists of 6 layers of merge attention networks (Yang et al., 2020). Concatenating patch-level embeddings from images and token-level embeddings from texts, it then feeds these embeddings into a vanilla transformer model.

utilising six layers of cross attention, which is a technique that is frequently utilised in image-text pretrained models, has been shown to be less effective than utilising this structure, according to empirical tests. Cross attention works for ranking tasks, but merge attention preserves more information from both modalities, improving approach integration recall scores (Yang et al., 2020).

Search click records are used to train the model during the training phase. When a user clicks on a product, the item tower receives the details (text and photos) and sends them to the query tower. Both towers are trained simultaneously using the proposed loss functions and training procedures, which will be explained in full below.

The vector-based approximate nearest neighbour (ANN) retrieval method is utilised in this configuration to facilitate image-to-product recall. Training Procedures for the MIEM System A MIEM is trained separately for each country/region with PyTorch, and the training procedure consists of three major parts. AdamW as the optimiser are employed for all three steps, conforming to the efforts that came before (Hoosian et al., 2023).

Achieving the Acquiring of Training Data When training MIEM, make use of the click logs of users. ▨query image, clicked item title, clicked item imagine list⟩ is the triplet that represents each log entry. In this case, the clicked item title and clicked item image lists show the names and pictures of the goods that users clicked on after searching with the query image. Although consumers might theoretically click on totally unrelated products, manual examination and analysis revealed that about half of the triplets contain identical query-item combinations, half are on comparable items, and less than five percent are on irrelevant noisy things. In light of this, the dataset is beneficial to objectives.

Based on assumptions, MIEM should be able to learn from item triplets that are very similar. Following is a list of the arguments:

a. When seen from the full system's point of view, these comparable items are products that people are interested in purchasing. retrieve them during the recall step even if they are not identical to one another.
b. From a psychological point of view, even while similar item triplets do not always precisely match, the (query image, clicked item title) pairs frequently correspond correctly, with the only difference being in the photographs.

Consequently, the model is still able to acquire valuable correlations between the enquiries and the products by reading through these samples. Consequently, save this section of the data even though it contains item triplets that are comparable. No specific cleanup has been performed on the 5% of data that is totally irrelevant at this time. It's possible that this could be a point of prospective extension in the future. The process of developing and deploying applications Shopee Image Search Engine serves Southeast Asia, Taiwan, and Brazil using MIEM since March 2023. The procedure that is depicted in Figure 2 is followed during the deployment. Along the course of creation and carrying out, a suite of technologies has been crafted to address realistic needs. Feature Extraction from Online Queries They changed the image encoder (a PyTorch) into a TensorRT (Hwang & Kim, 2021) model and added it to the online feature extraction service to make it work better for delivering services online.

TensorRT is able to optimise neural networks by utilising the GPU, which ultimately results in a reduction in service latency. Extraction of Features from Offline Items T he item tower service is also based on the TensorRT architecture. Images of the items do not need boundary boundaries anymore in this scenario. Pre-calculate the embeddings for products in the database to improve the efficiency of online services. Considering the huge size of the product database and the large number of things that are added and removed every day, created the following pipeline (Figure 4).

There is a full-featured Hive table that keeps for all of the items, and it is partitioned by day. The MIEM Elasticsearch (ES) Index is eventually updated with the features that have been gathered. On a daily basis, this procedure is carried out as follows:

1. The current day partition is initially cloned with the full-feature partition from the previous day. things that have been deleted or things that have had their information altered (such as photographs or titles) are not replicated. The up-

stream product information table is compared with the full-feature table from the previous day in order to accomplish this goal.

2. The information about things that have been recently added or updated is gathered and then provided to a PySpark (Kashyap, 2023) job. Uses gRPC calls to the item embedding service to efficiently get embeddings and post them to the current day partition.

Figure 4. MIEM item embedding pre-calculation

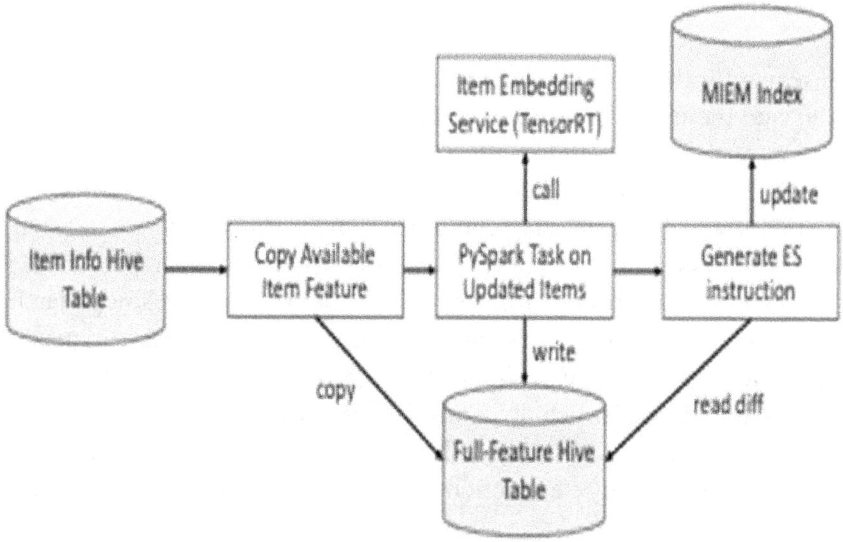

Items that are present in the old day partition but not in the current day partition are removed when the delete action is performed. Newly added or updated items for which the service was able to successfully obtain features are included in the update action list. Each of these directives is transmitted to the Index service in order to bring the ES index up to date. It is important to note that while though the full-feature Hive table looks to be unnecessary in conjunction with the ES index, it is, in fact, necessary for two reasons. First and foremost, to examine item features in the ES index, which makes debugging more difficult. Second, the HNSW algorithm has some restrictions, which means that the ES index needs to be reconstructed on a frequent basis. A decrease in the recall score occurs when there is an increase in the number of items that have been updated. Keeping the Hive table with all of its features updated makes the rebuilding process easier.

B. LLM With Multi Modal Analysis:

There is a display of the findings in Table 1. Furthermore, when contrasted with the image embedding model, MIEM brings about a significant reduction in the amount of storage space that is required. For the online ES index, MIEM uses roughly 61.17% less storage space than the previously used I2I index. Analysis of Qualitative Data Table 3 provides samples of the top four cases that have been found online. In the first illustration, the inquiry pertains to traditional clothing from in Indonesia. When it comes to protective apparel, the I2I model produces findings that are accurate. On the other hand, after implementing MIEM, this problem has demonstrated a significant improvement, and more pertinent results have been obtained. In the second illustration, the inquiry pertains to a body spray, in the form of Figure 3.

Returned by the I2I model are outcomes that resemble cake boxes. Improved search accuracy is being achieved using MIEM, which takes into account both visual and semantic characteristics to correctly identify the right product. Regarding the third scenario, the inquiry is directed at a speaker. MIEM effectively provides the top four results that correspond to the query image's appearance. This occurs because the multi-modal technique is not utilised. MIEM's multi-modal feature helps solve these kinds of problems by looking at both text and picture data. This makes suggestions that are more accurate and relevant to the situation, as shown in Tables 1, Table 2, and Table 3.

Table 1. offine evaluation results on a Shopee product test

Model	Category Accuracy	Recall@1	Recall@5	Recall@10	Recall@50	Recall@100
I2I	0.874	0.820	0.922	0.951	0.979	0.985
I2T	0.876	0.395	0.632	0.714	0.856	0.896
MIEM	0.881	0.812	0.927	0.952	0.984	0.988
MIEM (1 emb/img)	**0.894**	0.819	0.939	0.964	0.988	0.990
MIEM+I2I	0.879	**0.872**	**0.953**	**0.969**	**0.984**	**0.985**

Table 2. results of the Shopee Image Search Engine

	A/B Test Period	Group	Clicks/User	ΔClicks/User	Orders/User	ΔOrders/User
Shopee Indonesia	31/03/2023 -10/04/2023	I2I	3.84		0.0804	
		MIEM+I2I	4.22	+9.90%	0.0838	+4.23%
Shopee Brazil	20/04/2023 -05/05/2023	I2I	4.00		0.0364	
		MIEM+I2I	4.24	+6.00%	0.0382	+4.95%

Table 3. A/B test results on Same & Similar Item

Model	Same Item Recall@4	Similar Item Recall@4	Top 4 Irrelevant Rate
I2I	50.55%	93.26%	13.58%
MIEM+I2I	**53.66%**	**95.60%**	**10.71%**

V. PERFORMANCE ANALYSIS

Based on LLM strategy, data warehouse makes the total cost construction as contains Data Dimension Cost (DDC) and Import Data Cost (IDC).

Total Cost (TC) = Data Dimension Cost (DDC) + Import Data Cost (IDC)

A. Analysis of the OLAP Process:

As there are two OLAP query requests, various data dimension is required based on value query of fact information as it gets H Base get() operation and Hbase Scan () as represented in Table 4 and Table 5.

Table 4. Time cost based on Get () operation

No of Rows	HBase	Oracle
1000	4	22
10000	3.6	34
100000	2.8	45

Table 5. Time cost based on Scan () operation

No of Rows	HBase	Oracle
1000	20	25.4
10000	12.5	24.6
100000	19.2	26.6

B. Analysis of LLM process:

Here 1000, 10,000 and 1,00,000 data entries are considered as the HBase and traditional oracle are analysed as represented in Table 6, Table 7 and Table 8.

Table 6. DATA Process based on 1000 Datasets (ms)

No of Rows	HBase	Oracle
1	104	34
2	109	16
3	100	15
4	116	12
5	109	13
6	111	25
7	116	12
8	128	13.5
9	120	13.8
10	98	14.2

Table 7. LLM Process based on 10,000 Datasets (ms)

No of Rows	HBase	Oracle
1	650	190
2	600	96
3	625	60
4	680	45
5	800	48
6	790	54
7	765	51
8	600	53
9	605	170
10	790	68

Table 8. LLM Process based on 1,00,000 Datasets (ms)

No of Rows	HBase	Oracle
1	2900	509
2	2850	450
3	2950	465
4	2980	445
5	2450	451
6	2800	458
7	2750	462
8	2950	710
9	3450	462
10	2800	491

VI. CONCLUSION

The different advantages that artificial intelligence offers to corporate finance are highlighted in this research. Machine learning algorithms help financial experts get useful information from very large files. This lets them make very accurate and quick decisions based on data. Through the identification of patterns, trends, and anomalies in financial data, artificial intelligence improves the accuracy of forecasting and risk management. This, in turn, optimises resource allocation and assists in the growth of organisations. In addition, the use of natural language processing makes it possible to conduct an efficient analysis of unstructured data sources, such as regulatory filings, news articles, and the emotion expressed on social media.

When it comes to corporate governance, artificial intelligence offers extraordinary transparency. This lets them be fixed before they happen and encourages people to follow the rules and act in an honest way. LLM process is deployed as it performs certain process such as, data extraction, cleaning the data, data conforming and data delivery & loading. The data content profiling and analysing the data source are performed in the data extraction process. The data's are integrated in the distributed environment as it perform the database with different strategy i.e. merge, merge-union and union. The data conformation is created based on the analysing the data source, data refinement based on structure hierarchy. The data dimension and fact tables are associated in the process of LLM loading. In the analysis, Hbase data warehouse takes reduce time in the process of LLM than the traditional oracle. Ithe HBase takes faster query response by varying the datasets 1000, 10000, 100000 data entries. If the data value is larger, memory consumption is high and the query optimization gets reduced as the data value is smaller and it needs some better data partition in the data value.

REFERENCES

Amini, S., Elmore, R., Öztekin, Ö., & Strauss, J. (2021). Can machines learn capital structure dynamics? *Journal of Corporate Finance*, *70*, 102073.

Asatiani, A., & Penttinen, E. (2016). Turning robotic process automation into commercial success–Case OpusCapita. *Journal of Information Technology Teaching Cases*, *6*(2), 67–74.

Aziz, S., Dowling, M., Hammami, H., & Piepenbrink, A. (2022). Machine learning in finance: A topic modeling approach. *European Financial Management*, *28*(3), 744–770.

Cao, Y., & Zhai, J. (2023). Bridging the gap–the impact of ChatGPT on financial research. *Journal of Chinese Economic and Business Studies*, 1–15.

Gormley, C., & Tong, Z. (2015). *Elasticsearch: the definitive guide: a distributed real-time search and analytics engine*. O'Reilly Media, Inc.

Chen, B., Wu, Z., & Zhao, R. (2023). From fiction to fact: The growing role of generative AI in business and finance. *Journal of Chinese Economic and Business Studies*, *21*(4), 471–496.

Cheng, Z., Xiao, S., Zhai, Z., Zeng, X., & Huang, W. (2023). Mixer: Image to Multi-Modal Retrieval Learning for Industrial Application. arXiv preprint arXiv:2305.03972. Chicco, D. 2021. Siamese neural networks: An overview. Artifcial Neural Networks, 73–94.

Devlin, J., Chang, M.-W., Lee, K., & Toutanova, K. (2018). BERT: Pre-training of deep bidirectional transformers for language understanding. arXiv preprint arXiv:1810.04805.

DOGUC, O. (2021). Applications of robotic process automation in finance and accounting. *Beykent Üniversitesi Fen ve Mühendislik Bilimleri Dergisi*, *14*(1), 51–59.

. Dong, M. M., Stratopoulos, T. C., & Wang, V. X. (2023). A Scoping Review of ChatGPT Research in Accounting and Finance. Theophanis C. and Wang, Victor Xiaoqi, A Scoping Review of ChatGPT Research in Accounting and Finance (December 30, 2023).

Dosovitskiy, A., Beyer, L., Kolesnikov, A., Weissenborn, D., Zhai, X., Unterthiner, T., Dehghani, M., Minderer, M., Heigold, G., Gelly, S., ... (2020). An image is worth 16x16 words: Transformers for image recognition at scale. arXiv preprint arXiv:2010.11929.

Dou, Z.-Y., Xu, Y., Gan, Z., Wang, J., Wang, S., Wang, L., Zhu, C., Zhang, P., Yuan, L., & Peng, N.. (2022). An empirical study of training end-to-end vision-and-language transformers. In *Proceedings of the 2022 IEEE/CVF Conference on Computer Vision and Pattern Recognition (CVPR'22)*, 18166–18176.

Dowling, M., & Lucey, B. (2023). ChatGPT for (finance) research: The Bananarama conjecture. *Finance Research Letters*, *53*, 103662.

. Drabas, T.; and Lee, D. (2017). Learning PySpark. Packt Publishing Ltd. Fix, E.; and Hodges, J. L. 1989. Discriminatory analysis. Nonparametric discrimination: Consistency properties. International Statistical Review/Revue Internationale de Statistique, 57(3): 238–247.

Gan, L., Wang, H., & Yang, Z. (2020). Machine learning solutions to challenges in finance: An application to the pricing of financial products. *Technological Forecasting and Social Change*, *153*, 119928.

Goebel, R., Yu, H., Faltings, B., Fan, L., & Xiong, Z. (2023). *Trustworthy Federated Learning* (Vol. 13448). Springer.

Goodell, J. W., Kumar, S., Lim, W. M., & Pattnaik, D. (2021). Artificial intelligence and machine learning in finance: Identifying foundations, themes, and research clusters from bibliometric analysis. *Journal of Behavioral and Experimental Finance*, *32*, 100577.

Hwang, S., & Kim, J. (2021). Toward a Chatbot for Financial Sustainability. *Sustainability*, *13*, 3173. DOI: 10.3390/su13063173

Ibrahimi, S., Sors, A., de Rezende, R. S., & Clinchant, S. (2022). Learning with label noise for image retrieval by selecting interactions. In Proceedings of the 2022 IEEE/CVF Winter Conference on Applications of Computer Vision (WACV'22), 2181–2190. Li, J.; Li, D.

Jha, M., Qian, J., Weber, M., & Yang, B. (2023). ChatGPT and corporate policies. Chicago Booth Research Paper, (23-15).

Kashyap, K. (2023). The benefits of customer experience ai for financial institutions, https://www.forbes.com/sites/forbestechcouncil/2023/07/07/the-benefits-of-customer-experience-ai-for-financial-institutions/?sh=12b8f6d010a8, last accessed 2023/09/29.

. Kim, H. (2021). Machine Learning Applications in Finance Research. Fintech with Artificial Intelligence, Big Data, and Blockchain, 205-220.

Kokina, J., & Blanchette, S. (2019). Early evidence of digital labor in accounting: Innovation with Robotic Process Automation. *International Journal of Accounting Information Systems*, *35*, 100431.

Li, J., Li, D., Xiong, C., & Hoi, S. (2022). Blip: Bootstrapping language-image pre-training for unifed visionlanguage understanding and generation. In International Conference on Machine Learning, 12888–12900. PMLR. Li, J.

Liu, C., Yu, H., Li, B., Shen, Z., Gao, Z., Ren, P., Xie, X., Cui, L., & Miao, C. (2021a). Noise-resistant deep metric learning with ranking-based instance selection. In *Proceedings of the 2021 IEEE/CVF Conference on Computer Vision and Pattern Recognition (CVPR'21)*, 6811–6820.

Loshchilov, I., & Hutter, F. (2019). Decoupled weight decay regularization. In ICLR. Malkov, Y. A.; and Yashunin, D. A. 2018. Effcient and robust approximate nearest neighbor search using hierarchical navigable small world graphs. *IEEE Transactions on Pattern Analysis and Machine Intelligence*, *42*(4), 824–836.

. Met, İ., Kabukçu, D., Uzunoğulları, G., Soyalp, Ü., & Dakdevir, T. (2020). Transformation of business model in finance sector with artificial intelligence and robotic process automation. Digital Business Strategies in Blockchain Ecosystems: Transformational Design and Future of Global Business, 3-29.

Oord, A. d., Li, Y., & Vinyals, O. (2018). Representation learning with contrastive predictive coding. arXiv preprint arXiv:1807.03748.

Paszke, A., Gross, S., Massa, F., Lerer, A., Bradbury, J., Chanan, G., Killeen, T., Lin, Z., Gimelshein, N., & Antiga, L.. (2019). Pytorch: An imperative style, high-performance deep learning library. *Advances in Neural Information Processing Systems*.

Qian, Q., Shang, L., Sun, B., Hu, J., Li, H., & Jin, R. (2019). Softtriple loss: Deep metric learning without triplet sampling. In *Proceedings of the 2019 IEEE/CVF International Conference on Computer Vision (ICCV'19)*, 6450–6458.

Radford, A., Kim, J. W., Hallacy, C., Ramesh, A., Goh, G., Agarwal, S., Sastry, G., Askell, A., Mishkin, P., & Clark, J.. (2021). Learning transferable visual models from natural language supervision. In *Proceedings of the 38th International Conference on Machine Learning (ICML'21)*, 8748– 8763.

Rane, N. (2023). Role and Challenges of ChatGPT and Similar Generative Artificial Intelligence in Finance and Accounting. Available at *SSRN* 4603206.

Rizinski, M., Jankov, A., Sankaradas, V., Pinsky, E., Mishkovski, I., & Trajanov, D. (2024). Comparative Analysis of NLP-Based Models for Company Classification. *Information (Basel)*, *15*(2), 77.

Savarese, S., & Hoi, S. (2023). Blip-2: Bootstrapping language-image pre-training with frozen image encoders and large language models. arXiv preprint arXiv:2301.12597.

Selvaraju, R., Gotmare, A., Joty, S., Xiong, C., & Hoi, S. C. H. (2021). Align before fuse: Vision and language representation learning with momentum distillation. *Advances in Neural Information Processing Systems*, *34*, 9694–9705.

Smeets, M., Erhard, R., & Kaußler, T. (2021). *Robotic Process Automation (RPA) in the Financial Sector*. Springer Fachmedien Wiesbaden.

Song, L., Pan, P., Zhao, K., Yang, H., Chen, Y., Zhang, Y., Xu, Y., & Jin, R. (2020). Large-scale training system for 100-million classifcation at alibaba. In *Proceedings of the 26th ACM SIGKDD International Conference on Knowledge Discovery & Data Mining (KDD'20)*, 2909–2930.

Sun, Y., Cheng, C., Zhang, Y., Zhang, C., Zheng, L., Wang, Z., & Wei, Y. (2020). Circle loss: A unifed perspective of pair similarity optimization. In *Proceedings of the 2020 IEEE/CVF Conference on Computer Vision and Pattern Recognition (CVPR'20)*, 6398–6407.

Thekkethil, M. S., Shukla, V. K., Beena, F., & Chopra, A. (2021). Robotic process automation in banking and finance sector for loan processing and fraud detection. In 2021 9th international conference on reliability, infocom technologies and optimization (trends and future directions)(ICRITO) (pp. 1-6). IEEE.

Villar, A. S., & Khan, N. (2021). Robotic process automation in banking industry: A case study on Deutsche Bank. *Journal of Banking and Financial Technology*, *5*(1), 71–86.

Wang, H., Wang, Y., Zhou, Z., Ji, X., Gong, D., Zhou, J., & Liu, W. (2018). Cosface: Large margin cosine loss for deep face recognition. In *Proceedings of the IEEE conference on computer vision and pattern recognition* (pp. 5265-5274).

Wang, X., Han, X., Huang, W., Dong, D., & Scott, M. R. (2019). Multi-similarity loss with general pair weighting for deep metric learning. In *Proceedings of the IEEE/CVF conference on computer vision and pattern recognition* (pp. 5022-5030).

Wang, D. N., Li, L., & Zhao, D. (2022). Corporate finance risk prediction based on LightGBM. *Information Sciences*, *602*, 259–268.

Wang, X., Zhang, H., Huang, W., & Scott, M. R. (2020). Cross-batch memory for embedding learning. In *Proceedings of the 2020 IEEE/CVF Conference on Computer Vision and Pattern Recognition (CVPR'20)*, 6388–6397.

Wang, X., Zhao, H., & Zhu, J. (1993). GRPC: A communication cooperation mechanism in distributed systems. *Operating Systems Review*, *27*(3), 75–86.

Wyrobek, J. (2020). Application of machine learning models and artificial intelligence to analyze annual financial statements to identify companies with unfair corporate culture. *Procedia Computer Science*, *176*, 3037–3046.

Yang, Q., Liu, Y., Cheng, Y., Kang, Y., Chen, T., & Yu, H. (Eds.). (2020). *Federated Learning*. Springer.

KEY TERMS AND DEFINITIONS

Large Language Models (LLMs): These are advanced computer programs that understand and generate human language. They've read tons of text and can respond intelligently to questions or generate written content.

Imaging Integration: This means combining images with other data (like text) so that computers can understand and use both types of information at the same time.

Multimodal Analysis: This refers to studying and using multiple kinds of information together, such as images and text, to understand things better than using just one type.

Advanced Diagnostics: This means using technology to help experts find out what's wrong in complex situations, like in medicine or engineering, with more accuracy and speed.

Real-time Processing: This is the ability of a computer to handle information as it comes in, without delays, making decisions or providing information quickly.

Intelligent Systems: These are computer systems that can learn, reason, and make decisions—often helping people in tasks that require thinking.

Chapter 8
Future Directions and Innovations in AI and Imaging

Induni Nayodhara Weerarathna
https://orcid.org/0009-0007-6996-8270
Datta Meghe Institute of Higher Education and Research, India

Matteo Hirushan Jayakody Arachchige
University of Birmingham, UK

Austin Jojo Jallah
https://orcid.org/0009-0004-0941-0281
Datta Meghe Institute of Higher Education and Research, India

Mohammad Affan Kareem
https://orcid.org/0009-0008-0303-8262
Datta Meghe Institute of Higher Education and Research, India

Kidus Manaye Mulugeta
https://orcid.org/0009-0006-4872-0076
Datta Meghe Institute of Higher Education and Research, India

ABSTRACT

Radiology has been significantly impacted by artificial intelligence (AI), which has increased imaging capabilities, workflow efficiency, and diagnostic accuracy. With an emphasis on technologies like explainable AI, generative adversarial networks, and deep learning, this book chapter examines developments in AI applications in Imaging. These tools have changed medical Imaging by making automatic segmentation, picture reconstruction, and multimodal data integration possible. AI has also

DOI: 10.4018/979-8-3373-0903-3.ch008

improved theranostic techniques, predictive analytics, and point-of-care diagnostics. Even though these developments mark a new age in radiography, issues including data privacy, moral dilemmas, and integration barriers still exist. This chapter highlights the revolutionary potential of AI-powered Imaging in both clinical and non-clinical applications while speculating about its future paths.

1. INTRODUCTION

Contextually, the continuous evolution of artificial intelligence methods to enhance and extend imaging technology is key to this field, explicitly employing AI-powered technologies to automate or improve medical imaging processes and developing more sophisticated computer vision models to analyze and interpret image and video data correctly. Since rule-based expert systems were developed in the 1980s to mimic human diagnostic reasoning, artificial intelligence has advanced dramatically in Medical Imaging. The advent of machine learning methods, particularly supervised learning, in the early 2000s made it possible to extract features from radiography data automatically. Convolutional neural networks (CNNs) have been used in radiology to diagnose breast cancer from mammograms and classify chest X-rays using ImageNet-trained models, marking a significant advancement in the field. The first autonomous AI system utilized for clinical diagnostics was IDx-DR, which was approved by the Food and Drug Administration (FDA) in 2018 (Hosny et al., 2018a).

Neural networks have long been studied for their ability to classify and interpret medical imaging data. Early systems in the 1990s used backpropagation algorithms for tumor classification. The availability of large annotated datasets, such as ImageNet, NIH ChestX-ray14, and MIMIC-CXR, catalyzed the development of more robust AI models. Landmark studies have shown that AI systems can match or even outperform radiologists in specific diagnostic tasks, increasing interest in clinical adoption (*Segmentation and Classification on Chest Radiography: A Systematic Survey | The Visual Computer*, n.d.). Through intelligent image processing, emerging breakthroughs may use deep learning, generative adversarial networks, and other AI techniques to create synthetic medical pictures, enhance image quality and resolution, and provide more precise illness identification and diagnosis (Khalifa & Albadawy, 2024a). Medical technology advancement has enhanced disease diagnosis, prevention, monitoring, treatment, and care. Imaging technologies such as computer tomography (CT), medical imaging resonance (MRI), ultrasonography (USG), positron emission tomography (PET), and others, along with digital pathology, make it easy for medical practitioners to assess and treat any disorder (Akhter et al., 2023).

AI has impacted cardiac CT in recent years, and cutting-edge techniques like machine learning (ML) and deep learning (DL) have expanded the field's use. Large datasets are used in AI-driven methods to create and train algorithms for accurate assessments and predictions (Costantini et al., 2024). With developments in computer-aided detection, automated image analysis, and predictive modeling, AI is significantly influencing radiodiagnosis. By accelerating the detection of possible anomalies, optimizing workflow, and enhancing diagnostic precision and uniformity across medical imaging modalities, AI algorithms can help radiologists. Beyond practical applications, generative AI is driving innovation and creativity. Imaging is revolutionized by diffusion models and Generative Adversarial Networks (GANs), making it possible to create incredibly lifelike synthetic pictures and animations. AI also reshapes radiology workflows, enhancing efficiency and accuracy at multiple stages, including imaging requests, scan scheduling, and image interpretation. By automating routine and time-consuming tasks, AI enhances workflow efficiency, allowing radiologists to focus on more complex cases (*Revolutionizing Radiology With Artificial Intelligence - PMC*, n.d.). This comprehensive review scrutinizes the interplay of AI and ML in radiology, exploring their foundational principles, historical progression, practical applications, inherent challenges, and ethical dilemmas (Najjar, 2023a). By enriching the understanding of AI and ML's contributions to radiology, the review seeks to stimulate meaningful conversations among doctors, researchers, and politicians to improve patient outcomes and ultimately shape the direction of the profession. The investigation explores the core ideas of AI and ML, their expanding impact on radiology, practical integration techniques, and case studies that serve as examples in various medical specialties.

Additionally, it discusses issues including data quality, moral dilemmas, and possible future paths for AI-powered radiography. A vital component of the complex machinery of multidisciplinary medical teams is radiology. By providing accurate and timely imaging results, radiologists improve communication between experts and help shape crucial decisions, supporting a patient-centered, holistic approach to healthcare (Najjar, 2023a). After decades of study and application, AI has been widely used in critical clinical functions such as computerized electrocardiogram (ECG) analysis and arterial blood gas interpretation. However, AI has only been used in radiology, which has been made possible by creating computer programs capable of complex picture processing. As technology progresses, computers may eventually replace radiologists, eliminating human error. However, some contend that AI should never serve as more than a supplement to the clinical expertise of radiologists, even if computer systems develop to such a degree and earn a profit (Fazal et al., 2018). This chapter is organized as follows: Authors begin by exploring AI's historical context and development in radiology. Next, outline current capabilities and applications, followed by key challenges and ethical considerations. Finally, it discusses emerging trends and concludes with a future outlook on AI's evolving role in medical Imaging.

2. THE CURRENT STATE OF AI AND IMAGING

The creation of visual heatmaps that illustrate the impact of individual pixels on the classification outcome is likely the most widely used set of techniques for elucidating and interpreting image-based classification methods. The most straightforward method involves visualizing the internal activations of a model, which means that one or more combinations of intermediate, two-dimensional activation values are scaled to input size and visualized. Other popular techniques rely on attributing the classification results to the individual pixels, which is accomplished in practice using techniques like Layerwise-Relevance Propagation (LRP), Gradient Input, Grad-CAM, Integrated Gradient, DeepLift, or techniques based on mathematical decomposition like LRP Agglomerative Contextual Decomposition (ACD) (Lucieri et al., 2020). As well as SHapley Additive exPlanations(SHAP). These techniques need knowledge of the model architecture and access to the model parameters. In recent years, there has been an explosion in the number of research articles on the interpretability and explainability of AI, which has led to a rise in the use and modification of AI techniques in specific medical fields. In the following sections, we highlight studies with the most application to clinical decision support systems (Panayides et al., 2020). This is a significant advancement considering the high incidence of these illnesses and AI's ability to assist radiologists in identifying and ranking patients with the most severe or complicated conditions. The study also showed how AI may be used as a second reader with a radiologist by improving lesion localization, for instance.

According to different research, AI-based computer-aided design software detected fewer false positives per picture in digital mammograms than FDA-approved software while maintaining sensitivity. Additionally, there have been notable advancements in AI in other fields, such as detecting catheters and tubes in pediatric X-ray pictures and planning therapy for brain tumors (Alexander et al., 2020). Table 1 describes the comparison of AI and Imaging.

Table 1. Artificial Intelligence and Imaging

Serial No.	category	AI Techniques Used	Current Applications	Benefits	Challenges	Future Potential	References
1.	Image Analysis & Diagnosis	Deep Learning (CNN), Computer Vision, NLP (for report)	Detection of tumors (breast, lung, bring), Identification of fractures, cardiac Imaging and detection of COVID-19 From x-ray/ CTs.	Faster, more Accurate diagnosis, reduced workload or radiologists, early detection	Data privacy, Lack of generalization, Limited interpretability	Fully autonomous Image analysis, reduced need for human oversight	("X-Ray and CT-Scan-Based Automated Detection and Classification of Covid-19 Using Convolutional Neural Networks (CNN) I Request PDF," 2024)
2.	Segmentation & Annotation	CNNs, U-Nets, Transformer Model	Organ segmentation (liver, brain, heart) For treatment planning, radiotherapy planning, surgical planning	Automation of time-consuming tasks, increased accuracy, improved planning for surgeries	Need for large, Annotated datasets, variability in anatomical feature	Real-time Segmentation During surgical procedures, integration with AR/VR	(Ramesh et al., 2023)
3.	Image Reconstruction & Enhancement	GANs, Variational Autoencoders (VAEs), Super-Resolution models	MRI, CT, and PET image reconstruction, noise reduction, super-resolution imaging	Fear imaging (fewer scans needed), lower radiation exposure, better image quality	Lack of explainability, Risk of introduction artifacts	Low-dose Imaging with full diagnostic Power improved patient safety	(Chira et al., 2022)
4.	Predictive Analytics & prognosis	Machine learning (XGBoost, Random forest), Deep learning (RNNs, LSTMs)	Predict disease Progression (e.g., Alzheimer's cancer), mortality prediction, readmission risk	Early identification of high-risk patients, proactive care, personalized treatment	Data bias, difficulty in model validation, limited generalization	Precision medicine, Personalized Health care Pathway, risk forecasting	(Nguyen et al., 2020)
5.	Workflow Automation & triage	Natural language processing (NLP), RPA(robotic process automation)	Automated reporting, prioritization of urgent cases, workflow optimization	Reduce workload on Radiologists, Improves efficiency and response times	Ethical issues (e.g., bypassing human oversight), need for workflow integration	Autonomous triage Systems, seamless Integration with hospital workflows	(*Revolutionizing Radiology with Natural Language Processing and Chatbot Technologies: A Narrative Umbrella Review on Current Trends and Future Directions*, n.d.)
6.	Multimodal Integration	Multimodal Deep learning, Data fusion	Combining CT, MRI, EHR, and pathology slides for holistic analysis	Comprehensive Patient understanding, holistic decision support	Complex data Integration, computational power, and privacy concerns	Unified patient profiles for personalized care and precision medicine	(Krones et al., 2025)

continued on following page

Table 1. Continued

Serial No.	category	AI Techniques Used	Current Applications	Benefits	Challenges	Future Potential	References
7.	Radiology Reporting	NLP, Large language models (LLMs)	Automated generation of radiology reports from imaging finding	Saves time, consistent reporting reduces human error	Limited to simple cases, may require human edits, language barriers	Fully automated, real-time, and multilingual report generation	(*Large Language Models for Structured Reporting in Radiology: Past, Present, and Future* | *European Radiology*, n.d.)
8.	AI-Driven clinical trails	AI-powered image analysis predictive modeling	Identification of trail participants, analysis of imaging biomarkers	Faster recruitment, better participant targeting, predictive trial outcomes	Regulatory Hurdles, reproducibility, data privacy	Use of imaging biomarkers for personalized drug development	(*AI in Clinical Trials*, 2024)
9.	Education and Training	Virtual Reality, AI tutors	Simulation and training for Radiologists	Improve learning Experience	High setup cost	Allowing trainees to practice interpreting rare and complex cases	(*(PDF) Healthcare Applications of Augmented Reality(AR) and Virtual Reality (VR)*, 2024)
10.	Decision Support	Ensemble learning, NLP	Assisting Radiologist with diagnosis	Reduce Workload	Risk of over-reliance.	Reducing human bias in training evaluation.	(*(PDF) Healthcare Applications of Augmented Reality(AR) and Virtual Reality (VR)*, 2024)

AI will significantly impact the medical imaging industry and, consequently, radiologists' jobs, enabling them to accurately diagnose patients, expedite scan times, and reduce burden. With the growing value of AI in Medical Imaging, it is not easy to think that AI will not eventually revolutionize radiology (Alexander et al., 2020).

This Characterization broadly captures the segmentation, diagnosis, and staging of tumors. It can also include prognostication based on a given ailment and outcome prediction based on specific treatment modalities. Segmentation defines the extent of an abnormality. This can range from basic 2-dimensional (2D) measurements of the maximal in-plane tumor diameter to more involved volumetric segmentations in which the entire tumor and possibly surrounding tissues are assessed (Bi et al., 2019). Figure 1 shows the workflow process of using the suggested machine-learning algorithms for diagnosis.

Figure 1. The workflow process of using the suggested machine learning algorithms for diagnosis

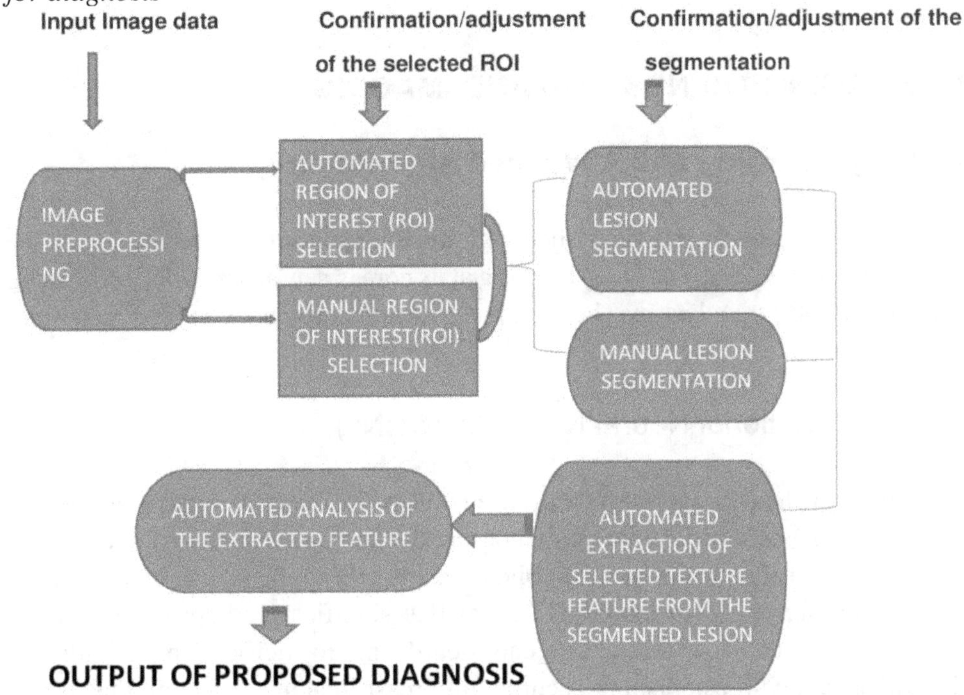

Even with AI's potential in radiology, certain intrinsic drawbacks still exist that might result in expensive diagnostic mistakes, most notably the inability to combine crucial clinical data with long-term imaging data. To overcome these constraints, AI models must be trained on various information, such as comprehensive clinical data and patient histories. Open communication between experts is essential to patient care as modern clinical medicine grows more specialized (Katal et al., 2024). Global healthcare expenses are constantly rising; therefore, making efficient use of the little resources available is crucial. AI may help with this in both non-clinical and clinical ways. AI software may help schedule imaging appointments before patients arrive at the radiology department. It could also forecast no-shows for helpful reminders or more effective scheduling. A model was developed by Chong et al. to identify patients who were most likely to skip their appointments. The no-show percentage dropped from 19.3% to 15.9% when these patients got a phone call reminder. Most of these solutions focus on boundary circumstances like patient management rather than necessarily detecting or diagnosing the illness. Thus, there is less danger associated with the applications. As well as have fewer requirements to meet before being used in therapeutic settings. However, the sector has space to develop because such software is unavailable and deployed (Alhussain et al., 2022a).

3. EMERGING TRENDS IN AI AND IMAGING

3.1 Deep Learning and Advanced Algorithms

AI-driven radiology has flourished with the emergence of deep learning as the backbone of image analysis. Deep learning at its core is neural networks, processing and learning off large datasets showing patterns humans cannot notice (Nakamura et al., 2024).

3.1.1 Convolutional Neural Networks (CNNs):

Modern medical image analysis is based on CNNs. These architectures are outstanding in image classification, segmentation, and anomaly detection. For example, existing state-of-the-art CNNs are applied to early-stage lung cancer identification by searching for small nodules in CT scans that significantly improve diagnostic sensitivity. We also find that CNNs can identify microcalcifications, a hallmark of malignancy, with astonishing accuracy in breast imaging, reducing the risk of missing such a diagnosis.

3.1.2 Transformers in Imaging:

Now, transformer models are transforming imaging analysis, which is borrowed from natural language processing. Transformers have become successful by employing attention mechanisms that facilitate multi-scale feature extraction capacity and, hence, discovering the complex relationship in imaging datasets. For instance, Vision Transformers (ViTs) have shown superior performance on chest radiographs in a few problem areas, such as pneumothorax and fractures.

3.1.3 Self-Supervised Learning (SSL):

SSL represents a change in the paradigm of AI learning methodologies, where algorithms can learn from large amounts of unlabeled data. This innovation decreases reliance on manually annotated datasets, a significant bottleneck for radiology. For instance, we use SSL to pre-train models on large public datasets of brain MRI scans and then fine-tune them on a specific diagnostic task, such as tumor detection or multiple sclerosis characterization.

3.2 Explainable AI (XAI)

While having unparalleled capabilities, diagnosis with AI is also opaque regarding how it reaches its conclusions, making it challenging to trust and adopt. This challenge requires a critical response in which Explainable AI (XAI) prioritizes transparency and interpretability with no loss in performance.

XAI systems use visualization tools to show the picture elements that shape an AI's prediction. For example, heatmaps over the suspected areas of abnormality allow radiologists to have insightful clues about how the AI is reasoning. It promotes collaboration in decision-making and increases confidence in the diagnosis. LRP outlines AI predictions and which input features contribute to the outcome. LRP is a technique that brings out explainability and is used to interpret the predictions made by highly complex deep learning models. For example, LRP can help close that gap between the algorithmic output and the clinical reasoning of brain tumor grading by showing how tiny changes in MRI signal intensity across different MRI regions can underlie how an AI model classifies.

XAI builds trust through its recommendations by enabling us to provide clear justifications. Aidoc's AI platform for intracranial hemorrhage detection includes explainability features that have helped it get regulatory approvals and adoption in high-stakes clinical settings (Neri et al., 2023).

3.3 Multimodal Imaging

Multimodal AI is not a new approach to medical Imaging. It is a holistic approach to combining a multitude of imaging modalities along with clinical data, which is a leap for patient care. At the same time, the integration of complementary datasets provides unprecedented diagnostic insights offered by AI systems.

Precision diagnostics are driven by AI models that combine genetic and proteomic data to image data. Combining MRI-derived radiomic features with genomic profiles can help provide a nuanced view of the behavior of the tumor in glioblastoma analysis and guide personalized treatment strategies. Multimodal AI is good at tracking disease progression over time. Models combining PET imaging and cognitive and biochemical data can predict disease trajectory in Alzheimer's research and enable clinicians to make informed therapeutic decisions. In cancer care, multimodal AI is changing tumor classification and prognosis. For example, PET/CT data and molecular markers facilitate more precise non-small cell lung carcinoma staging and mandate more accurate treatment planning. The principles of precision medicine highlighted above, tailoring care to individual patient profiles while resulting in this integration paradigm, also enhance diagnostic accuracy(Kitamura & Topol, 2023).

3.4 Predictive and personalized diagnostics

AI can forecast potential health issues based on historical data and make early diagnoses and interventions. AI can become a proactive health strategy in predictive analytics as it recognizes risks before they become severe. Additionally, AI's application is also possible in personalized medicine, which allows the diagnostic approaches to be tailored to each patient's characteristics to achieve more accurate diagnoses and customized treatment plans (Khalifa & Albadawy, 2024b).

4. INNOVATIONS IN IMAGING TECHNOLOGIES ENHANCED BY AI

4.1 3D and 4D Imaging: AI's Role in Improving Spatial and Temporal Resolution

With 3D and 4D imaging technologies, diagnostic radiology has revolutionized to incorporate comprehensive information about anatomical and physiological processes in a spatial and temporal context. However, AI significantly enhances these modalities, with spatial and temporal resolution information bounds approaching perfection. With these deep learning algorithms, image reconstruction reduces noise and artifacts, leading to a profound ability to visualize intricate anatomical details with unprecedented clarity. Studies have shown that using AI-based denoising methods, such as CNN, has proven to increase the diagnostic quality from low-dose CT scans by lowering the noise while maintaining fine structural quality (Shao et al., 2024).

Similarly, in dynamic MRI applications, clinical evaluations have demonstrated that AI-driven reconstruction techniques significantly reduce imaging times while not affecting image fidelity. These improvements mean better images and more accuracy in diagnosis and, therefore, better patient outcomes. For example, AI-enhanced CNN-based reconstruction algorithms perform better in artifact correction and noise reduction in cardiac MRI, resulting in better diagnostic capability (Prasad et al., 2024). In 4D Imaging, AI aids real-time analysis by managing the massive volumes of data obtained during dynamic imaging studies, like respiratory-gated CT scans. This capability enables accurate motion tracking for applications like radiation therapy planning and Functional Imaging.

Beyond resolution, AI helps with faster workflow in 3D and 4D Imaging. AI-powered automated segmentation tools help delineate anatomical structures for radiologists, saving time and effort. In cardiac MRI studies, an application for AI algorithms is automatic segmentation of the heart and the major vessels, allowing accurate quantification of specific criteria like ejection fraction and myocardial strain. Studies have proved that in cardiac Imaging, AI-powered segmentation tools like U-Net and DeepMedic architectures are precise and efficient and have also demonstrated near-human performance in delineating myocardial boundaries and ventricular volumes, improving reproducibility, and reducing inter-observer variability (Morales et al., 2024). In addition, research states that AI segmentation can increase diagnostic reliability while shortening analysis times by as much as 70%, thereby streamlining workflows. Continued advances in image registration with AI have led to easy alignment of sequential images (in 4D studies) to track disease progression or response to treatment over time (Bissell et al., 2023).

AI-driven motion estimation techniques in 4D optical coherence tomography (OCT) can provide robust tracking of dynamic changes in tissues, which is critical for implementing OCT applications such as cardiovascular Imaging (Bengs et al., 2020). With AI-based reconstruction, cine-MRI has yielded high-resolution anatomical Imaging from under-sampled datasets even quickly enough to accelerate Imaging without losing diagnostic quality (Shao et al., 2024). Additionally, AI-enabled technologies develop predictive models that mimic temporal patient-specific physiological changes to support personalized treatment planning and research activities.

4.2 Augmented and Virtual Reality (AR/VR): Applications in radiology training and diagnosis

Radiology has found AR and VR to be transformative tools for training and improving diagnostic accuracy by merging real-world and virtual environments. AI-enhanced AR/VR applications bring immersive, risk-free experiences of complex medical procedures, such as interventional radiology, to medical trainees. Platforms like Osso VR and Touch Surgery have successfully provided realistic procedural simulation, including interactive feedback. These technologies also permit the secure combination of 3D anatomical models with patient images during preoperative planning, thus allowing surgeons to have remarkable spatial awareness. Similarly, HoloLens from Microsoft has been incorporated into radiology workflows to visualize complex anatomical structures in AR, enhancing surgical precision and radiological interpretation.

AR and VR platforms with AI-driven analytics added to radiology training provide personalized feedback to trainees to enhance their skills iteratively. In particular, these tools help teach complex tasks, such as navigating catheter-based interventions or interpreting subtle imaging findings. AI-enabled AR can help adequately identify regions of interest within an imaging dataset, extending radiologists during the diagnosis process faster and more accurately. For example, AI-featured AR headsets can project real-time enhanced imaging data onto the physical patient during procedures, leading to real-time decision-making during interventional radiology.

Using VR platforms with AI-powered diagnostic systems has accelerated training efficiency and diagnostic accuracy by simulating real-life scenarios such as fracture assessment and tumor localization (D. Wang et al., 2024). Table 2 describes the difference between AR and VR.

Table 2. Difference Between Augmented Reality (AR) and Virtual Reality (VR)

Sr.No	Features	AR	VR	References
1	**Definition**	Enhances the real-world environment by overlaying digital information	Creates a complete, immersive, computer-generated virtual environment.	(Neri et al., 2023; D. Wang et al., 2024)
2	**Interaction with reality**	Integrates virtual objects into the real-world view.	Replaces the real-world environment entirely with a virtual one.	(D. Wang et al., 2024)
3	**Application in Radiology**	Preoperative planning, guiding interventional procedures.	Training in complex procedures such as tumors, etc.; simulating diagnostic scenarios.	(D. Wang et al., 2024)
4	**Uses beyond Radiology**	Used in rehabilitation, anatomy education, and telemedicine.	In surgical simulation, pain management, and phobia treatment.	(Neri et al., 2023; D. Wang et al., 2024)
5	**Examples**	AR glasses/headsets (e.g., Microsoft HoloLens).	VR headsets (e.g., Oculus Rift, HTC Vive).	(D. Wang et al., 2024)
6	**Level of Immersion**	Partial immersion: users remain aware of the real world.	Complete immersion: users are isolated from the real-world environment.	(D. Wang et al., 2024)
7	**Key advantages**	Enhances spatial awareness and real-time interaction.	It gives risk-free training in a controlled virtual space.	(D. Wang et al., 2024)

4.3 AI-Assisted Image Reconstruction: Speeding Up and Enhancing Imaging Techniques Like MRI and CT

AI has transformed image reconstruction processes in MRI and CT. Traditional reconstruction techniques are typically computationally intensive and time-consuming iterative processes. However, AI-based algorithms, such as CNNs, accelerate these processes by learning the pattern from the trained datasets to generate high-quality images from raw data.

For example, AI-aided techniques such as deep learning reconstruction (DLR) facilitate ultra-fast MRI scans with improved image quality without patient discomfort or scanner occupancy. In particular, these advancements are important in settings where patient movement can negatively impact image quality, such as in pediatric Imaging and patients with movement disorders. In CT, AI boosts low-dose

Imaging by preserving diagnostic accuracy while lowering radiation dose to critical groups such as pediatric and high-risk patients. Additionally, AI has made spectral CT possible, which uses AI algorithms to process multi-energy data to create material-specific images, allowing new possibilities for tissue characterization and quantitative Imaging.

In low-dose CT imaging, deep learning-based reconstruction achieves a diagnostic quality similar to standard dose techniques and up to 80% reduction in radiation exposure (Brady, 2023). Chen et al. demonstrated that AI-based reconstructions could preserve diagnostic accuracy comparable to the standard dose while obtaining. A significant reduction in noise and preservation of edge details using a deep learning algorithm. The algorithms studied were tested via a multicenter design to ensure that the results were robust over different scanners and patient populations and shown to be likely capable of reducing radiation exposure without loss of diagnostic utility. AI-driven reconstructions have been shown in MRI to improve spatial resolution and reduce acquisition times with no compromise in image clarity (Lin et al., 2021). Additionally, the use of generative adversarial networks (GANs) for additional improvement in reconstruction fidelity is explored to achieve sharper and more accurate images in challenging cases.

4.4 Hybrid Imaging Modalities: AI applications combining PET/CT, SPECT/MRI, etc.

PET/CT and Single Photon Emission Computed Tomography (SPECT) /MRI have revolutionized medical diagnostics by developing hybrid imaging technologies that integrate two powerful Imaging approaches into one unified imaging system. These sophisticated tools combine anatomical Imaging (using MRI to show the body's structures) with functional Imaging (using SPECT to show processes within the body), thus yielding a picture of the body's form and function. With AI, these modalities are integrated and enhanced by automating the image registration and fusion steps, ensuring data for different modalities are precisely aligned. AI-driven approaches register much more quickly and accurately than existing traditional manual methods. AI reduces the human errors that can happen at the critical stage when aligning two images from different modalities, for example, trying to perfectly overlay two transparent sheets, with a tiny misalignment leading to incorrect interpretation. Studies revealed that AI performs imaging fusion with greater precision and less variability among operators, increasing hybrid imaging reliability in clinical settings (El-Bejou et al., 2020). What makes AI powerful in hybrid Imaging is that it can find things where we cannot, a combination of multiple types of imaging data that might be very subtle. For example, AI can also look at anatomical structures (from CT or MRI) and metabolic activity (from PET or SPECT) co-occurring and spot correlations that help physicians become more certain when diagnosing a cancer patient. In the case of complex medical fields such as oncology and neurology, where it is important to understand structure and function to diagnose and plan treatment, this multi-layered analysis becomes quite valuable.

AI-enabled analysis of PET/CT scans can quantify tumor metabolic activity and structural changes in the same scan, providing a better characterization of the tumor and assessing tumor responsiveness to therapy. This capability is significant for oncology, where accurate quantification of tumor metabolism and morphology provides input for the planning of treatment and prognosis. In SPECT/MRI, AI can enable the integration of functional and structural data to improve diagnostic accuracy for epilepsy and Parkinson's disease. AI algorithms can also detect more subtle patterns throughout multimodal datasets that might escape conventional analysis, allowing early detection of diseases like Alzheimer's.

Machine learning algorithms for PET/CT and SPECT/MRI datasets applied to cardiac Imaging for handling vessel pathology have improved the accuracy of myocardial viability assessments, which can provide a new understanding of ischemic heart disease (Leiner et al., 2019). Furthermore, AI is evolving quantitative Imaging, which can be applied to precise volumetric and texture analysis to advance clinical decision-making and other research. Table 2 represents the comparison of AI applications in imaging modalities.

Table 3. Comparison of AI Applications in Imaging Modalities

Sr No.	Imaging Modality	Traditional Methods	AI-Driven Advancements	References
1	**3D/4D Imaging**	Time-consuming manual reconstruction	AI speeds up reconstruction and improves noise reduction.	(Prasad et al., 2024; Shao et al., 2024)
2	**Hybrid Imaging**	Manual image fusion is prone to errors	AI automates and improves fusion accuracy	(El-Bejou et al., 2020; Leiner et al., 2019)
3	**Low-Dose CT**	Higher radiation exposure	AI enables low-dose Imaging with diagnostic quality.	(Brady, 2023)

5. FUTURE APPLICATIONS AND TRANSFORMATION

5.1 Point-of-Care Imaging

Point of care imaging represents the process of Imaging at the patient's bedside without transporting the patient to centralized radiology departments. AI has transformed traditional medical Imaging into a new era with a significant impact on how we deliver diagnostic care, especially in resource-constrained environments where expertise is scarce or unavailable. These portable systems were not as sophisticated as the bulkier centralized infrastructure in hospitals, and previous diagnoses heavily relied on the operator's expertise. However, the combination of AI and portable imaging technology has rocked this area. Currently, AI-augmented portable ultrasound can offer automatic image interpretation and the ability to detect potential abnormalities while making specialist-level expertise available when these remote sites have no radiologist on board (Rubin, 2019).

AI's application in point-of-care Imaging is not limited to image interpretation. Najjar's (2023) studies demonstrated that AI algorithms redefine the diagnostic workflow by allowing real-time analysis. Today, these systems can execute AI-based edge computing locally on images, enabling a portable X-ray machine to quickly identify a fracture or pneumothorax without an Internet connection or by shipping images away to a remote specialist in central facilities. This capability can become life-saving (Najjar, 2023b). AI-enhanced imaging tools are redefining emergency and trauma care. For instance, these tools can immediately evaluate CT scans for intracranial hemorrhage in a patient complaining of a suspected brain injury, processing a critical diagnostics decision within moments instead of waiting the usual time for a specialist to interpret them (Wismüller & Stockmaster, 2020). This advancement is beneficial in situations without fast access to specialists, such as outlying or low-asset environments.

Though some of these advances are genuinely remarkable, point-of-care Imaging augmented by AI still has issues to overcome. The initial cost of advanced hardware and, more generally, the associated infrastructure and the supported maintenance of such sophisticated systems in remote locations also present unique challenges regarding ensuring consistent image quality. Innovation is being made in edge computing architecture, lower-priced hardware and software, and the creation of robust training data sets relevant to the patient population and clinical settings.

5.2 AI-Driven Clinical Decision Systems

AI's presence in diagnostic precision and patient management is a massive leap in clinical decision support systems (CDSS). AI works seamlessly with electronic health records (EHRs), enabling clinicians with real-time information, streamlining workflows, decreasing errors, and developing more personal care.

The power of these AI-driven systems is that they can synthesize many streams of medical data. Instead of looking at Imaging in isolation, they combine all the radiological findings with the medical history, laboratory, and genetic findings for a holistic diagnosis. It is beneficial when you have an emergency. Imagine a scenario where a patient arrives at the emergency department. Using this AI system, important abnormal findings on imaging studies are immediately identified and linked to relevant patient EHR information and provide evidence-based recommendations for further action, including ordering more tests and immediate treatment (Farič et al., 2024).

Although it has benefits, implementing AI-driven CDSS is not a piece of cake. A significant area of concern rests in algorithmic bias: if an AI has been trained on data that does not reflect all patients, it may, in turn, only perpetuate or exacerbate healthcare disparities. Additionally, patient privacy and data security are still a priority when combined with AI. These challenges are addressed by healthcare providers, tech developers, and regulatory bodies working together towards transparency, growing diversity in training data, and installing strong security mechanisms (Dikici et al., 2019).

Interoperability – the seamless work of different systems performing functions simply and efficiently is critical to the success of AI deployment in clinical settings. AI solutions must be embedded naturally within the existing EHR systems and imaging platforms to avoid disruptions. For example, in radiology departments, the smoother transitions experienced when using interoperable AI tools are reported with reduced implementation costs and improved clinician satisfaction. By selecting systems programmed for compatibility with the facilities, workflows, and scalability are efficient and possible within facilities of varying capacities (Jorg et al., 2024).

The Enhancement of AI in clinical decision support systems is based on the setup of good feedback loops. These loops enable clinicians to give real-time validation of the insights delivered by AI and the systems to continue to learn and adapt to real-world clinical scenarios. The system continually goes through this ongoing refinement process as we build trust among healthcare providers and continually make the system so much more reliable and effective (Dikici et al., 2019).

The future looks extremely exciting for AI-driven clinical decision support systems. These are increasingly predictive systems that leverage population health data to predict disease trends and prevent outcomes that could happen. While this improvement in diagnostic accuracy is undoubtedly a success, it symbolizes a significant step toward more complete and fair healthcare delivery, where sophisticated clinical decision support will eventually be available to all healthcare providers, regardless of geographical area or resources.

5.3 Automated Reporting and Annotations:

AI-powered automated reporting and annotation systems have become an advanced version of radiology workflow. These tools examine the medical imaging data, pinpoint the critical findings, and produce structured diagnostic reports. These systems limit radiologists' workload by automatically annotating abnormalities such as lesions, fractures, or masses in the images and provide powerful assistive points of view to radiologists, increasing the consistency and accuracy of diagnostic reporting.

The prompt for structured and automated reports depends upon complex AI algorithms and natural language processing. These systems assess imaging data, conduct them carefully, compile preliminary findings, and finely point out areas that require attention. Wang and colleagues, in 2024, demonstrate that through tools such as CopilotCAD, which shows how reporting tools can automate reporting processes and standardize reporting across multiple healthcare institutions for pragmatic consistency of diagnostic communication (S. Wang et al., 2024).

The annotating capacities of these reporting systems efficiently improve workflow in radiology departments. These intelligent tools precisely identify and mark important imaging findings (tumors, calcifications, fractures) that go into more accurate, more uniform radiology reports. This capability is particularly adjuvant in emergency departments, where making fast, correct decisions can be a matter of life and death. Sloan and colleagues 2024 stated that automated systems for quickly identifying critical findings like intracranial hemorrhages or pulmonary embolisms in CT scans could speed up patient care by dramatically shortening the radiological review time (Sloan et al., 2024).

These AI-driven reporting systems are built on natural language processing. One of the studies explained the use of Natural Language Processing (NLP) in these systems to understand complex clinical terms and contexts and produce accurate reports that seamlessly integrate with more general patient information. Because of the flexibility of technology in evolving with changing medical terminology, it is very relevant in this ever-changing healthcare environment. Leveraging NLP, these solutions generate highly precise, clinically relevant narratives, which radiologists can further refine to standardize reporting formats, reduce errors, and increase the quality of diagnostic communication in general (Syed & Zoga, 2018).

You need to understand that these automated reporting tools are genuine complements and not replacements of radiologists. These systems free up valuable time for radiologists to discuss complex cases with the referring physicians and make critical clinical decisions.

These systems have the potential to bring significant benefits to patients when implemented. This significantly reduces the diagnostic waiting time, which gets especially critical in time-sensitive conditions such as trauma or stroke. Moreover, these systems also increase diagnostic accuracy based on consistency and eliminate errors between several healthcare providers.

5.4 Theranostics in Radiology

Theranostic is a combination of diagnostic Imaging and therapeutic intervention that personalizes medical treatment for an individual patient. Radiology uses imaging techniques like PET-CT or SPECT to identify disease sites and then apply targeted therapies, often via radiopharmaceuticals, to diagnose, treat, and follow disease progression. AI enhances this process by assessing imaging data to suggest the appropriate therapy decisions.

AI in theranostics can examine imaging data to identify specific disease markers, accurately measure tumor burden, and predict patient treatment response. In oncology, for example, AI systems can scan through PET-CT scans, looking for the pinpoint details of elevated metabolic activity that correlates with suspicious malignancies. These insights help physicians to deliver competent radiopharmaceuticals like Lutetium 177, explicitly targeting cancer cells but spare healthy tissue, better treatment delivery, and regulating therapy effectiveness. This precision of diagnosis in targeting therapy now provides each patient with a therapy specific to their condition that may improve treatment outcomes and decrease adverse effects (Belge Bilgin et al., 2024).

Theranostic is not limited to therapy but also treatment monitoring through real-time assessment of therapeutic effectiveness, all of which have been part of the contribution made by AI. Clinicians can monitor changes, such as tumor size, metabolic activity, and disease progression, to modify treatment protocol decisions. Such a robust approach to treatment monitoring and setting of treatment parameters improves precise interventions and better patient outcomes (Yazdani et al., 2024).

However, despite its promising potential, implementing AI-driven theranostics faces multiple important challenges. The key concerns necessary to build confidence for healthcare providers and patients include ensuring that AI algorithms are accurate, that the data used to train those systems are not biased, and that there is transparency in how treatment decisions are made. Indeed, integrating these advanced tools into existing healthcare systems depends upon ground-level collaborations and thorough technology validation (Burkett et al., 2023).

Theranostics will evolve as a broad approach to integrate genomic, proteomic, and clinical data to develop highly personalized treatment strategies. With ongoing research, this field has promising potential to combine AI with emerging technologies, such as theranostic nanoparticles. Table 4 shows the AI-featured imaging technologies.

Table 4. AI-featured Imaging Technologies

Sr. No	Features	Definition	Examples	References
1	**3D/4D Imaging**	AI enhances spatial and temporal resolution, enabling noise reduction, artifact correction, and real-time analysis in dynamic imaging studies.	AI-driven motion tracking in respiratory-gated CT; AI-enhanced cardiac MRI reconstruction.	(Morales et al., 2024; Prasad et al., 2024; Shao et al., 2024)
2	**AR**	AR overlays digital information onto real-world environments to assist with surgical planning and interventional radiology.	Microsoft HoloLens is used for surgical precision, and AI-enhanced AR is used to identify regions of interest.	(Neri et al., 2023; S. Wang et al., 2024)
3	**VR**	VR creates immersive virtual environments for radiology training and preoperative simulations.	Osso VR is used for procedural training, and touch surgery is used for interventional skills.	(S. Wang et al., 2024)
4	**Hybrid Imaging**	AI integrates modalities like PET/CT and SPECT/MRI by automating image registration and fusion, enabling comprehensive diagnostic insights.	AI-based tumor metabolism quantification in PET/CT; AI-assisted SPECT/MRI for neurological diseases.	(El-Bejou et al., 2020; Leiner et al., 2019)
5	**Image Reconstruction**	AI accelerates MRI and CT reconstruction processes, reducing acquisition times and enhancing image quality, particularly in low-dose settings.	Deep learning reconstruction (DLR) for MRI; AI in spectral CT for tissue characterization.	(Brady, 2023; Lin et al., 2021)
6	**Multimodal Imaging**	Combines imaging data with clinical datasets to drive precision diagnostics and personalized treatment strategies.	PET and genomic data integration for Alzheimer's research; MRI and proteomic data for glioblastoma.	(Kitamura & Topol, 2023; Yazdani et al., 2024)

continued on following page

Table 4. Continued

Sr. No	Features	Definition	Examples	References
7	**Explainable AI (XAI)**	Provides transparency in AI predictions through tools like heat maps and Layer-Wise Relevance Propagation (LRP).	Aidoc for hemorrhage detection with explainability features.	(Neri et al., 2023)
8	**Point-of-Care Imaging**	Portable imaging systems enhanced by AI enable bedside diagnostics with rapid analysis and interpretation.	AI-based portable X-ray for pneumothorax detection; AI-augmented ultrasound for remote settings.	(Najjar, 2023b; Rubin, 2019)
9	**Predictive Diagnostics**	AI forecasts health risks using historical data, enabling early detection and personalized care plans.	Predicting disease trajectory in Alzheimer's; early detection of cardiac risks from Imaging.	(Khalifa & Albadawy, 2024b)
10	**Theranostics**	Combines Diagnostic Imaging with targeted therapeutic interventions, leveraging AI for precise delivery and monitoring of radiopharmaceuticals.	PET/CT guides Lutetium-177 therapy, and tumor response tracking is done with AI.	(Belge Bilgin et al., 2024; Yazdani et al., 2024)
11	**Automated Reporting**	AI-driven tools streamline radiology reporting by auto-annotating critical findings and generating structured diagnostic reports.	CopilotCAD is used for report standardization; automated fracture annotation is used in emergency CT.	(Sloan et al., 2024; S. Wang et al., 2024)
12	**Clinical Decision Support**	AI integrates imaging data with EHRs for holistic diagnoses and actionable recommendations, enhancing decision-making processes.	Linking imaging findings to EHR in emergency scenarios; AI-driven evidence-based recommendations.	(Dikici et al., 2019; Jorg et al., 2024)

6. ETHICAL AND REGULATORY CONSIDERATIONS

As AI becomes increasingly integral to Imaging, ethical and regulatory challenges must be addressed to ensure its safe and equitable deployment. Data privacy, algorithmic bias, and the transparency of AI decision-making processes will require robust frameworks to ensure fairness and accountability(Geis et al., 2019). For instance, ensuring compliance with standards like HIPAA for patient data or implementing explainable AI (XAI) models that allow clinicians to understand and trust AI recommendations will be critical.

Collaboration between technologists, clinicians, and policymakers will be essential in creating guidelines that balance innovation with patient safety(Litjens et al., 2017). Future AI systems must be explainable, providing clinicians with clear insights into their decision-making processes to build trust and ensure ethical use. Additionally, mechanisms for continuous monitoring and validation of AI systems post-deployment will be necessary to maintain performance and safety standards.

Education and training will also play a vital role in addressing ethical concerns. Equipping healthcare professionals with the knowledge to interpret and scrutinize AI-driven insights will foster a culture of accountability and ensure that these technologies augment rather than replace human judgment. (Patel et al., 2024)

While healthcare remains a primary focus, the implications of AI in Imaging extend to other domains, such as environmental monitoring, security, and entertainment(Zech et al., 2018). For example, AI-powered imaging systems are used in wildlife conservation to track and monitor endangered species using drone-captured images. These systems can analyze animal behavior, habitat changes, and population dynamics with unprecedented precision, aiding conservation efforts.

In astronomy, AI helps process terabytes of data from telescopes, enabling the identification of extrasolar or distant galaxies. By automating data analysis and pattern recognition, AI accelerates previously unattainable discoveries, deepening our understanding of the universe. (Kumar, 2022) Similarly, in urban planning, AI-driven imaging systems can analyze real-time traffic patterns, optimizing city infrastructure for efficiency and sustainability. These applications illustrate the transformative potential of AI in addressing global challenges and advancing scientific discovery.

In the creative industries, AI-enhanced Imaging is revolutionizing fields like film, gaming, and virtual reality. By enabling hyper-realistic visuals and dynamic scene generation, these technologies push the boundaries of storytelling and immersive experiences, offering new avenues for artistic expression (Z. Zhang, 2024).

7. CHALLENGES AND POTENTIAL SOLUTIONS

AI has revolutionized the field of Imaging, transforming how we capture, process, and interpret visual information across industries. From medical diagnostics and remote sensing to entertainment and industrial automation, AI-driven imaging technologies have demonstrated their potential to enhance precision, efficiency, and decision-making. Despite these advancements, the journey toward fully realizing the potential of AI in Imaging is fraught with challenges. Data scarcity, ethical concerns, interpretability, and scalability pose significant barriers to innovation and widespread adoption. Addressing these challenges is critical for advancing the state of the art and ensuring that these technologies are equitable, reliable, and aligned with societal needs.

Annotating medical imaging data is time-consuming and costly, limiting the size of training datasets. Models trained on one population may not generalize well to others, raising concerns about equity and bias. Algorithmic transparency, or the lack thereof, also affects clinician trust. Meanwhile, trends such as multimodal models, federated learning, and real-time inference are shaping the future of AI in this field. Ethical debates persist over whether AI should replace or augment radiologists.

To bridge the gap between current challenges and future possibilities, it is essential to develop innovative solutions that address the limitations of AI in Imaging. Overcoming hurdles such as biased datasets, computational inefficiencies, and regulatory disparities will require a synergistic approach that combines technological advancements with policy-making and public engagement. Equally important is fostering transparency and trust by creating explainable AI systems that empower users to understand and validate the decisions made by these technologies. By tackling these issues head-on, the field can establish a solid foundation for integrating AI in Imaging, paving the way for groundbreaking innovations that will define the future of this domain.

Looking ahead, the future of AI in Imaging is both inspiring and complex. Emerging trends such as multimodal data integration, explainable AI, and real-time processing are shaping the next generation of imaging technologies. The convergence of AI with cutting-edge fields like quantum computing, neuroscience, and synthetic biology promises transformative possibilities. However, realizing this vision will require interdisciplinary collaboration, robust policy frameworks, and a steadfast commitment to ethical practices. This chapter explores the challenges and potential solutions in AI and Imaging while envisioning a future where these technologies seamlessly integrate into diverse applications, driving innovation and societal progress. Table 5 describes the challenges and potential solutions for each.

Table 5. Challenges and potential solutions related to AI in Medical Imaging

Sr.No	Challenge	Description	Potential Solution	Reference
1	**Data Availability and Quality**	• AI models rely on large, high-quality datasets for training. However, many industries, especially healthcare, face challenges in collecting diverse, representative, and annotated datasets. Biases in datasets can lead to skewed outcomes and reduced model reliability.	• Implement federated learning to access decentralized and secure data from multiple sources without violating privacy laws. • Data augmentation techniques are used to expand the size and diversity of datasets artificially. • Leverage generative adversarial networks (GANs) to produce high-quality synthetic data to fill real-world data gaps.	(Goodfellow et al., 2016)
2	**Ethical and Privacy Concerns**	• Using sensitive data, such as medical images or personal photos, raises concerns about privacy violations, data misuse, and potential discrimination. Additionally, the proliferation of deepfakes threatens societal trust in digital media.	• Apply privacy-preserving methods such as differential privacy and homomorphic encryption to protect individual data. • Develop robust frameworks for detecting and mitigating misuse, including deep fake identification systems. • Advocate for comprehensive regulations and ethical guidelines governing the use of AI in sensitive domains.	(Zhu et al., 2024)
3	**High Computational Costs**	• Training and deploying AI models, intense learning models, require significant computational resources, often leading to high energy consumption and environmental impact. This also creates a barrier for smaller organizations.	• Optimize AI models by pruning unnecessary parameters, applying quantization, and using knowledge distillation to reduce model complexity. • Transition to edge computing for local processing to minimize dependency on large-scale data centers. • Explore emerging technologies like quantum computing and neuromorphic hardware to enhance energy efficiency.	(LeCun et al., 2015)
4	**Lack of Interpretability**	• AI models often operate as black boxes, making it difficult for users to understand their decision-making process. This lack of transparency undermines trust and limits the adoption of AI in critical areas like healthcare.	• Develop explainable AI (XAI) tools, such as saliency maps, attention mechanisms, and feature importance visualizations, to help users interpret AI decisions. • Encourage the adoption of inherently interpretable models like decision trees or linear models where possible. • Standardize reporting of AI decision rationale to ensure consistency and reliability.	(Russell & Norvig, 2016)
5	**Integration Challenges**	• Many existing imaging systems are not designed to accommodate AI integration. This results in compatibility issues, high costs of retrofitting, and technical challenges in merging old and new systems.	• Develop open-source libraries and APIs to bridge gaps between legacy systems and AI platforms. • Encourage collaboration between hardware manufacturers and AI developers to ensure forward compatibility. • Introduce modular AI solutions that can be seamlessly incorporated into existing infrastructure.	(Esteva et al., 2019)
6	**Bias and Fairness Issues**	• AI models trained on biased data can perpetuate and amplify disparities, leading to unfair healthcare, hiring, and law enforcement outcomes.	• Regularly audit AI models for bias and fairness using diverse validation datasets. • Ensure datasets are representative of different demographics and conditions. • Develop algorithms that can detect and correct biases during training and inference.	(Kaushal et al., 2020)

continued on following page

Table 5. Continued

Sr.No	Challenge	Description	Potential Solution	Reference
7	**Legal and Regulatory Hurdles**	• Variations in AI regulations across regions create challenges in deploying imaging technologies globally. Regulatory frameworks often lag behind technological advancements, creating uncertainty for developers and users.	• Advocate for the creation of harmonized global AI standards to streamline deployment. • Work closely with policymakers during the AI development process to ensure compliance. • Implement robust documentation and transparency measures to simplify regulatory approval processes.	(Zaidan & Ibrahim, 2024)
8	**Limited Domain Expertise in AI Teams**	• Many AI development teams lack specialized knowledge in domains such as medical Imaging or industrial inspection, leading to poorly tailored solutions.	• Foster interdisciplinary collaboration by integrating domain experts into AI development teams. • Provide domain-specific training to AI researchers and engineers. • Develop publicly available benchmarks and guidelines for specialized imaging applications.	(Hong et al., 2023)
9	**Overfitting and Generalization Issues**	• AI models trained on limited or overly specific datasets may overfit, performing well on training data but poorly on new, unseen data.	• Implement regularization techniques, such as dropout, weight decay, and early stopping, to prevent overfitting. • Train models on larger, more diverse datasets and conduct cross-validation to assess generalization. • Use ensemble methods to combine predictions from multiple models for greater robustness.	(Liu et al., 2023)
10	**Real-Time Processing Limitations**	• Real-time applications, such as autonomous vehicles or emergency medical imaging, require high-speed processing with minimal latency, which current AI models sometimes struggle to achieve.	• Design lightweight AI architectures optimized for speed, such as MobileNets. • Use hardware accelerators like GPUs, TPUs, and FPGAs to enhance processing efficiency. • Implement asynchronous and distributed processing to handle real-time workloads effectively.	(Park et al., 2023)
11	**Scalability Challenges**	Scaling AI solutions from prototypes to real-world deployment involves addressing performance, cost, and reliability issues at scale.	• Adopt scalable cloud-based platforms with elastic computing resources. • Implement robust testing frameworks to validate performance across diverse environments. • Use containerization technologies like Docker and Kubernetes to simplify scaling.	(Esmaeilzadeh, 2024)
12	**Transferability of AI Models**	• AI models often fail to adapt to new domains or datasets due to differences in data characteristics or application requirements.	• Apply transfer learning techniques to fine-tune pre-trained models for new tasks. • Use domain adaptation methods to align feature distributions between datasets. • Train models on diverse, multi-domain datasets to improve versatility.	(Y. Zhang et al., 2024)
13	**Cultural and Social Acceptance**	• Public skepticism about AI's capabilities and impact on jobs and privacy can hinder adoption, even when technologies are beneficial.	• Conduct public outreach and education programs to raise awareness of AI's positive potential. • Develop AI systems with clear safeguards to address ethical and societal concerns. • Highlight success stories and demonstrate tangible benefits of AI adoption.	(Wu et al., 2023)

continued on following page

Table 5. Continued

Sr.No	Challenge	Description	Potential Solution	Reference
14	**Adversarial Vulnerabilities**	• AI models can be intentionally misled through adversarial attacks, posing risks to security-critical applications like medical diagnostics and autonomous systems.	• Develop robust algorithms that are resistant to adversarial attacks. • Regularly test systems against adversarial scenarios to identify vulnerabilities. • Use adversarial training to improve model resilience.	(Li et al., 2021)
15	**Limited Long-Term Data Storage Solutions**	• Imaging datasets are often vast, creating challenges for storage, retrieval, and long-term archiving, especially in industries like healthcare and astronomy.	• Develop advanced compression techniques that preserve critical features while reducing storage needs. • Utilize distributed storage networks and cloud-based solutions for scalable data management. • Explore emerging storage technologies like DNA-based data storage for long-term archiving.	(Zhou et al., 2023)
16	**Cross-Modality Integration**	• Combining data from different imaging modalities, such as CT, MRI, and PET, is challenging due to differences in resolution, format, and scale.	• Develop advanced AI algorithms for multimodal data fusion that extract complementary information from various modalities. • Standardize data formats and protocols to facilitate interoperability. • Use ontologies and unified representations for seamless integration.	(Sun et al., 2024)

8. VISION FOR THE FUTURE

AI increasingly plays a significant role in various healthcare applications, including virtual assistants, wearable technology, risk management, medical diagnostics and Imaging, remote patient monitoring, medication development, and hospital administration. AI is also anticipated to be beneficial in several big data-related fields, including DNA and RNA sequencing data analysis. AI techniques have already started to help medical specialties that depend on image data, such as radiology, pathology, dermatology, and ophthalmology (Hosny et al., 2018b). The Covid-19 epidemic has increased the use of digital technologies in healthcare and education. A promising advancement in health technology is AI, which may be described as intelligence demonstrated by computers to mimic human cognitive processes, including learning, pattern recognition, planning, and decision-making. There is much excitement about AI's potential to increase workflow efficiency and lessen harm from human mistakes, despite worries about how it may affect doctor-patient communication and the preservation of clinical supervision (Alhussain et al., 2022b). AI and imaging technologies are on the cusp of transformative advancements, poised to redefine industries ranging from healthcare to entertainment. This chapter explores the future trajectory of these fields, focusing on emerging trends, potential breakthroughs, and the implications of these innovations for society (Hosny et al., 2018b).

AI-powered decision support systems are built on a solid data collection and analysis foundation. These systems use data from various sources, including electronic health records, claims data, patient-reported outcomes, social determinants of health data, wearable technology data, and remote monitoring tools. Advanced data analytics methods glean valuable insights from these enormous databases, including machine learning algorithms, natural language processing, and predictive modeling. Normalization, cleansing, and preprocessing guarantee data integrity and quality. Moreover, stringent implementation of data privacy and security measures is necessary to safeguard confidential patient data and adhere to legal mandates like HIPAA. Establishing cooperative relationships with medical facilities, research institutes, and technology suppliers is essential for accessing a variety of datasets and guaranteeing the generalizability and representativeness of the analysis; recognizing Inequalities in AI-powered decision support systems can detect differences in health outcomes, care quality, and access to care among various demographic groups once the data has been gathered and examined. These systems use machine learning algorithms and statistical techniques to find data trends, patterns, and discrepancies (Molli, 2024).

Healthcare resource allocation has also improved due to the introduction of computerized diagnostics and robotic surgery. Robotic technologies enable surgeons to complete more procedures in less time, boosting surgical units' throughput. Automated diagnoses make better use of human resources possible, freeing medical personnel from more arduous duties. This is especially crucial when there is a lack of qualified medical personnel since automation may fill the gap and guarantee high-quality treatment. Automation in healthcare is not without its difficulties, however. Automated technology, such as robotic surgical units, might be prohibitively expensive for smaller healthcare facilities, raising worries about the high expenses involved.

Furthermore, data security is questioned, particularly when sensitive health data is stored via networked automated systems. Healthcare organizations must make significant investments in strong cybersecurity measures to guard against unwanted access or data breaches and ensure the privacy and security of this data. AI-powered automation has started transforming several industries, including radiology, particularly in emergency care situations. Given the organized form of imaging data, radiology is a field that is especially well-suited for the use of AI. The application of AI in this field has broad ramifications, affecting radiologists' workflow and diagnosis accuracy (Aoun & Sandhu, 2019).

Additionally, AI has demonstrated potential in identifying and treating renal calculi. CT and ultrasound imaging algorithms can accurately identify renal calculi. Predicting the composition of stones, their recurrence rates, and the results of procedures like extracorporeal shockwave lithotripsy and percutaneous nephrolithotomy are also being done with machine learning models. These resources support individualized therapy planning, which improves patient outcomes (Bhandari, n.d.). To sum up, combining AI with medical Imaging has significantly improved healthcare. AI has shown promise in transforming medical practice, from early illness detection to individualized diagnosis and treatment. Medical practitioners may use AI to give precise diagnoses, customize treatment regimens, and enhance patient outcomes by utilizing abundant information in Medical Imaging. We may anticipate many more groundbreaking discoveries as technology develops, which will significantly change the field of AI and Medical Imaging in the future (Pinto-Coelho, 2023).

8.1 Enhanced Diagnostic Precision

One of AI's most significant advancements in Imaging is enhanced diagnostic accuracy (Hosny et al., 2018c). Machine learning algorithms, intense learning ones, have demonstrated remarkable proficiency in detecting abnormalities across various imaging modalities. For example, CNNs have been utilized to identify early-stage lung cancers in CT scans and detect diabetic retinopathy in fundus images with accuracy comparable to or exceeding that of expert clinicians. These developments underscore the transformative potential of AI in advancing medical diagnostics.

Future developments are expected to focus on multimodal imaging systems where data from different imaging sources, such as MRI, CT, and PET scans, are integrated. For instance, AI systems could combine the functional Imaging of PET scans with the structural detail of MRI to detect neurodegenerative diseases like Alzheimer's at earlier stages. By combining these modalities, AI systems can provide comprehensive insights that surpass the limitations of individual techniques. This integrative approach will not only enhance diagnostic precision but also enable personalized treatment plans tailored to the unique characteristics of each patient, ensuring more effective interventions and improved health outcomes (Kale et al., 2024).

Moreover, as computational power and algorithmic sophistication increase, detecting rare and subtle diseases will become more feasible. These advancements will empower healthcare professionals to address diagnostic challenges more confidently, reducing misdiagnoses and unnecessary procedures. Such innovations are crucial for advancing global healthcare and ensuring equitable access to cutting-edge diagnostic tools.

8.2 Real-Time Imaging and Decision Support

AI-driven imaging systems of the future will likely emphasize real-time capabilities, offering unprecedented support during critical medical procedures. Intraoperative Imaging, for instance, can benefit immensely from AI algorithms that are capable of instant analysis and feedback. For example, during tumor resection surgeries, AI could assist by identifying tumor margins in real-time using augmented reality overlays, helping surgeons achieve complete tumor removal while preserving healthy tissue (Lundervold & Lundervold, 2019). This real-time guidance can improve surgical outcomes and significantly reduce complications.

Moreover, AI is expected to evolve into a robust decision-support tool that integrates seamlessly with broader healthcare systems. By combining imaging data with EHRs, AI systems can provide context-aware recommendations, aiding clinicians in choosing the best course of action. For example, an AI system could analyze CT perfusion imaging alongside EHR data in a patient with a suspected stroke to prioritize thrombectomy candidates within the critical therapeutic window. This symbiosis of imaging and data analytics will redefine patient care by fostering more informed and timely decisions, ultimately improving prognosis and quality of life (Mohsen et al., 2022).

Applications in emergency treatment, where time is of the essence, may be added in the future. AI systems with real-time processing capabilities can analyze imaging data in seconds, assisting first responders and emergency physicians in making life-saving decisions. These systems could also provide remote support to healthcare professionals in under-resourced settings, bridging gaps in expertise and infrastructure.

8.3 Automation and Workflow Optimization

Automation is a key area where AI will continue to make strides, addressing one of the most pressing challenges in healthcare: the increasing workload of radiologists and imaging specialists. These professionals often face substantial workloads, leading to burnout and potential errors. AI has already shown promise in automating routine tasks, such as image segmentation and preliminary reporting. For instance, AI-driven CAD (Computer-Aided Diagnosis) systems can automatically flag suspicious lesions in mammograms, reducing the time spent on routine screenings (G. Wang, 2016).

Future innovations will likely expand these capabilities to include end-to-end automation of imaging workflows. AI systems could handle tasks such as scheduling imaging studies, ensuring optimal machine utilization, and preprocessing images for analysis. For example, intelligent scheduling algorithms could minimize patient wait times and maximize equipment use by predicting no-show rates and overbooking accordingly. By automating these processes, healthcare providers can enhance efficiency and redirect human expertise to more complex tasks requiring critical thinking and judgment (Erickson et al., 2017).

Additionally, AI-enabled automation can facilitate greater standardization in imaging practices. By reducing variability introduced by human factors, these systems can improve the consistency and reliability of imaging results, further boosting diagnostic confidence and patient trust.

8.4 Innovations in Imaging Hardware

Advancements in imaging hardware are expected to complement AI innovations, creating a synergistic ecosystem of intelligent tools and devices. Next-generation imaging devices will likely incorporate AI at the hardware level, enabling on-device processing and analysis. For instance, portable ultrasound machines integrated with AI could assist in diagnosing conditions like deep vein thrombosis in real-time, even in remote or resource-limited settings. Such devices could revolutionize point-of-care diagnostics, making high-quality Imaging accessible to underserved populations (Akkus et al., 2019).

Additionally, AI-driven design optimization can lead to the development of more compact, energy-efficient, and cost-effective imaging equipment. A prime example is AI-enabled MRIs that use compressed sensing algorithms to accelerate scan times without compromising image quality. These innovations will democratize access to high-quality Imaging, particularly in underserved regions, bridging the gap in global healthcare equity. Enhanced portability and affordability of imaging hardware will play a pivotal role in addressing disparities and fostering a more inclusive healthcare landscape.

Moreover, integrating AI into imaging hardware paves the way for more intelligent devices capable of self-calibration and adaptive learning. These features will ensure consistently high performance, even in challenging environments or with minimal user expertise, expanding the usability of advanced imaging technologies across diverse contexts (Rajpurkar et al., 2017).

9. CONCLUSION AND FUTURE PROSPECTIVE:

AI in Medical Imaging has advanced from theoretical instruments to systems that have been clinically verified. Its incorporation into diagnostic workflows is progressing despite ethical and regulatory obstacles. Developing explainable models, guaranteeing fair access, and establishing standardized evaluation procedures must be the main goals of future research. Cooperation between technologists, physicians, and legislators is necessary for AI in radiology to reach its full potential. In order to create more comprehensive and individualized healthcare systems, future advancements are also anticipated to involve the integration of AI with other digital health tools, such as wearable biosensors, telemedicine platforms, and EHRs. The development of foundation models trained on multimodal data, such as text, photos, and clinical notes, holds promise for expanding the capabilities of decision-making and diagnostic support. There is an increasing need for international cooperation on AI principles, validation standards, and ethical frameworks to guarantee that these tools are secure, open, and fair to all populations. The medical community must actively participate in developing governance frameworks that balance innovation, patient safety, and responsibility as AI systems become more autonomous.

REFERENCES

Akhter, Y., Singh, R., & Vatsa, M. (2023). AI-based radiodiagnosis using chest X-rays: A review. *Frontiers in Big Data*, *6*. Advance online publication. DOI: 10.3389/fdata.2023.1120989 PMID: 37091458

Akkus, Z., Cai, J., Boonrod, A., Zeinoddini, A., Weston, A. D., Philbrick, K. A., & Erickson, B. J. (2019). A Survey of Deep-Learning Applications in Ultrasound: Artificial Intelligence–Powered Ultrasound for Improving Clinical Workflow. *Journal of the American College of Radiology*, *16*(9, Part B), 1318–1328. DOI: 10.1016/j.jacr.2019.06.004 PMID: 31492410

Al-Hussain, G., Kelly, A., O'Flaherty, E. I., Quinn, D. P., & Flaherty, G. T. (2022a). The emerging role of artificial intelligence in global health care. *Health Policy and Technology*, *11*(3), 100661. DOI: 10.1016/j.hlpt.2022.100661 PMID: 35991006

Alexander, A., Jiang, A., Ferreira, C., & Zurkiya, D. (2020). An Intelligent Future for Medical Imaging: A Market Outlook on Artificial Intelligence for Medical Imaging. *Journal of the American College of Radiology*, *17*(1, Part B), 165–170. DOI: 10.1016/j.jacr.2019.07.019 PMID: 31918875

Alhussain, G., Kelly, A., O'Flaherty, E. I., Quinn, D. P., & Flaherty, G. T. (2022b). Emerging role of artificial intelligence in global health care. *Health Policy and Technology*, *11*(3), 100661. DOI: 10.1016/j.hlpt.2022.100661 PMID: 35991006

Aoun, M., & Sandhu, A. K. (2019). Understanding the Impact of AI-Driven Automation on the Workflow of Radiologists in Emergency Care Settings. *Journal of Intelligent Connectivity and Emerging Technologies*, *4*(6), 6. https://questsquare.org/index.php/JOUNALICET/article/view/11

Belge Bilgin, G., Bilgin, C., Burkett, B. J., Orme, J. J., Childs, D. S., Thorpe, M. P., Halfdanarson, T. R., Johnson, G. B., Kendi, A. T., & Sartor, O. (2024). Theranostics and artificial intelligence: New frontiers in personalized medicine. *Theranostics*, *14*(6), 2367–2378. DOI: 10.7150/thno.94788 PMID: 38646652

Bengs, M., Gessert, N., Schlüter, M., & Schlaefer, A. (2020). *Spatio-Temporal Deep Learning Methods for Motion Estimation Using 4D OCT Image Data* (arXiv:2004.10114). arXiv. https://doi.org//arXiv.2004.10114DOI: 10.48550

Bhandari, A. (n.d.). Revolutionizing Radiology With Artificial Intelligence. *Cureus*, *16*(10), e72646. DOI: 10.7759/cureus.72646 PMID: 39474591

Bi, W. L., Hosny, A., Schabath, M. B., Giger, M. L., Birkbak, N. J., Mehrtash, A., Allison, T., Arnaout, O., Abbosh, C., Dunn, I. F., Mak, R. H., Tamimi, R. M., Tempany, C. M., Swanton, C., Hoffmann, U., Schwartz, L. H., Gillies, R. J., Huang, R. Y., & Aerts, H. J. W. L. (2019). Artificial intelligence in cancer imaging: Clinical challenges and applications. *CA (Edinburgh)*, *69*(2), 127–157. DOI: 10.3322/caac.21552 PMID: 30720861

Bissell, M. M., Raimondi, F., Ait Ali, L., Allen, B. D., Barker, A. J., Bolger, A., Burris, N., Carhäll, C.-J., Collins, J. D., Ebbers, T., Francois, C. J., Frydrychowicz, A., Garg, P., Geiger, J., Ha, H., Hennemuth, A., Hope, M. D., Hsiao, A., Johnson, K., & Dyverfeldt, P. (2023). 4D Flow cardiovascular magnetic resonance consensus statement: 2023 update. *Journal of Cardiovascular Magnetic Resonance : Official Journal of the Society for Cardiovascular Magnetic Resonance*, *25*(1), 40. DOI: 10.1186/s12968-023-00942-z PMID: 37474977

Brady, S. L. (2023). Implementation of AI image reconstruction in CT—How is it validated and what dose reductions can be achieved. *The British Journal of Radiology*, *96*(1150), 20220915. DOI: 10.1259/bjr.20220915 PMID: 37102695

Burkett, B. J., Bartlett, D. J., McGarrah, P. W., Lewis, A. R., Johnson, D. R., Berberoğlu, K., Pandey, M. K., Packard, A. T., Halfdanarson, T. R., Hruska, C. B., Johnson, G. B., & Kendi, A. T. (2023). A Review of Theranostics: Perspectives on Emerging Approaches and Clinical Advancements. *Radiology. Imaging Cancer*, *5*(4), e220157. DOI: 10.1148/rycan.220157 PMID: 37477566

Chira, D., Haralampiev, I., Winther, O., Dittadi, A., & Liévin, V. (2022). *Image Super-Resolution With Deep Variational Autoencoders* (arXiv:2203.09445). arXiv. https://doi.org//arXiv.2203.09445DOI: 10.48550

Costantini, P., Groenhoff, L., Ostillio, E., Coraducci, F., Secchi, F., Carriero, A., Colarieti, A., & Stecco, A. (2024). Advancements in Cardiac CT Imaging: The Era of Artificial Intelligence. *Echocardiography (Mount Kisco, N.Y.)*, *41*(12), e70042. DOI: 10.1111/echo.70042 PMID: 39584228

Dikici, E., Bigelow, M., Prevedello, L. M., White, R. D., & Erdal, B. S. (2019). *Integrating AI into Radiology workflow: Levels of research, production, and feedback maturity* (arXiv:1910.06424). arXiv. https://doi.org//arXiv.1910.06424DOI: 10.48550

El-Bejou, S. M., Bouhali, O., Nortje, L. J., Almeida, A. I., Shabani, A., & Djekidel, M. (2020). Hybrid Imaging with SPECT-CT and SPECT-MR in Renal Scintigraphy. *Journal of Nuclear Medicine*, *61*(supplement 1), 1587–1587.

Erickson, B. J., Korfiatis, P., Akkus, Z., & Kline, T. L. (2017). Machine Learning for Medical Imaging. *Radiographics*, *37*(2), 505–515. DOI: 10.1148/rg.2017160130 PMID: 28212054

Esmaeilzadeh, P. (2024). Challenges and strategies for wide-scale artificial intelligence (AI) deployment in healthcare practices: A perspective for healthcare organizations. *Artificial Intelligence in Medicine*, *151*, 102861. DOI: 10.1016/j.artmed.2024.102861 PMID: 38555850

Esteva, A., Robicquet, A., Ramsundar, B., Kuleshov, V., DePristo, M., Chou, K., Cui, C., Corrado, G., Thrun, S., & Dean, J. (2019). A guide to deep learning in healthcare. *Nature Medicine*, *25*(1), 24–29. DOI: 10.1038/s41591-018-0316-z PMID: 30617335

Farič, N., Hinder, S., Williams, R., Ramaesh, R., Bernabeu, M. O., van Beek, E., & Cresswell, K. (2024). Early experiences of integrating an artificial intelligence-based diagnostic decision support system into radiology settings: A qualitative study. *Journal of the American Medical Informatics Association : JAMIA*, *31*(1), 24–34. DOI: 10.1093/jamia/ocad191 PMID: 37748456

Fazal, M. I., Patel, M. E., Tye, J., & Gupta, Y. (2018). The past, present and future role of artificial intelligence in Imaging. *European Journal of Radiology*, *105*, 246–250. DOI: 10.1016/j.ejrad.2018.06.020 PMID: 30017288

Geis, J. R., Brady, A. P., Wu, C. C., Spencer, J., Ranschaert, E., Jaremko, J. L., Langer, S. G., Borondy Kitts, A., Birch, J., Shields, W. F., van den Hoven van Genderen, R., Kotter, E., Wawira Gichoya, J., Cook, T. S., Morgan, M. B., Tang, A., Safdar, N. M., & Kohli, M. (2019). Ethics of Artificial Intelligence in Radiology: Summary of the Joint European and North American Multisociety Statement. *Radiology*, *293*(2), 436–440. DOI: 10.1148/radiol.2019191586 PMID: 31573399

Goodfellow, I., Bengio, Y., & Courville, A. (2016). *Deep Learning*. MIT Press.

Hong, G.-S., Jang, M., Kyung, S., Cho, K., Jeong, J., Lee, G. Y., Shin, K., Kim, K. D., Ryu, S. M., Seo, J. B., Lee, S. M., & Kim, N. (2023). Overcoming the Challenges in the Development and Implementation of Artificial Intelligence in Radiology: A Comprehensive Review of Solutions Beyond Supervised Learning. *Korean Journal of Radiology*, *24*(11), 1061–1080. DOI: 10.3348/kjr.2023.0393 PMID: 37724586

Hosny, A., Parmar, C., Quackenbush, J., Schwartz, L. H., & Aerts, H. J. W. L. (2018a). Artificial intelligence in radiology. *Nature Reviews. Cancer*, *18*(8), 500–510. DOI: 10.1038/s41568-018-0016-5 PMID: 29777175

Jorg, T., Halfmann, M. C., Stoehr, F., Arnhold, G., Theobald, A., Mildenberger, P., & Müller, L. (2024). A novel reporting workflow for automated integration of artificial intelligence results into structured radiology reports. *Insights Into Imaging, 15*(1), 80. DOI: 10.1186/s13244-024-01660-5 PMID: 38502298

Kale, M., Wankhede, N., Pawar, R., Ballal, S., Kumawat, R., Goswami, M., Khalid, M., Taksande, B., Upaganlawar, A., Umekar, M., Kopalli, S. R., & Koppula, S. (2024). AI-driven innovations in Alzheimer's disease: Integrating early diagnosis, personalized treatment, and prognostic modelling. *Ageing Research Reviews, 101*, 102497. DOI: 10.1016/j.arr.2024.102497 PMID: 39293530

Katal, S., York, B., & Gholamrezanezhad, A. (2024). AI in radiology: From promise to practice – A guide to effective integration. *European Journal of Radiology, 181*, 111798. DOI: 10.1016/j.ejrad.2024.111798 PMID: 39471551

Kaushal, A., Altman, R., & Langlotz, C. (2020). Health care AI systems are biased. *Scientific American, 11*, 17.

Khalifa, M., & Albadawy, M. (2024a). AI in diagnostic Imaging: Revolutionising accuracy and efficiency. *Computer Methods and Programs in Biomedicine Update, 5*, 100146. DOI: 10.1016/j.cmpbup.2024.100146

Khalifa, M., & Albadawy, M. (2024b). AI in diagnostic Imaging: Revolutionising accuracy and efficiency. *Computer Methods and Programs in Biomedicine Update, 5*, 100146. DOI: 10.1016/j.cmpbup.2024.100146

Kitamura, F. C., & Topol, E. J. (2023). The Initial Steps of Multimodal AI in Radiology. *Radiology, 309*(1), e232372. DOI: 10.1148/radiol.232372 PMID: 37787677

Krones, F., Marikkar, U., Parsons, G., Szmul, A., & Mahdi, A. (2025). Review of multimodal machine learning approaches in healthcare. *Information Fusion, 114*, 102690. DOI: 10.1016/j.inffus.2024.102690

Kumar, A. (2022). *Astronomy and AI Beyond conventional astronomy*. https://ir.iimcal.ac.in:8443/jspui/handle/123456789/4067

Large language models for structured reporting in radiology: Past, present, and future | European Radiology. (n.d.). Retrieved December 17, 2024, from https://link.springer.com/article/10.1007/s00330-024-11107-6

LeCun, Y., Bengio, Y., & Hinton, G. (2015). Deep learning. *Nature, 521*(7553), 436–444. DOI: 10.1038/nature14539 PMID: 26017442

Leiner, T., Rueckert, D., Suinesiaputra, A., Baeßler, B., Nezafat, R., Išgum, I., & Young, A. A. (2019). Machine learning in cardiovascular magnetic resonance: Basic concepts and applications. *Journal of Cardiovascular Magnetic Resonance : Official Journal of the Society for Cardiovascular Magnetic Resonance, 21*(1), 61. DOI: 10.1186/s12968-019-0575-y PMID: 31590664

Li, X., Pan, D., & Zhu, D. (2021). Defending Against Adversarial Attacks On Medical Imaging Ai System, Classification Or Detection? *2021 IEEE 18th International Symposium on Biomedical Imaging (ISBI)*, 1677–1681. https://doi.org/DOI: 10.1109/ISBI48211.2021.9433761

Lin, D. J., Johnson, P. M., Knoll, F., & Lui, Y. W. (2021). Artificial Intelligence for MR Image Reconstruction: An Overview for Clinicians. *Journal of Magnetic Resonance Imaging : JMRI, 53*(4), 1015–1028. DOI: 10.1002/jmri.27078 PMID: 32048372

Litjens, G., Kooi, T., Bejnordi, B. E., Setio, A. A. A., Ciompi, F., Ghafoorian, M., van der Laak, J. A. W. M., van Ginneken, B., & Sánchez, C. I. (2017). A survey on deep learning in medical image analysis. *Medical Image Analysis, 42*, 60–88. DOI: 10.1016/j.media.2017.07.005 PMID: 28778026

Liu, B., Yu, L., Che, C., Lin, Q., Hu, H., & Zhao, X. (2023). *Integration and Performance Analysis of Artificial Intelligence and Computer Vision Based on Deep Learning Algorithms* (arXiv:2312.12872). arXiv. https://doi.org//arXiv.2312.12872DOI: 10.48550

Lucieri, A., Bajwa, M. N., Dengel, A., & Ahmed, S. (2020). *Achievements and Challenges in Explaining Deep Learning based Computer-Aided Diagnosis Systems* (arXiv:2011.13169). arXiv. https://doi.org//arXiv.2011.13169DOI: 10.48550

Lundervold, A. S., & Lundervold, A. (2019). An overview of deep learning in medical Imaging focusing on MRI. *Zeitschrift für Medizinische Physik, 29*(2), 102–127. DOI: 10.1016/j.zemedi.2018.11.002 PMID: 30553609

Mohsen, F., Ali, H., El Hajj, N., & Shah, Z. (2022). Artificial intelligence-based methods for fusion of electronic health records and imaging data. *Scientific Reports, 12*(1), 17981. DOI: 10.1038/s41598-022-22514-4 PMID: 36289266

Molli, V. L. P. (2024). Enhancing Healthcare Equity through AI-Powered Decision Support Systems: Addressing Disparities in Access and Treatment Outcomes. *International Journal of Sustainable Development Through AI, ML and IoT, 3*(1), Article 1. https://ijsdai.com/index.php/IJSDAI/article/view/49

Morales, M. A., Manning, W. J., & Nezafat, R. (2024). Present and Future Innovations in AI and Cardiac MRI. *Radiology, 310*(1), e231269. DOI: 10.1148/radiol.231269 PMID: 38193835

Najjar, R. (2023a). Redefining Radiology: A Review of Artificial Intelligence Integration in Medical Imaging. *Diagnostics (Basel), 13*(17), 17. Advance online publication. DOI: 10.3390/diagnostics13172760 PMID: 37685300

Najjar, R. (2023b). Redefining Radiology: A Review of Artificial Intelligence Integration in Medical Imaging. *Diagnostics (Basel), 13*(17), 2760. DOI: 10.3390/diagnostics13172760 PMID: 37685300

Neri, E., Aghakhanyan, G., Zerunian, M., Gandolfo, N., Grassi, R., Miele, V., Giovagnoni, A., & Laghi, A. & SIRM expert group on Artificial Intelligence. (2023). Explainable AI in radiology: A white paper of the Italian Society of Medical and Interventional Radiology. *La Radiologia Medica, 128*(6), 755–764. https://doi.org/ DOI: 10.1007/s11547-023-01634-5

Nguyen, M., He, T., An, L., Alexander, D. C., Feng, J., & Yeo, B. T. T. (2020). Predicting Alzheimer's disease progression using deep recurrent neural networks. *NeuroImage, 222*, 117203. DOI: 10.1016/j.neuroimage.2020.117203 PMID: 32763427

Panayides, A. S., Amini, A., Filipovic, N. D., Sharma, A., Tsaftaris, S. A., Young, A., Foran, D., Do, N., Golemati, S., Kurc, T., Huang, K., Nikita, K. S., Veasey, B. P., Zervakis, M., Saltz, J. H., & Pattichis, C. S. (2020). AI in Medical Imaging Informatics: Current Challenges and Future Directions. *IEEE Journal of Biomedical and Health Informatics, 24*(7), 1837–1857. DOI: 10.1109/JBHI.2020.2991043 PMID: 32609615

Park, J., Bai, B., Ryu, D., Liu, T., Lee, C., Luo, Y., Lee, M. J., Huang, L., Shin, J., Zhang, Y., Ryu, D., Li, Y., Kim, G., Min, H., Ozcan, A., & Park, Y. (2023). Artificial intelligence-enabled quantitative phase imaging methods for life sciences. *Nature Methods, 20*(11), 1645–1660. DOI: 10.1038/s41592-023-02041-4 PMID: 37872244

Patel, M. R., Balu, S., & Pencina, M. J. (2024). Translating AI for the Clinician. *Journal of the American Medical Association, 332*(20), 1701–1702. DOI: 10.1001/jama.2024.21772 PMID: 39405321

(PDF) Healthcare Applications of Augmented Reality(AR) and Virtual Reality (VR): Immersive Simulation in Medical- Clinical Education. (2024, December 19). ResearchGate. https://www.researchgate.net/publication/336145610_Healthcare_Applications_of_Augmented_RealityAR_and_Virtual_Reality_VR_Immersive_Simulation_in_Medical-_Clinical_Education

Pinto-Coelho, L. (2023). How Artificial Intelligence Is Shaping Medical Imaging Technology: A Survey of Innovations and Applications. *Bioengineering (Basel, Switzerland), 10*(12), 12. Advance online publication. DOI: 10.3390/bioengineering10121435 PMID: 38136026

Prasad, V. K., Verma, A., Bhattacharya, P., Shah, S., Chowdhury, S., Bhavsar, M., Aslam, S., & Ashraf, N. (2024). Revolutionizing healthcare: A comparative insight into deep learning's role in medical Imaging. *Scientific Reports, 14*(1), 30273. DOI: 10.1038/s41598-024-71358-7 PMID: 39632902

Rajpurkar, P., Irvin, J., Zhu, K., Yang, B., Mehta, H., Duan, T., Ding, D., Bagul, A., Langlotz, C., Shpanskaya, K., Lungren, M. P., & Ng, A. Y. (2017). *CheXNet: Radiologist-Level Pneumonia Detection on Chest X-Rays with Deep Learning* (arXiv:1711.05225). arXiv. https://doi.org//arXiv.1711.05225DOI: 10.48550

Ramesh, K. K., Xu, K. M., Trivedi, A. G., Huang, V., Sharghi, V. K., Kleinberg, L. R., Mellon, E. A., Shu, H.-K. G., Shim, H., & Weinberg, B. D. (2023). A Fully Automated Post-Surgical Brain Tumor Segmentation Model for Radiation Treatment Planning and Longitudinal Tracking. *Cancers (Basel), 15*(15), 3956. DOI: 10.3390/cancers15153956 PMID: 37568773

Revolutionizing Radiology With Artificial Intelligence—PMC. (n.d.). Retrieved December 10, 2024, from https://pmc.ncbi.nlm.nih.gov/articles/PMC11521355/

Revolutionizing Radiology with Natural Language Processing and Chatbot Technologies: A Narrative Umbrella Review on Current Trends and Future Directions. (n.d.). Retrieved December 17, 2024, from https://www.mdpi.com/2077-0383/13/23/7337

Rubin, D. L. (2019). Artificial Intelligence in Imaging: The Radiologist's Role. *Journal of the American College of Radiology, 16*(9 Pt B), 1309–1317. DOI: 10.1016/j.jacr.2019.05.036 PMID: 31492409

Russell, S. J., & Norvig, P. (2016). *Artificial intelligence: A modern approach*. Pearson. https://thuvienso.hoasen.edu.vn/handle/123456789/8967

Segmentation and classification on chest radiography: A systematic survey | The Visual Computer. (n.d.). Retrieved May 23, 2025, from https://link.springer.com/article/10.1007/s00371-021-02352-7

Shao, H.-C., Mengke, T., Deng, J., & Zhang, Y. (2024). 3D cine-magnetic resonance imaging using spatial and temporal implicit neural representation learning (STINR-MR). *Physics in Medicine and Biology, 69*(9), 095007. DOI: 10.1088/1361-6560/ad33b7 PMID: 38479004

Sloan, P., Clatworthy, P., Simpson, E., & Mirmehdi, M. (2024). Automated Radiology Report Generation: A Review of Recent Advances. *IEEE Reviews in Biomedical Engineering*, •••, 1–20. DOI: 10.1109/RBME.2024.3408456 PMID: 38829752

Sun, K., Xue, S., Sun, F., Sun, H., Luo, Y., Wang, L., Wang, S., Guo, N., Liu, L., Zhao, T., Wang, X., Yang, L., Jin, S., Yan, J., & Dong, J. (2024). *Medical Multimodal Foundation Models in Clinical Diagnosis and Treatment: Applications, Challenges, and Future Directions* (arXiv:2412.02621). arXiv. https://doi.org//arXiv.2412.02621DOI: 10.48550

Syed, A. B., & Zoga, A. C. (2018). Artificial Intelligence in Radiology: Current Technology and Future Directions. *Seminars in Musculoskeletal Radiology*, *22*(5), 540–545. DOI: 10.1055/s-0038-1673383 PMID: 30399618

Wang, D., Huai, B., Ma, X., Jin, B., Wang, Y., Chen, M., Sang, J., & Liu, R. (2024). Application of artificial intelligence-assisted image diagnosis software based on volume data reconstruction technique in medical imaging practice teaching. *BMC Medical Education*, *24*(1), 405. DOI: 10.1186/s12909-024-05382-6 PMID: 38605345

Wang, G. (2016). A Perspective on Deep Imaging. *IEEE Access, 4*, 8914–8924. IEEE Access. https://doi.org/DOI: 10.1109/ACCESS.2016.2624938

Wang, S., Du, T., Fischer, K., Tasian, G. E., Ziemba, J., Garratt, J. M., Sagreiya, H., & Fan, Y. (2024). *CopilotCAD: Empowering Radiologists with Report Completion Models and Quantitative Evidence from Medical Image Foundation Models* (arXiv:2404.07424). arXiv. https://doi.org//arXiv.2404.07424DOI: 10.48550

Wismüller, A., & Stockmaster, L. (2020). *A Prospective Randomized Clinical Trial for Measuring Radiology Study Reporting Time on Artificial Intelligence-Based Detection of Intracranial Hemorrhage in Emergent Care Head CT* (arXiv:2002.12515). arXiv. https://doi.org//arXiv.2002.12515DOI: 10.48550

Wu, C., Xu, H., Bai, D., Chen, X., Gao, J., & Jiang, X. (2023). Public perceptions on the application of artificial intelligence in healthcare: A qualitative meta-synthesis. *BMJ Open*, *13*(1), e066322. DOI: 10.1136/bmjopen-2022-066322 PMID: 36599634

X-Ray and CT-Scan-Based Automated Detection and Classification of Covid-19 Using Convolutional Neural Networks (CNN) | Request PDF. (2024). *ResearchGate*. https://doi.org/DOI: 10.1016/j.bspc.2021.102920

Yazdani, E., Geramifar, P., Karamzade-Ziarati, N., Sadeghi, M., Amini, P., & Rahmim, A. (2024). Radiomics and Artificial Intelligence in Radiotheranostics: A Review of Applications for Radioligands Targeting Somatostatin Receptors and Prostate-Specific Membrane Antigens. *Diagnostics (Basel, Switzerland), 14*(2), 181. DOI: 10.3390/diagnostics14020181 PMID: 38248059

Zaidan, E., & Ibrahim, I. A. (2024). AI Governance in a Complex and Rapidly Changing Regulatory Landscape: A Global Perspective. *Humanities & Social Sciences Communications, 11*(1), 1–18. DOI: 10.1057/s41599-024-03560-x

Zech, J. R., Badgeley, M. A., Liu, M., Costa, A. B., Titano, J. J., & Oermann, E. K. (2018). Variable generalization performance of a deep learning model to detect pneumonia in chest radiographs: A cross-sectional study. *PLoS Medicine, 15*(11), e1002683. DOI: 10.1371/journal.pmed.1002683 PMID: 30399157

Zhang, Y., Zhang, J., Li, T., Yang, F., & Yin, Z. (2024). Transfer Learning of Reconstructing Imaging From Speckles Generated by Different Spatial Coherence Light. *IEEE Access, 12*, 153911–153921. IEEE Access. https://doi.org/DOI: 10.1109/ACCESS.2024.3483961

Zhang, Z. (2024). Exploring the Synergy Between AI and VR: Advancing Film, Gaming, and E-Learning. *SHS Web of Conferences, 188*, 03021. https://doi.org/DOI: 10.1051/shsconf/202418803021

Zhou, W., Guan, H., Li, Z., Shao, Z., & Delavar, M. R. (2023). Remote Sensing Image Retrieval in the Past Decade: Achievements, Challenges, and Future Directions. *IEEE Journal of Selected Topics in Applied Earth Observations and Remote Sensing, 16*, 1447–1473. *IEEE Journal of Selected Topics in Applied Earth Observations and Remote Sensing*. Advance online publication. DOI: 10.1109/JSTARS.2023.3236662

Zhu, Y., Yin, X., Liew, A. W.-C., & Tian, H. (2024). *Privacy-Preserving in Medical Image Analysis: A Review of Methods and Applications* (arXiv:2412.03924). arXiv. https://doi.org//arXiv.2412.03924DOI: 10.48550

Compilation of References

Abdelhalim, I., Alksas, A., Balaha, H. M., Badawy, M. A., El-Ghar, M. A., Alghamdi, N. S., Ghazal, M., Contractor, S., Van Bogaert, E., Gondim, D., Silva, S., Khalifa, F., & El-Baz, A. (2024). *Incorporating Imaging, Clinical, Pathology, and Demographic Markers for Hormonal Therapy Prediction in Prostate Cancer*. IEEE., DOI: 10.1109/ACCESS.2024.3520160

Abuzaid, M. M., Tekin, H. O., Reza, M., Elhag, I. R., & Elshami, W. (2021). Assessment of MRI technologists in acceptance and willingness to integrate artificial intelligence into practice. *Radiography*, *27*, S83–S87. PMID: 34364784

Adebayo, P. O., Jimoh, R. G., & Yahya, W. B. (2024). Hybridization of data-driven threshold algorithm with fuzzy particle swarm optimization technique for gene selection in microarray data. *Scientific African*, *23*. Advance online publication. DOI: 10.1016/j.sciaf.2023.e02012

Adegun, A. A., Ogundokun, R. O., Adebiyi, M. O., & Asani, E. O. (2020). CAD-based machine learning project for reducing human-factor-related errors in medical image analysis. In *Handbook of research on the role of human factors in IT project management* (pp. 164–172). IGI Global.

Adegun, A. A., & Viriri, S. (2020). Deep learning-based system for automatic melanoma detection. *IEEE Access : Practical Innovations, Open Solutions*, *8*, 7160–7172. DOI: 10.1109/ACCESS.2019.2962812

Adir, O., Poley, M., Chen, G., Froim, S., Krinsky, N., Shklover, J., & Schroeder, A. (2019). Integrating artificial intelligence and nanotechnology for precision cancer medicine. *Advanced Materials*, *32*(13), 1901989. PMID: 31286573

Ahn, J. S., Ebrahimian, S., McDermott, S., Lee, S., Naccarato, L., di Capua, J. F., Wu, M. Y., Zhang, E. W., Muse, V., Miller, B., Digumarthy, S. R., & Kalra, M. K. (2022). Association of Artificial Intelligence-Aided Chest Radiograph Interpretation with Reader Performance and Efficiency. *JAMA Network Open*, *5*(8), E2229289. DOI: 10.1001/jamanetworkopen.2022.29289 PMID: 36044215

Akhter, Y., Singh, R., & Vatsa, M. (2023). AI-based radiodiagnosis using chest X-rays: A review. *Frontiers in Big Data*, *6*, 1120989. PMID: 37091458

Akkus, Z., Cai, J., Boonrod, A., Zeinoddini, A., Weston, A. D., Philbrick, K. A., & Erickson, B. J. (2019). A Survey of Deep-Learning Applications in Ultrasound: Artificial Intelligence–Powered Ultrasound for Improving Clinical Workflow. *Journal of the American College of Radiology*, *16*(9, Part B), 1318–1328. DOI: 10.1016/j.jacr.2019.06.004 PMID: 31492410

Alahmari, S. S., Cherezov, D., Goldgof, D. B., Hall, L. O., Gillies, R. J., & Schabath, M. B. (2018). Delta Radiomics Improves Pulmonary Nodule Malignancy Prediction in Lung Cancer Screening. *IEEE Access : Practical Innovations, Open Solutions*, *6*, 77796–77806. DOI: 10.1109/ACCESS.2018.2884126 PMID: 30607311

Al-Azzawi, N. A. (2015). Medical image fusion based on shearlets and human feature visibility. *International Journal of Computer Applications*, *125*(12), 1–12.

Alexander, A., Jiang, A., Ferreira, C., & Zurkiya, D. (2020). An Intelligent Future for Medical Imaging: A Market Outlook on Artificial Intelligence for Medical Imaging. *Journal of the American College of Radiology*, *17*(1, Part B), 165–170. DOI: 10.1016/j.jacr.2019.07.019 PMID: 31918875

Al-Hussain, G., Kelly, A., O'Flaherty, E. I., Quinn, D. P., & Flaherty, G. T. (2022a). The emerging role of artificial intelligence in global health care. *Health Policy and Technology*, *11*(3), 100661. DOI: 10.1016/j.hlpt.2022.100661 PMID: 35991006

Aljabali, A. A. A., Qar, J., Al Zoubi, M. S., Al-Batanyeh, K. M., Al Trad, B., Alkaraki, A. K., Al Khateeb, W., Hussein, E. I., Alrababaa, A., Muhaidat, R., & El-Oqlah, A. (2021). A new frontier in switchable bioelectronics and bionanotechnology interfaces. *Functional Materials Processing for Switchable Device Modulation*, 25–42. https://doi.org/DOI: 10.1016/B978-0-12-823972-8.00010-1

Allam, A. H., Eltewacy, N. K., Alabdallat, Y. J., Owais, T. A., Salman, S., Ebada, M. A., Aldare, H. A., Rais, M. A., Salem, M., Al-Dabagh, J. D., Alakhrass, D. N., & Alkanj, S. (2024). Knowledge, attitude, and perception of Arab medical students towards artificial intelligence in medicine and radiology: A multi-national cross-sectional study. *European Radiology*, *34*(7), 1–14. DOI: 10.1007/s00330-023-10509-2 PMID: 38150076

Alwiyah, A., & Setyowati, W. (2023). A Comprehensive Survey of Machine Learning Applications in Medical Image Analysis for Artificial Vision. *International Transactions on Artificial Intelligence*, *2*(1), 90–98.

Amini, S., Elmore, R., Öztekin, Ö., & Strauss, J. (2021). Can machines learn capital structure dynamics? *Journal of Corporate Finance*, *70*, 102073.

Ampofo, J. W., Emery, C. V., & Ofori, I. N. (2023). Assessing the level of understanding (knowledge) and awareness of diagnostic imaging students in Ghana on Artificial Intelligence and its applications in Medical Imaging. *Radiology Research and Practice*, *2023*(1), 4704342. PMID: 37362195

Antun, V., Renna, F., Poon, C., Adcock, B., & Hansen, A. C. (2020). On instabilities of deep learning in image reconstruction and the potential costs of AI. *Proceedings of the National Academy of Sciences of the United States of America*, *117*(48), 30088–30095. https://pmc.ncbi.nlm.nih.gov/articles/PMC7720232/pdf/pnas.201907377.pdf PMID: 32393633

Aonpong, P., Iwamoto, Y., Han, X.-H., Lin, L., & Chen, Y.-W. (2021). Genotype-Guided Radiomics Signatures for Recurrence Prediction of Non-Small Cell Lung Cancer. *IEEE Access : Practical Innovations, Open Solutions*, *9*, 90244–90254. DOI: 10.1109/ACCESS.2021.3088234 PMID: 34892008

Aoun, M., & Sandhu, A. K. (2019). Understanding the Impact of AI-Driven Automation on the Workflow of Radiologists in Emergency Care Settings. *Journal of Intelligent Connectivity and Emerging Technologies*, *4*(6), 6. https://questsquare.org/index.php/JOUNALICET/article/view/11

Aoyagi, H., Tsujinaga, S., Takahashi, Y., Naito, S., Sato, T., Otsuka, T., Tamaki, Y., Motoi, K., Ishizaka, S., & Chiba, Y. (2023). Multimodal Imaging of Constrictive Pericarditis Induced by Long-term Pergolide Treatment for Parkinson's Disease. *Internal Medicine (Tokyo, Japan)*, *62*(24), 3637–3641. https://pmc.ncbi.nlm.nih.gov/articles/PMC10781551/pdf/1349-7235-62-3637.pdf PMID: 37005266

Asani, F., Patel, B., Srikanthan, S., & Agu, E. (2023). BioscoreNet: Traumatic Brain Injury (TBI) detection using a multimodal self-attention fusion neural network and a passive bioscore monitoring framework from smartphone sensor data. *Smart Health (Amsterdam, Netherlands)*, *27*. Advance online publication. DOI: 10.1016/j.smhl.2022.100352

Asatiani, A., & Penttinen, E. (2016). Turning robotic process automation into commercial success–Case OpusCapita. *Journal of Information Technology Teaching Cases*, *6*(2), 67–74.

Attenberger, U. I., Biber, S., & Wichtmann, B. D. (2020). Technological Advances of Magnetic Resonance Imaging in Today's Health Care Environment. *Investigative Radiology*, *55*(9), 531–542. DOI: 10.1097/RLI.0000000000000678 PMID: 32487969

Attenberger, U. I., Morelli, J., Budjan, J., Henzler, T., Sourbron, S., Bock, M., & Schoenberg, S. O. (2015). Fifty years of technological innovation: Potential and limitations of current technologies in abdominal magnetic resonance imaging and computed tomography. *Investigative Radiology*, *50*(9), 584–593. PMID: 26039773

Auloge, P., Garnon, J., Robinson, J. M., Dbouk, S., Sibilia, J., Braun, M., Vanpee, D., Koch, G., Cazzato, R. L., & Gangi, A. (2020). Interventional radiology and artificial intelligence in radiology: Is it time to enhance the vision of our medical students? *Insights Into Imaging*, *11*(1). Advance online publication. DOI: 10.1186/s13244-020-00942-y PMID: 33252702

Avanzo, M., Stancanello, J., Pirrone, G., Drigo, A., & Retico, A. (2024). The Evolution of Artificial Intelligence in Medical Imaging: From Computer Science to Machine and Deep Learning. *Cancers (Basel)*, *16*(21), 3702. DOI: 10.3390/CANCERS16213702 PMID: 39518140

Azizi, S., Culp, L., Freyberg, J., Mustafa, B., Baur, S., Kornblith, S., Chen, T., MacWilliams, P., Mahdavi, S. S., Wulczyn, E., Babenko, B., Wilson, M., Loh, A., Chen, P.-H. C., Liu, Y., Bavishi, P., McKinney, S. M., Winkens, J., Roy, A. G., & Natarajan, V. (2022). *Robust and Efficient Medical Imaging with Self-Supervision*. http://arxiv.org/abs/2205.09723

Aziz, S., Dowling, M., Hammami, H., & Piepenbrink, A. (2022). Machine learning in finance: A topic modeling approach. *European Financial Management*, *28*(3), 744–770.

Bafiti, V., Ouzounis, S., Chalikiopoulou, C., Grigorakou, E., Grypari, I. M., Gregoriou, G., Theofanopoulos, A., Panagiotopoulos, V., Prodromidi, E., Cavouras, D., Zolota, V., Kardamakis, D., & Katsila, T. (2022). A 3-miRNA Signature Enables Risk Stratification in Glioblastoma Multiforme Patients with Different Clinical Outcomes. *Current Oncology (Toronto, Ont.)*, *29*(6), 4315–4331. DOI: 10.3390/curroncol29060345 PMID: 35735454

Balaji, T. S., & Srinivasan, S. (2023). Detection of safety wearable's of the industry workers using deep neural network. *Materials Today: Proceedings*, *80*, 3064–3068. DOI: 10.1016/j.matpr.2021.06.464

Baniecki, H., Sobieski, B., Szatkowski, P., Bombinski, P., & Biecek, P. (2025). Interpretable machine learning for time-to-event prediction in medicine and healthcare. *Artificial Intelligence in Medicine, 159*. Advance online publication. DOI: 10.1016/j.artmed.2024.103026 PMID: 39579416

Bansal, M., Goyal, A., & Choudhary, A. (2022). A comparative analysis of K-nearest neighbor, genetic, support vector machine, decision tree, and long short term memory algorithms in machine learning. *Decision Analytics Journal, 3*, 100071.

Bansal, S. (2021). Determining disease using machine learning algorithm in medical image processing: A gentle review. *Biomedical Statistics and Informatics, 6*(4), 84.

Barragán-Montero, A., Javaid, U., Valdés, G., Nguyen, D., Desbordes, P., Macq, B., Willems, S., Vandewinckele, L., Holmström, M., & Löfman, F. (2021). Artificial intelligence and machine learning for medical imaging: A technology review. *Physica Medica, 83*, 242–256. https://pmc.ncbi.nlm.nih.gov/articles/PMC8184621/pdf/nihms-1702435.pdf PMID: 33979715

Begum, S. H., & Vidyullatha, P. (2022). A Study of Deep Learning Models in Diagnosis and Prediction of Chronic Diseases. *2022 3rd International Conference on Issues and Challenges in Intelligent Computing Techniques, ICICT 2022*. https://doi.org/DOI: 10.1109/ICICT55121.2022.10064613

Belcari, N., Del Guerra, A., & Panetta, D. (2021). High-Resolution and Animal Imaging Instrumentation and Techniques. In *Handbook of Particle Detection and Imaging* (pp. 1497–1535). Springer.

Belge Bilgin, G., Bilgin, C., Burkett, B. J., Orme, J. J., Childs, D. S., Thorpe, M. P., Halfdanarson, T. R., Johnson, G. B., Kendi, A. T., & Sartor, O. (2024). Theranostics and artificial intelligence: New frontiers in personalized medicine. *Theranostics, 14*(6), 2367–2378. DOI: 10.7150/thno.94788 PMID: 38646652

Bengs, M., Gessert, N., Schlüter, M., & Schlaefer, A. (2020). *Spatio-Temporal Deep Learning Methods for Motion Estimation Using 4D OCT Image Data* (arXiv:2004.10114). arXiv. https://doi.org//arXiv.2004.10114DOI: 10.48550

Bhandari, A. (n.d.). Revolutionizing Radiology With Artificial Intelligence. *Cureus, 16*(10), e72646. DOI: 10.7759/cureus.72646 PMID: 39474591

Bhattacharyya, A., Bhaik, D., Kumar, S., Thakur, P., Sharma, R., & Pachori, R. B. (2022). A deep learning based approach for automatic detection of COVID-19 cases using chest X-ray images. *Biomedical Signal Processing and Control, 71*. Advance online publication. DOI: 10.1016/j.bspc.2021.103182 PMID: 34580596

Bhuva, A. N., Moralee, R., Moon, J. C., & Manisty, C. H. (2020). Making MRI available for patients with cardiac implantable electronic devices: Growing need and barriers to change. *European Radiology, 30*(3), 1378–1384. DOI: 10.1007/s00330-019-06449-5 PMID: 31776746

Bissell, M. M., Raimondi, F., Ait Ali, L., Allen, B. D., Barker, A. J., Bolger, A., Burris, N., Carhäll, C.-J., Collins, J. D., Ebbers, T., Francois, C. J., Frydrychowicz, A., Garg, P., Geiger, J., Ha, H., Hennemuth, A., Hope, M. D., Hsiao, A., Johnson, K., & Dyverfeldt, P. (2023). 4D Flow cardiovascular magnetic resonance consensus statement: 2023 update. *Journal of Cardiovascular Magnetic Resonance : Official Journal of the Society for Cardiovascular Magnetic Resonance, 25*(1), 40. DOI: 10.1186/s12968-023-00942-z PMID: 37474977

Bi, W. L., Hosny, A., Schabath, M. B., Giger, M. L., Birkbak, N. J., Mehrtash, A., Allison, T., Arnaout, O., Abbosh, C., Dunn, I. F., Mak, R. H., Tamimi, R. M., Tempany, C. M., Swanton, C., Hoffmann, U., Schwartz, L. H., Gillies, R. J., Huang, R. Y., & Aerts, H. J. W. L. (2019). Artificial intelligence in cancer imaging: Clinical challenges and applications. *CA (Edinburgh), 69*(2), 127–157. DOI: 10.3322/caac.21552 PMID: 30720861

Blamire, A. M. (2008). The technology of MRI—The next 10 years? *The British Journal of Radiology, 81*(968), 601–617. PMID: 18628329

Block, V. A. J., Pitsch, E., Tahir, P., Cree, B. A. C., Allen, D. D., & Gelfand, J. M. (2016). Remote physical activity monitoring in neurological disease: A systematic review. *PLoS One, 11*(4). Advance online publication. DOI: 10.1371/journal.pone.0154335 PMID: 27124611

Bonfanti-Gris, M., Garcia-Cañas, A., Alonso-Calvo, R., Salido Rodriguez-Manzaneque, M. P., & Pradies Ramiro, G. (2022). Evaluation of an Artificial Intelligence web-based software to detect and classify dental structures and treatments in panoramic radiographs. *Journal of Dentistry, 126*. Advance online publication. DOI: 10.1016/j.jdent.2022.104301 PMID: 36150430

Bortulev, P. I., Baskaeva, T. V., Vissarionov, S. V., Barsukov, D. B., Pozdnikin, I. Yu., Poznovich, M. S., Baskov, V. E., & Kornyakov, P. N. (2023). The choice of pelvic osteotomy technique in young children with hip dysplasia. Pediatric Traumatology. *Orthopaedics and Reconstructive Surgery, 11*(1), 5–16. DOI: 10.17816/PTORS138629

Borys, K., Schmitt, Y. A., Nauta, M., Seifert, C., Krämer, N., Friedrich, C. M., & Nensa, F. (2023). Explainable AI in medical imaging: An overview for clinical practitioners – Saliency-based XAI approaches. *European Journal of Radiology*, *162*, 110787. DOI: 10.1016/J.EJRAD.2023.110787 PMID: 37001254

Boudabbous, S., Neroladaki, A., Bagetakos, I., Hamard, M., Delattre, B. M., & Vargas, M. I. (2018). Feasibility of synthetic MRI in knee imaging in routine practice. *Acta Radiologica Open*, *7*(5), 2058460118769686. https://pmc.ncbi.nlm.nih.gov/articles/PMC5952291/pdf/10.1177_2058460118769686.pdf PMID: 29780615

Brady, S. L. (2023). Implementation of AI image reconstruction in CT—How is it validated and what dose reductions can be achieved. *The British Journal of Radiology*, *96*(1150), 20220915. DOI: 10.1259/bjr.20220915 PMID: 37102695

Brajtburg, J., & Bolard, J. (1996). Lipid-based formulas of amphotericin B. *Drugs*, *51*(6), 1025–1044.

Brutzman, K., Burns, Q., Cammisa, V., Peracchio, J., Phillips, C., Sarpong, K., & Liu, L. (2024). Integrating AI and ChatGPT in Wearable Devices for Enhanced Abnormal Activity Reporting: A Mixture of Experts Approach. *2024 4th IEEE International Conference on Software Engineering and Artificial Intelligence, SEAI 2024*, 231–235. https://doi.org/DOI: 10.1109/SEAI62072.2024.10674191

Burkett, B. J., Bartlett, D. J., McGarrah, P. W., Lewis, A. R., Johnson, D. R., Berberoğlu, K., Pandey, M. K., Packard, A. T., Halfdanarson, T. R., Hruska, C. B., Johnson, G. B., & Kendi, A. T. (2023). A Review of Theranostics: Perspectives on Emerging Approaches and Clinical Advancements. *Radiology. Imaging Cancer*, *5*(4), e220157. DOI: 10.1148/rycan.220157 PMID: 37477566

Cai, Z., Li, S., Xiong, Z., Lin, J., & Sun, Y. (2024). Multimodal MRI-based deep-radiomics model predicts response in cervical cancer treated with neoadjuvant chemoradiotherapy. *Scientific Reports 2024 14:1, 14*(1), 1–11. https://doi.org/DOI: 10.1038/s41598-024-70055-9

Cai, C., Xiao, J. F., Cai, R., Ou, D., Wang, Y. W., Chen, J. Y., & Xu, H. P. (2024). Longitudinal dynamic MRI radiomic models for early prediction of prognosis in locally advanced cervical cancer treated with concurrent chemoradiotherapy. *Radiation Oncology (London, England)*, *19*(1), 1–12. DOI: 10.1186/S13014-024-02574-8/FIGURES/9 PMID: 39707484

Cai, J., Luo, J., Wang, S., & Yang, S. (2018). Feature selection in machine learning: A new perspective. *Neurocomputing*, *300*, 70–79. DOI: 10.1016/J.NEUCOM.2017.11.077

Calivà, F., Namiri, N. K., Dubreuil, M., Pedoia, V., Ozhinsky, E., & Majumdar, S. (2022). Studying osteoarthritis with artificial intelligence applied to magnetic resonance imaging. *Nature Reviews. Rheumatology*, *18*(2), 112–121. PMID: 34848883

Cao, Y., & Zhai, J. (2023). Bridging the gap–the impact of ChatGPT on financial research. *Journal of Chinese Economic and Business Studies*, ●●●, 1–15.

Capobianco, E. (2019). Next generation networks: Featuring the potential role of emerging applications in translational oncology. *Journal of Clinical Medicine*, *8*(5), 664. https://pmc.ncbi.nlm.nih.gov/articles/PMC6572295/pdf/jcm-08-00664.pdf PMID: 31083565

Castro, D. C., Walker, I., & Glocker, B. (2020). Causality matters in medical imaging. *Nature Communications*, *11*(1), 3673. https://pmc.ncbi.nlm.nih.gov/articles/PMC7376027/pdf/41467_2020_Article_17478.pdf PMID: 32699250

Cau, R., Cherchi, V., Micheletti, G., Porcu, M., Mannelli, L., Bassareo, P., & Saba, L. (2021). Potential role of artificial intelligence in cardiac magnetic resonance imaging: Can it help clinicians in making a diagnosis? *Journal of Thoracic Imaging*, *36*(3), 142–148. PMID: 33769416

Chaddad, A., Kucharczyk, M. J., Desrosiers, C., Okuwobi, I. P., Katib, Y., Zhang, M., Rathore, S., Sargos, P., & Niazi, T. (2020). Deep radiomic analysis to predict gleason score in prostate cancer. *IEEE Access : Practical Innovations, Open Solutions*, *8*, 167767–167778. DOI: 10.1109/ACCESS.2020.3023902

Chavez, C., Gangadharan, K., & Zhang, Q. (2023). Knowledge Transferring in Deep Learning of Wearable Dynamics. *Digest of Technical Papers - IEEE International Conference on Consumer Electronics, 2023-Janua*. https://doi.org/DOI: 10.1109/ICCE56470.2023.10043543

Chen, B., Cui, J., Li, C., Xu, P., Xu, G., Jiang, J., Xue, P., Sun, Y., & Cui, Z. (2024). Application of radiomics model based on lumbar computed tomography in diagnosis of elderly osteoporosis. *Journal of Orthopaedic Research : Official Publication of the Orthopaedic Research Society*, *42*(6), 1356–1368. DOI: 10.1002/JOR.25789 PMID: 38245854

Chen, B., Wu, Z., & Zhao, R. (2023). From fiction to fact: The growing role of generative AI in business and finance. *Journal of Chinese Economic and Business Studies*, *21*(4), 471–496.

Cheng, Z., Xiao, S., Zhai, Z., Zeng, X., & Huang, W. (2023). Mixer: Image to Multi-Modal Retrieval Learning for Industrial Application. arXiv preprint arXiv:2305.03972. Chicco, D. 2021. Siamese neural networks: An overview. Artifcial Neural Networks, 73–94.

Chen, L., Zhang, J., & Huang, W. (2020). Real-time imaging and minimally invasive surgery: Improving outcomes and safety. *Surgical Innovation*, *27*(2), 123–132. DOI: 10.1177/1553350619898193

Chen, Q., Fu, C., Qiu, X., He, J., Zhao, T., Zhang, Q., Hu, X., & Hu, H. (2024). Machine-learning-based performance comparison of two-dimensional (2D) and three-dimensional (3D) CT radiomics features for intracerebral haemorrhage expansion. *Clinical Radiology*, *79*(1), e26–e33. DOI: 10.1016/J.CRAD.2023.10.002 PMID: 37926647

Chen, Q.-Y., Xie, J.-W., Zhong, Q., Wang, J.-B., Lin, J.-X., Lu, J., Cao, L.-L., Lin, M., Tu, R.-H., & Huang, Z.-N. (2020). Safety and efficacy of indocyanine green tracer-guided lymph node dissection during laparoscopic radical gastrectomy in patients with gastric cancer: A randomized clinical trial. *JAMA Surgery*, *155*(4), 300–311. PMID: 32101269

Chen, R., Zhou, B., Liu, W., Gan, H., Liu, X., & Zhou, L. (2024). Association of Pathological Features and Multiparametric MRI-Based Radiomics With TP53-Mutated Prostate Cancer. *Journal of Magnetic Resonance Imaging*, *60*(3), 1134–1145. DOI: 10.1002/JMRI.29186 PMID: 38153859

Chen, Y., & Wu, M. (2023). Artificial Intelligence-enabled contactless sensing for medical diagnosis. *Medical Review (Berlin, Germany)*, *3*(3), 195–197. DOI: 10.1515/mr-2023-0022

Chen, Z., Liu, X., Kojima, M., Huang, Q., & Arai, T. (2021). A wearable navigation device for visually impaired people based on the real-time semantic visual slam system. *Sensors (Basel)*, *21*(4), 1–14. DOI: 10.3390/s21041536 PMID: 33672146

Chhatlani, J., Mahajan, T., Rijhwani, R., Bansode, A., & Bhatia, G. (2022). DermaGenics - Early Detection of Melanoma using YOLOv5 Deep Convolutional Neural Networks. *2022 IEEE Delhi Section Conference. DELCON, 2022*. Advance online publication. DOI: 10.1109/DELCON54057.2022.9753227

Chidambaram, S., Sounderajah, V., Maynard, N., & Markar, S. R. (2022). Diagnostic Performance of Artificial Intelligence-Centred Systems in the Diagnosis and Postoperative Surveillance of Upper Gastrointestinal Malignancies Using Computed Tomography Imaging: A Systematic Review and Meta-Analysis of Diagnostic Accuracy. *Annals of Surgical Oncology*, *29*(3), 1977–1990. DOI: 10.1245/s10434-021-10882-6 PMID: 34762214

Chow, D. C., Johannes, M. S., Lee, W. K., Clark, R. L., Zauscher, S., & Chilkoti, A. (2005). Nanofabrication with biomolecules. *Materials Today*, *8*(12, SUPPL. 1), 30–39. DOI: 10.1016/S1369-7021(05)71287-6

Chowdhary, C. L., & Acharjya, D. P. (2020). Segmentation and Feature Extraction in Medical Imaging: A Systematic Review. *Procedia Computer Science*, *167*, 26–36. DOI: 10.1016/J.PROCS.2020.03.179

Chudobiński, C., Świderski, B., Antoniuk, I., & Kurek, J. (2024). Enhancements in Radiological Detection of Metastatic Lymph Nodes Utilizing AI-Assisted Ultrasound Imaging Data and the Lymph Node Reporting and Data System Scale. *Cancers (Basel)*, *16*(8). Advance online publication. DOI: 10.3390/cancers16081564 PMID: 38672646

Clement, C. (2024, February 29). Real-world examples and applications of AI in healthcare. OpenLoop Health.

Cohen, R. Y., & Kovacheva, V. P. (2021). A methodology for a scalable, collaborative, and resource-efficient platform to facilitate healthcare AI research. arXiv preprint arXiv:2112.06883.

Collewet, G., Strzelecki, M., & Mariette, F. (2004). Influence of MRI acquisition protocols and image intensity normalization methods on texture classification. *Magnetic Resonance Imaging*, *22*(1), 81–91. DOI: 10.1016/J.MRI.2003.09.001 PMID: 14972397

Combs, C. D., & Combs, P. F. (2019). Emerging roles of virtual patients in the age of AI. *AMA Journal of Ethics*, *21*(2), E153–E159. PMID: 30794125

Coroller, T. P., Agrawal, V., Huynh, E., Narayan, V., Lee, S. W., Mak, R. H., & Aerts, H. J. (2017). Radiomic-based pathological response prediction from primary tumors and lymph nodes in NSCLC. *Journal of Thoracic Oncology*, *12*(3), 467–476. https://pmc.ncbi.nlm.nih.gov/articles/PMC5318226/pdf/nihms-832642.pdf PMID: 27903462

Coroller, T. P., Grossmann, P., Hou, Y., Rios Velazquez, E., Leijenaar, R. T. H., Hermann, G., & Aerts, H. J. (2017). CT-based radiomic signature predicts distant metastasis in lung adenocarcinoma. *Radiotherapy and Oncology : Journal of the European Society for Therapeutic Radiology and Oncology, 123*(3), 480–486. DOI: 10.1016/j.radonc.2017.04.006 PMID: 25746350

Costantini, P., Groenhoff, L., Ostillio, E., Coraducci, F., Secchi, F., Carriero, A., Colarieti, A., & Stecco, A. (2024). Advancements in Cardiac CT Imaging: The Era of Artificial Intelligence. *Echocardiography (Mount Kisco, N.Y.), 41*(12), e70042. DOI: 10.1111/echo.70042 PMID: 39584228

Cui, Y., Li, L., Tao, Z., Chen, M., & Wei, T. (2023). Filtering Out High Noise Data for Distributed Deep Neural Networks. *IEEE Transactions on Automation Science and Engineering, 20*(1), 101–111. DOI: 10.1109/TASE.2022.3208027

Dadkhah, A., & Jiao, S. (2020). Integrating photoacoustic microscopy, optical coherence tomography, OCT angiography, and fluorescence microscopy for multimodal imaging. *Experimental Biology and Medicine, 245*(4), 342–347. https://pmc.ncbi.nlm.nih.gov/articles/PMC7370601/pdf/10.1177_1535370219897584.pdf PMID: 31914810

Darbandi, M. R., Darbandi, M., Darbandi, S., Bado, I., Hadizadeh, M., & Khorram Khorshid, H. R. (2024). Artificial intelligence breakthroughs in pioneering early diagnosis and precision treatment of breast cancer: A multimethod study. *European Journal of Cancer, 209*, 114227. DOI: 10.1016/J.EJCA.2024.114227 PMID: 39053289

de Haën, C. (2001). Conception of the first magnetic resonance imaging contrast agents: A brief history. *Topics in Magnetic Resonance Imaging, 12*(4), 221–230. PMID: 11687712

Dell'Aria, A., Tack, D., Saddiki, N., Makdoud, S., Alexiou, J., de Hemptinne, F.-X., Berkenbaum, I., Neugroschl, C., & Tacelli, N. (2024). Radiographic Detection of Post-Traumatic Bone Fractures: Contribution of Artificial Intelligence Software to the Analysis of Senior and Junior Radiologists. *Journal of the Belgian Society of Radiology, 108*(1). Advance online publication. DOI: 10.5334/jbsr.3574 PMID: 38680721

Deng, M., Song, G., Zhong, K., Wang, Z., Xia, X., & Tian, Y. (2022). Wearable fluorescent contact lenses for monitoring glucose via a smartphone. *Sensors and Actuators. B, Chemical, 352*. Advance online publication. DOI: 10.1016/j.snb.2021.131067

Deng, Z., Liu, X., Wu, R., Yan, H., Gou, L., Hu, W., Wan, J., Song, C., Chen, J., Ma, D., Zhou, H., & Tian, D. (2024). Ultrasound-based radiomics machine learning models for diagnosing cervical lymph node metastasis in patients with non-small cell lung cancer: A multicentre study. *BMC Cancer, 24*(1), 1–11. DOI: 10.1186/S12885-024-12306-6/FIGURES/5 PMID: 38678211

Devlin, J., Chang, M.-W., Lee, K., & Toutanova, K. (2018). BERT: Pre-training of deep bidirectional transformers for language understanding. arXiv preprint arXiv:1810.04805.

Dhinagar, N. J., Speier, W., Sarma, K. V., Raman, A., Kinnaird, A., Raman, S. S., Marks, L. S., & Arnold, C. W. (2020). Semi-automated PIRADS scoring via mpMRI analysis. *Journal of Medical Imaging (Bellingham, Wash.), 7*(6). Advance online publication. DOI: 10.1117/1.JMI.7.6.064501 PMID: 33392358

Dicle, O. (2023). Artificial intelligence in diagnostic ultrasonography. *Diagnostic and Interventional Radiology, 29*(1), 40–45. DOI: 10.4274/dir.2022.211260 PMID: 36959754

DOGUC, O. (2021). Applications of robotic process automation in finance and accounting. *Beykent Üniversitesi Fen ve Mühendislik Bilimleri Dergisi, 14*(1), 51–59.

Doi, K. (2006). Diagnostic imaging over the last 50 years: Research and development in medical imaging science and technology. *Physics in Medicine and Biology, 51*(13), R5. PMID: 16790920

Dong, D., Hui, H., Yang, C., Guo, J., Yang, Y., Shi, L., Mu, W., & Tian, J. (2014). Preliminary design of a multimodality molecular imaging system. 2014 IEEE 11th International Symposium on Biomedical Imaging (ISBI)

Dosovitskiy, A., Beyer, L., Kolesnikov, A., Weissenborn, D., Zhai, X., Unterthiner, T., Dehghani, M., Minderer, M., Heigold, G., Gelly, S., ... (2020). An image is worth 16x16 words: Transformers for image recognition at scale. arXiv preprint arXiv:2010.11929.

Dou, Z.-Y., Xu, Y., Gan, Z., Wang, J., Wang, S., Wang, L., Zhu, C., Zhang, P., Yuan, L., & Peng, N.. (2022). An empirical study of training end-to-end vision-and-language transformers. In *Proceedings of the 2022 IEEE/CVF Conference on Computer Vision and Pattern Recognition (CVPR'22)*, 18166–18176.

Dowling, M., & Lucey, B. (2023). ChatGPT for (finance) research: The Bananarama conjecture. *Finance Research Letters, 53*, 103662.

Dremin, V., Marcinkevics, Z., Zherebtsov, E., Popov, A., Grabovskis, A., Kronberga, H., Geldnere, K., Doronin, A., Meglinski, I., & Bykov, A. (2021). Skin Complications of Diabetes Mellitus Revealed by Polarized Hyperspectral Imaging and Machine Learning. *IEEE Transactions on Medical Imaging*, *40*(4), 1207–1216. DOI: 10.1109/TMI.2021.3049591 PMID: 33406038

Dubey, A. K., Chabert, G. L., Carriero, A., Pasche, A., Danna, P. S. C., Agarwal, S., & Mohanty, L., Nillmani, Sharma, N., Yadav, S., Saba, L., & Suri, J. S. (2023). Ensemble Deep Learning Derived from Transfer Learning for Classification of COVID-19 Patients on Hybrid Deep-Learning-Based Lung Segmentation: A Data Augmentation and Balancing Framework. *Diagnostics (Basel)*, *13*(11). Advance online publication. DOI: 10.3390/diagnostics13111954 PMID: 37296806

Du, Y., Guo, W., Xiao, Y., Chen, H., Yao, J., & Wu, J. (2024). Ultrasound-based deep learning radiomics model for differentiating benign, borderline, and malignant ovarian tumours: A multi-class classification exploratory study. *BMC Medical Imaging*, *24*(1), 1–16. DOI: 10.1186/S12880-024-01251-2/FIGURES/6 PMID: 38622546

Du, Y., Xiao, Y., Guo, W., Yao, J., Lan, T., Li, S., Wen, H., Zhu, W., He, G., Zheng, H., & Chen, H. (2024). Development and validation of an ultrasound-based deep learning radiomics nomogram for predicting the malignant risk of ovarian tumours. *Biomedical Engineering Online*, *23*(1), 1–21. DOI: 10.1186/S12938-024-01234-Y/FIGURES/8 PMID: 38594729

Ebrahimpour, L., Després, P., & Manem, V. S. K. (2024). Differential Radiomics-Based Signature Predicts Lung Cancer Risk Accounting for Imaging Parameters in NLST Cohort. *Cancer Medicine*, *13*(20). Advance online publication. DOI: 10.1002/CAM4.70359 PMID: 39463128

Ehman, E. C., Shin, H., Farjat, A. E., Lowe, V. J., & McGee, K. P. (2024). Head-to-head comparison of the diagnostic performance of FDG PET/CT and FDG PET/MRI in patients with cancer: A systematic review and meta-analysis. *AJR. American Journal of Roentgenology*. Advance online publication. DOI: 10.2214/AJR.24.31519 PMID: 39016450

Ek, S., Presotto, R., Civitarese, G., Portet, F., Lalanda, P., & Bettini, C. (2024). *Comparing Self-Supervised Learning Techniques for Wearable Human Activity Recognition*. http://arxiv.org/abs/2404.15331

El-Bejou, S. M., Bouhali, O., Nortje, L. J., Almeida, A. I., Shabani, A., & Djekidel, M. (2020). Hybrid Imaging with SPECT-CT and SPECT-MR in Renal Scintigraphy. *Journal of Nuclear Medicine*, *61*(supplement 1), 1587–1587.

Elouerghi, A., Bellarbi, L., Khomsi, Z., Jbari, A., Errachid, A., & Yaakoubi, N. (2022). A Flexible Wearable Thermography System Based on Bioheat Microsensors Network for Early Breast Cancer Detection: IoT Technology. *Journal of Electrical and Computer Engineering, 2022*. Advance online publication. DOI: 10.1155/2022/5921691

Erickson, B. J., Korfiatis, P., Akkus, Z., & Kline, T. L. (2017). Machine Learning for Medical Imaging. *Radiographics, 37*(2), 505–515. DOI: 10.1148/rg.2017160130 PMID: 28212054

Esmaeilzadeh, P. (2024). Challenges and strategies for wide-scale artificial intelligence (AI) deployment in healthcare practices: A perspective for healthcare organizations. *Artificial Intelligence in Medicine, 151*, 102861. DOI: 10.1016/j.artmed.2024.102861 PMID: 38555850

Esteva, A., Robicquet, A., Ramsundar, B., Kuleshov, V., DePristo, M., Chou, K., Cui, C., Corrado, G., Thrun, S., & Dean, J. (2019). A guide to deep learning in healthcare. *Nature Medicine, 25*(1), 24–29. PMID: 30617335

Fabrizio, C., & Termine, A. (2023). Artificial Intelligence Applications for Traumatic Brain Injury Research and Clinical Management. *Contemporary Clinical Neuroscience*, (Part F276), 391–402. DOI: 10.1007/978-3-031-24930-3_18

Failmezger, H., Hessel, H., Kapil, A., Schmidt, G., & Harder, N. (2022). Spatial heterogeneity of cancer associated protein expression in immunohistochemically stained images as an improved prognostic biomarker. *Frontiers in Oncology, 12*, 964716. https://pmc.ncbi.nlm.nih.gov/articles/PMC9806230/pdf/fonc-12-964716.pdf PMID: 36601480

Fang, T., Liu, N., Nie, S., Jia, S., & Ye, X. (2024). A deep learning and radiomics based Alberta stroke program early CT score method on CTA to evaluate acute ischemic stroke. *Journal of X-Ray Science and Technology, 32*(1), 17–30. DOI: 10.3233/XST-230119 PMID: 37980594

Fan, L., Wu, H., Wu, Y., Wu, S., Zhao, J., & Zhu, X. (2024). Preoperative prediction of rectal Cancer staging combining MRI deep transfer learning, radiomics features, and clinical factors: Accurate differentiation from stage T2 to T3. *BMC Gastroenterology, 24*(1), 1–12. DOI: 10.1186/S12876-024-03316-6/FIGURES/7 PMID: 39103772

Farič, N., Hinder, S., Williams, R., Ramaesh, R., Bernabeu, M. O., van Beek, E., & Cresswell, K. (2024). Early experiences of integrating an artificial intelligence-based diagnostic decision support system into radiology settings: A qualitative study. *Journal of the American Medical Informatics Association : JAMIA*, *31*(1), 24–34. DOI: 10.1093/jamia/ocad191 PMID: 37748456

Farouk, S., Osman, A. M., Awadallah, S. M., & Abdelrahman, A. S. (2023). The added value of using artificial intelligence in adult chest X-rays for nodules and masses detection in daily radiology practice. *The Egyptian Journal of Radiology and Nuclear Medicine*, *54*(1). Advance online publication. DOI: 10.1186/s43055-023-01093-y

Fatahi, M., & Speck, O. (2015). Magnetic resonance imaging (MRI): A review of genetic damage investigations. *Mutation Research/Reviews in Mutation Research*, *764*, 51–63. PMID: 26041266

Fatima, N. (2020). AI in Photography: Scrutinizing Implementation of Super-Resolution Techniques in Photo-Editors. *International Conference Image and Vision Computing New Zealand, 2020-Novem*. https://doi.org/DOI: 10.1109/IVCNZ51579.2020.9290737

Fazal, M. I., Patel, M. E., Tye, J., & Gupta, Y. (2018). The past, present and future role of artificial intelligence in Imaging. *European Journal of Radiology*, *105*, 246–250. DOI: 10.1016/j.ejrad.2018.06.020 PMID: 30017288

Fazal, M. I., Patel, M. E., Tye, J., & Gupta, Y. (2018). The past, present and future role of artificial intelligence in imaging. *European Journal of Radiology*, *105*, 246–250. DOI: 10.1016/J.EJRAD.2018.06.020 PMID: 30017288

Ferrari, M. (2005). Cancer nanotechnology: Opportunities and challenges. *Nature Reviews. Cancer*, *5*(3), 161–171. PMID: 15738981

Filice, R. W., Stein, A., Pan, I., & Shih, G. (2022). Federated Deep Learning to More Reliably Detect Body Part for Hanging Protocols, Relevant Priors, and Workflow Optimization. *Journal of Digital Imaging*, *35*(2), 335–339. DOI: 10.1007/s10278-021-00547-x PMID: 35018541

Forghani, N., Maghooli, K., Dabanloo, N. J., Farahani, A. V., & Forouzanfar, M. (2022). DeepPAD: Detection of Peripheral Arterial Disease Using Deep Learning. *IEEE Sensors Journal*, *22*(16), 16254–16262. DOI: 10.1109/JSEN.2022.3188810

Forte, E., Fiorenza, D., Torino, E., Costagliola di Polidoro, A., Cavaliere, C., Netti, P. A., Salvatore, M., & Aiello, M. (2019). Radiolabeled PET/MRI nanoparticles for tumor imaging. *Journal of Clinical Medicine*, *9*(1), 89. https://pmc.ncbi.nlm.nih.gov/articles/PMC7019574/pdf/jcm-09-00089.pdf PMID: 31905769

Fotaki, A., Puyol-Antón, E., Chiribiri, A., Botnar, R., Pushparajah, K., & Prieto, C. (2022). Artificial intelligence in cardiac MRI: Is clinical adoption forthcoming? *Frontiers in Cardiovascular Medicine*, *8*, 818765. PMID: 35083303

Fowler, G. E., Blencowe, N. S., Hardacre, C., Callaway, M. P., Smart, N. J., & MacEfield, R. (2023). Artificial intelligence as a diagnostic aid in cross-sectional radiological imaging of surgical pathology in the abdominopelvic cavity: A systematic review. *BMJ Open*, *13*(3). Advance online publication. DOI: 10.1136/bmjopen-2022-064739 PMID: 36878659

Frank, A. M., & Trappe, A. E. (1990). The role of magnetic resonance imaging (MRI) in the diagnosis of spondylodiscitis. *Neurosurgical Review*, *13*, 279–283. PMID: 2280839

Fu, Y., Zhang, H., Morris, E. D., Glide-Hurst, C. K., Pai, S., Traverso, A., Wee, L., Hadzic, I., Lønne, P.-I., & Shen, C. (2021). Artificial intelligence in radiation therapy. *IEEE Transactions on Radiation and Plasma Medical Sciences*, *6*(2), 158–181. PMID: 35992632

Gadde, S. S., & Kalli, V. D. R. (2020). Applications of artificial intelligence in medical devices and healthcare. [IJCST]. *International Journal of Computer Science Trends and Technology*, *8*(2), 182–188.

Galati, F., Luciani, M. L., Caruso, D., Catalano, C., De Vincentiis, L., Bonomo, L., & Laghi, A. (2022). Multiparametric MRI in breast cancer: A radiomic approach for differentiating benign and malignant lesions. *European Journal of Radiology*, *146*, 110065. DOI: 10.1016/j.ejrad.2021.110065

Galati, F., Rizzo, V., Trimboli, R. M., Kripa, E., Maroncelli, R., & Pediconi, F. (2022). MRI as a biomarker for breast cancer diagnosis and prognosis. *BJR Open*, *4*(1), 20220002. DOI: 10.1259/bjro.20220002 PMID: 36105423

Gamal, A., Sharafeldeen, A., Alnaghy, E., Alghandour, R., Saleh Alghamdi, N., Ali, K. M., Shamaa, S., Aboueleneen, A., Elsaid Tolba, A., Elmougy, S., Ghazal, M., Contractor, S., & El-Baz, A. (2024). A Novel Machine Learning Approach for Predicting Neoadjuvant Chemotherapy Response in Breast Cancer: Integration of Multimodal Radiomics With Clinical and Molecular Subtype Markers. *IEEE Access : Practical Innovations, Open Solutions*, *12*, 104983–105003. DOI: 10.1109/ACCESS.2024.3432459

Gan, L., Wang, H., & Yang, Z. (2020). Machine learning solutions to challenges in finance: An application to the pricing of financial products. *Technological Forecasting and Social Change*, *153*, 119928.

Gao, S., Peng, C., Wang, G., Deng, C., Zhang, Z., & Liu, X. (2024). Cartilage T2 mapping-based radiomics in knee osteoarthritis research: Status, progress and future outlook. *European Journal of Radiology*, *181*. Advance online publication. DOI: 10.1016/J.EJRAD.2024.111826 PMID: 39522425

Geis, J. R., Brady, A. P., Wu, C. C., Spencer, J., Ranschaert, E., Jaremko, J. L., Langer, S. G., Borondy Kitts, A., Birch, J., Shields, W. F., van den Hoven van Genderen, R., Kotter, E., Wawira Gichoya, J., Cook, T. S., Morgan, M. B., Tang, A., Safdar, N. M., & Kohli, M. (2019). Ethics of Artificial Intelligence in Radiology: Summary of the Joint European and North American Multisociety Statement. *Radiology*, *293*(2), 436–440. DOI: 10.1148/radiol.2019191586 PMID: 31573399

Gitto, S., Annovazzi, A., Nulle, K., Interlenghi, M., Salvatore, C., Anelli, V., Baldi, J., Messina, C., Albano, D., Di Luca, F., Armiraglio, E., Parafioriti, A., Luzzati, A., Biagini, R., Castiglioni, I., & Sconfienza, L. M. (2024). X-rays radiomics-based machine learning classification of atypical cartilaginous tumour and high-grade chondrosarcoma of long bones. *EBioMedicine*, *101*. Advance online publication. DOI: 10.1016/J.EBIOM.2024.105018 PMID: 38377797

Glover, G. H. (2011). Overview of functional magnetic resonance imaging. *Neurosurgery Clinics*, *22*(2), 133–139. PMID: 21435566

Glover, J., & Young, A. (2022). Autonomous surgical robotic systems and the liability dilemma. *Frontiers in Surgery*, *9*, 1015367. PMID: 36277285

Goebel, R., Yu, H., Faltings, B., Fan, L., & Xiong, Z. (2023). *Trustworthy Federated Learning* (Vol. 13448). Springer.

Gomi, T., Sakai, R., Hara, H., Watanabe, Y., & Mizukami, S. (2019). Development of a denoising convolutional neural network-based algorithm for metal artifact reduction in digital tomosynthesis for arthroplasty: A phantom study. *PLoS One*, *14*(9). Advance online publication. DOI: 10.1371/journal.pone.0222406 PMID: 31518374

Gong, Q. Y., Hu, G. Y., Yu, S. Q., Qian, T. W., & Xu, X. (2022). Comprehensive assessment of growth factors, inflammatory mediators, and cytokines in vitreous from patients with proliferative diabetic retinopathy. *International Journal of Ophthalmology*, *15*(11), 1736–1742. PMID: 36404978

Goodell, J. W., Kumar, S., Lim, W. M., & Pattnaik, D. (2021). Artificial intelligence and machine learning in finance: Identifying foundations, themes, and research clusters from bibliometric analysis. *Journal of Behavioral and Experimental Finance*, *32*, 100577.

Goodfellow, I., Bengio, Y., & Courville, A. (2016). *Deep Learning*. MIT Press.

Goossens, S., Navickaite, G., Monasterio, C., Gupta, S., Piqueras, J. J., Pérez, R., Burwell, G., Nikitskiy, I., Lasanta, T., Galán, T., Puma, E., Centeno, A., Pesquera, A., Zurutuza, A., Konstantatos, G., & Koppens, F. (2017). Broadband image sensor array based on graphene-CMOS integration. *Nature Photonics*, *11*(6), 366–371. DOI: 10.1038/nphoton.2017.75

Gormley, C., & Tong, Z. (2015). *Elasticsearch: the definitive guide: a distributed real-time search and analytics engine*. O'Reilly Media, Inc.

Gou, F., Liu, J., Xiao, C., & Wu, J. (2024). Research on artificial-intelligence-assisted medicine: A survey on medical artificial intelligence. *Diagnostics (Basel)*, *14*(14), 1472. PMID: 39061610

Green, M. M., & Wittcoff, H. A. (2003). Chapter 9: Polymers: The Fourth Dimension of Chemistry. In Organic Chemistry Principles and Industrial Practice (pp. 275–312).

Gross, M., Huber, S., Arora, S., Ze'evi, T., Haider, S. P., Kucukkaya, A. S., Iseke, S., Kuhn, T. N., Gebauer, B., Michallek, F., Dewey, M., Vilgrain, V., Sartoris, R., Ronot, M., Jaffe, A., Strazzabosco, M., Chapiro, J., & Onofrey, J. A. (2024). Automated MRI liver segmentation for anatomical segmentation, liver volumetry, and the extraction of radiomics. *European Radiology*, *34*(8), 5056–5065. DOI: 10.1007/S00330-023-10495-5/FIGURES/4 PMID: 38217704

Gunia, A., Varma, P., Zhang, J., Fehervari, M., & Ashrafian, H. (2024). Artificial Intelligence in Surgery: The Future Is Now. *European Surgical Research*, *65*(1), 22–39.

Guo, K., Orban, M., Lu, J., Al-Quraishi, M. S., Yang, H., & Elsamanty, M. (2023). Empowering Hand Rehabilitation with AI-Powered Gesture Recognition: A Study of an sEMG-Based System. *Bioengineering (Basel, Switzerland)*, *10*(5). Advance online publication. DOI: 10.3390/bioengineering10050557 PMID: 37237627

Guo, X., He, Y., Yuan, Z., Nie, T., Liu, Y., & Xu, H. (2025). Association Analysis Between Intratumoral and Peritumoral MRI Radiomics Features and Overall Survival of Neoadjuvant Therapy in Rectal Cancer. *Journal of Magnetic Resonance Imaging*, *61*(1), 452–465. DOI: 10.1002/JMRI.29396 PMID: 38733601

Guo, Y., Wang, X., Xiao, P., & Xu, X. (2020). An ensemble learning framework for convolutional neural network based on multiple classifiers. *Soft Computing*, *24*(5), 3727–3735. DOI: 10.1007/s00500-019-04141-w

Gurev, S. (2023, September 15). EVEScape: Predicting Virus Evolution with AI. *Time*.

Hagen, F., Walder, L., Fritz, J., Gutjahr, R., Schmidt, B., Faby, S., Bamberg, F., Schoenberg, S., Nikolaou, K., & Horger, M. (2022). Image quality and radiation dose of contrast-enhanced chest-CT acquired on a clinical photon-counting detector CT vs. second-generation dual-source CT in an oncologic cohort: Preliminary results. *Tomography : a Journal for Imaging Research*, *8*(3), 1466–1476. https://pmc.ncbi.nlm.nih.gov/articles/PMC9227736/pdf/tomography-08-00119.pdf PMID: 35736867

Han, J., & Cha, J. (2020). Advances in intraoperative MRI for brain tumor surgery: Navigating the challenges of real-time imaging. *Neurosurgery Clinics of North America*, *31*(3), 327–338. DOI: 10.1016/j.nec.2020.03.004

Han, J.-H., & Cha, J. (2020). Intraoperative imaging based on common-path time-domain reflectometry for brain tumor surgery. *Optica Applicata*, *50*(2).

Hasei, J., Nakahara, R., Otsuka, Y., Nakamura, Y., Hironari, T., Kahara, N., Miwa, S., Ohshika, S., Nishimura, S., Ikuta, K., Kunisada, T., & Ozaki, T. (2024). High-quality expert annotations enhance artificial intelligence model accuracy for osteosarcoma X-ray diagnosis. *Cancer Science*, *115*(11), 3695–3704. DOI: 10.1111/cas.16330 PMID: 39223070

Hashimoto, D. A., Rosman, G., Rus, D., & Meireles, O. R. (2018). Artificial intelligence in surgery: Promises and perils. *Annals of Surgery*, *268*(1), 70. DOI: 10.1097/SLA.0000000000002693 PMID: 29389679

Hassantabar, S., Zhang, J., Yin, H., & Jha, N. K. (2022). MHDeep: Mental Health Disorder Detection System Based on Wearable Sensors and Artificial Neural Networks. *ACM Transactions on Embedded Computing Systems*, *21*(6). Advance online publication. DOI: 10.1145/3527170

Heise, H. M., Delbeck, S., & Marbach, R. (2021). Noninvasive monitoring of glucose using near-infrared reflection spectroscopy of skin—Constraints and effective novel strategy in multivariate calibration. *Biosensors (Basel)*, *11*(3). Advance online publication. DOI: 10.3390/bios11030064 PMID: 33673679

Hendi, A. A. (2023). Development of Medical Imaging Techniques: A Review of Technological Advances in the Field of Medical Imaging, Such as Magnetic Resonance Imaging (MRI), Computed Tomography (CT), and Ultrasound Imaging (Ultrasound). *Journal of Positive Psychology and Wellbeing*, *7*(3), 569–578.

Herpe, G., Nelken, H., Vendeuvre, T., Guenezan, J., Giraud, C., Mimoz, O., Feydy, A., Tasu, J.-P., & Guillevin, R. (2024). Effectiveness of an Artificial Intelligence Software for Limb Radiographic Fracture Recognition in an Emergency Department. *Journal of Clinical Medicine*, *13*(18). Advance online publication. DOI: 10.3390/jcm13185575 PMID: 39337062

He, Z., Lv, W., & Hu, J. (2020). A Simple Method to Train the AI Diagnosis Model of Pulmonary Nodules. *Computational and Mathematical Methods in Medicine*, *2020*. Advance online publication. DOI: 10.1155/2020/2812874 PMID: 32802147

Hill, C. E., Biasiolli, L., Robson, M. D., Grau, V., & Pavlides, M. (2021). Emerging artificial intelligence applications in liver magnetic resonance imaging. *World Journal of Gastroenterology*, *27*(40), 6825. PMID: 34790009

Hirano, Y., Hanaoka, S., Nakao, T., Miki, S., Kikuchi, T., Nakamura, Y., Nomura, Y., Yoshikawa, T., & Abe, O. (2024). GPT-4 Turbo with Vision fails to outperform text-only GPT-4 Turbo in the Japan Diagnostic Radiology Board Examination. *Japanese Journal of Radiology*, *42*(8), 918–926. DOI: 10.1007/s11604-024-01561-z PMID: 38733472

Hong, G.-S., Jang, M., Kyung, S., Cho, K., Jeong, J., Lee, G. Y., Shin, K., Kim, K. D., Ryu, S. M., Seo, J. B., Lee, S. M., & Kim, N. (2023). Overcoming the Challenges in the Development and Implementation of Artificial Intelligence in Radiology: A Comprehensive Review of Solutions Beyond Supervised Learning. *Korean Journal of Radiology*, *24*(11), 1061–1080. DOI: 10.3348/kjr.2023.0393 PMID: 37724586

Hosny, A., Bitterman, D. S., Guthier, C. V., Qian, J. M., Roberts, H., Perni, S., Saraf, A., Peng, L. C., Pashtan, I., Ye, Z., Aerts, H. J. W. L., & Mak, R. H. (2022). Clinical validation of deep learning algorithms for radiotherapy targeting of non-small-cell lung cancer: An observational study. *The Lancet. Digital Health*, *4*(9), e657–e666. DOI: 10.1016/S2589-7500(22)00129-7 PMID: 36028289

Hosny, A., Parmar, C., Quackenbush, J., Schwartz, L. H., & Aerts, H. J. W. L. (2018a). Artificial intelligence in radiology. *Nature Reviews. Cancer*, *18*(8), 500–510. DOI: 10.1038/s41568-018-0016-5 PMID: 29777175

Huang, B., Yang, F., Yin, M., Mo, X., & Zhong, C. (2020). A review of multimodal medical image fusion techniques. *Computational and Mathematical Methods in Medicine*, *2020*(1), 8279342. PMID: 32377226

Huang, L., Ruan, S., & Denœux, T. (2023). Application of belief functions to medical image segmentation: A review. *Information Fusion*, *91*, 737–756. DOI: 10.1016/J.INFFUS.2022.11.008

Huang, T., Ma, L., Zhang, B., & Liao, H. (2023). Advances in deep learning: From diagnosis to treatment. *Bioscience Trends, 17*(3), 190–192. https://www.jstage.jst.go.jp/article/bst/17/3/17_2023.01148/_pdf PMID: 37394613

Huang, Y., Qian, H., Zheng, Y., Song, H., & Liu, X. (2024). A radiomics model based on transrectal ultrasound for predicting prostate cancer. *Medical Ultrasonography, 26*(2), 138–146. DOI: 10.11152/MU-4329 PMID: 38537183

Hu, H., Huang, H., Li, M., Gao, X., Yin, L., Qi, R., Wu, R. S., Chen, X., Ma, Y., Shi, K., Li, C., Maus, T. M., Huang, B., Lu, C., Lin, M., Zhou, S., Lou, Z., Gu, Y., Chen, Y., & Xu, S. (2023). A wearable cardiac ultrasound imager. *Nature, 613*(7945), 667–675. DOI: 10.1038/s41586-022-05498-z PMID: 36697864

Huisman, M., Ranschaert, E., Parker, W., Mastrodicasa, D., Koci, M., Pinto de Santos, D., Coppola, F., Morozov, S., Zins, M., Bohyn, C., Leiner, T., & Willemink, M. J. (2021). An international survey on AI in radiology in 1041 radiologists and radiology residents part 2: Expectations, hurdles to implementation, and education. *European Radiology, 31*(11), 8797–8806. DOI: 10.1007/s00330-021-07782-4 PMID: 33974148

Hu, X., & Norris, D. G. (2004). Advances in high-field magnetic resonance imaging. *Annual Review of Biomedical Engineering, 6*(1), 157–184. PMID: 15255766

Hwang, S., & Kim, J. (2021). Toward a Chatbot for Financial Sustainability. *Sustainability, 13*, 3173. DOI: 10.3390/su13063173

Hyun, D., Brickson, L., Zhuang, L., Simson, W. A., Pinton, G., & Dahl, J. (2022). Applications of ultrasound image reconstruction using deep learning. *The Journal of the Acoustical Society of America, 152*(4, Supplement), A113–A113. DOI: 10.1121/10.0015721

Ibrahimi, S., Sors, A., de Rezende, R. S., & Clinchant, S. (2022). Learning with label noise for image retrieval by selecting interactions. In Proceedings of the 2022 IEEE/CVF Winter Conference on Applications of Computer Vision (WACV'22), 2181–2190. Li, J.; Li, D.

Indoria, A., Kulanthaivelu, K., Prasad, C., Srinivas, D., Rao, S., Sinha, N., Potluri, V., Netravathi, M., Nalini, A., & Saini, J. (2024). Radiomics features for the discrimination of tuberculomas from high grade gliomas and metastasis: A multimodal study. *Neuroradiology, 66*(11), 1979–1992. DOI: 10.1007/S00234-024-03435-7/FIGURES/3 PMID: 39102087

Jackson, L. R., Masi, M. R., Selman, B. M., Sandusky, G. E., Zarrinmayeh, H., Das, S. K., Maharjan, S., Wang, N., Zheng, Q.-H., & Pollok, K. E. (2022). Use of multi-modality imaging, histology, and treatment feasibility to characterize a transgenic Rag2-null rat model of glioblastoma. *Frontiers in Oncology*, *12*, 939260. https://pmc.ncbi.nlm.nih.gov/articles/PMC9722958/pdf/fonc-12-939260.pdf PMID: 36483050

jagsi, R., & Lehmann, L. S. (2004). The ethics of medical education. BMJ, 329(7461), 332–334.

Jain, K. K. (2008). Nanomedicine: Application of nanobiotechnology in medical practice. *Medical Principles and Practice : International Journal of the Kuwait University, Health Science Centre*, *17*(2), 89–101. PMID: 18287791

Jee, C. (2020, February 11). Robot-assisted high-precision surgery has passed its first test in humans. *MIT Technology Review*.

Jeong, S., Yu, H., Park, S. H., Woo, D., Lee, S. J., Chong, G. O., Han, H. S., & Kim, J. C. (2024). Comparing deep learning and handcrafted radiomics to predict chemoradiotherapy response for locally advanced cervical cancer using pretreatment MRI. *Scientific Reports 2024 14:1, 14*(1), 1–11. https://doi.org/DOI: 10.1038/s41598-024-51742-z

Jha, M., Qian, J., Weber, M., & Yang, B. (2023). ChatGPT and corporate policies. Chicago Booth Research Paper, (23-15).

Jiang, B., Bao, L., He, S., Chen, X., Jin, Z., & Ye, Y. (2024). Deep learning applications in breast cancer histopathological imaging: Diagnosis, treatment, and prognosis. *Breast Cancer Research : BCR*, *26*(1), 1–17. DOI: 10.1186/S13058-024-01895-6/TABLES/2 PMID: 39304962

Jiang, F., Jiang, Y., Zhi, H., Dong, Y., Li, H., Ma, S., Wang, Y., Dong, Q., Shen, H., & Wang, Y. (2017). Artificial intelligence in healthcare: Past, present and future. *Stroke and Vascular Neurology*, *2*(4), 230–243. PMID: 29507784

Jiang, Y., Edwards, A. V., & Newstead, G. M. (2021). Artificial intelligence applied to breast MRI for improved diagnosis. *Radiology*, *298*(1), 38–46. PMID: 33078996

Jia, W., Li, F., Cui, Y., Wang, Y., Dai, Z., Yan, Q., Liu, X., Li, Y., Chang, H., & Zeng, Q. (2024). Deep Learning Radiomics Model of Contrast-Enhanced CT for Differentiating the Primary Source of Liver Metastases. *Academic Radiology*, *31*(10), 4057–4067. DOI: 10.1016/j.acra.2024.04.012 PMID: 38702214

Jin, C. Y. (2019). A review of AI Technologies for Wearable Devices. *IOP Conference Series. Materials Science and Engineering*, *688*(4). Advance online publication. DOI: 10.1088/1757-899X/688/4/044072

Jing, X., Wielema, M., Monroy-Gonzalez, A. G., Stams, T. R. G., Mahesh, S. V. K., Oudkerk, M., Sijens, P. E., Dorrius, M. D., & van Ooijen, P. M. A. (2024). Automated Breast Density Assessment in MRI Using Deep Learning and Radiomics: Strategies for Reducing Inter-Observer Variability. *Journal of Magnetic Resonance Imaging*, *60*(1), 80–91. DOI: 10.1002/JMRI.29058 PMID: 37846440

Jones, M. T., Smith, R. A., & Wilson, D. J. (2024). Intraoperative imaging and nerve-sparing prostatectomy: Enhancing functional outcomes. [Note: Journal title may be fictional—verify source]. *Urology Today*, *59*(1), 45–52.

Jorg, T., Halfmann, M. C., Stoehr, F., Arnhold, G., Theobald, A., Mildenberger, P., & Müller, L. (2024). A novel reporting workflow for automated integration of artificial intelligence results into structured radiology reports. *Insights Into Imaging*, *15*(1), 80. DOI: 10.1186/s13244-024-01660-5 PMID: 38502298

Joyce, K. A. (2006). From numbers to pictures: The development of magnetic resonance imaging and the visual turn in medicine. *Science as culture*, *15*(01), 1–22.

Joyce, K. A. (2008). *Magnetic appeal: MRI and the myth of transparency*. Cornell University Press.

Juang, W.-C., Hsu, M.-H., Cai, Z.-X., & Chen, C.-M. (2022). Developing an AI-assisted clinical decision support system to enhance in-patient holistic health care. *PLoS One*, *17*(10), e0276501. PMID: 36315554

Kale, M., Wankhede, N., Pawar, R., Ballal, S., Kumawat, R., Goswami, M., Khalid, M., Taksande, B., Upaganlawar, A., Umekar, M., Kopalli, S. R., & Koppula, S. (2024). AI-driven innovations in Alzheimer's disease: Integrating early diagnosis, personalized treatment, and prognostic modelling. *Ageing Research Reviews*, *101*, 102497. DOI: 10.1016/j.arr.2024.102497 PMID: 39293530

Kanakarajan, H., De Baene, W., Hanssens, P., & Sitskoorn, M. (2024). Predicting local control of brain metastases after stereotactic radiotherapy with clinical, radiomics and deep learning features. *Radiation Oncology 2024 19:1, 19*(1), 1–15. https://doi.org/DOI: 10.1186/S13014-024-02573-9

Kashyap, K. (2023). The benefits of customer experience ai for financial institutions, https://www.forbes.com/sites/forbestechcouncil/2023/07/07/the-benefits-of-customer-experience-ai-for-financial-institutions/?sh=12b8f6d010a8, last accessed 2023/09/29.

Kassay, A., & De Silva, A. (2022). Necessity of Diagnostic Imaging and its Lacking Availability. *University of Western Ontario Medical Journal*, *90*(1). Advance online publication. DOI: 10.5206/uwomj.v90i1.13506

Katal, S., York, B., & Gholamrezanezhad, A. (2024). AI in radiology: From promise to practice – A guide to effective integration. *European Journal of Radiology*, *181*, 111798. DOI: 10.1016/j.ejrad.2024.111798 PMID: 39471551

Katti, G., Ara, S. A., & Shireen, A. (2011). Magnetic resonance imaging (MRI)–A review. *International Journal of Dental Clinics*, *3*(1), 65–70.

Kaushal, A., Altman, R., & Langlotz, C. (2020). Health care AI systems are biased. *Scientific American*, *11*, 17.

Keel, S., Lee, P. Y., Scheetz, J., Li, Z., Kotowicz, M. A., MacIsaac, R. J., & He, M. (2018). Feasibility and patient acceptability of a novel artificial intelligence-based screening model for diabetic retinopathy at endocrinology outpatient services: A pilot study. *Scientific Reports*, *8*(1), 4330. https://pmc.ncbi.nlm.nih.gov/articles/PMC5847544/pdf/41598_2018_Article_22612.pdf PMID: 29531299

Keenan, K. E., Biller, J. R., Delfino, J. G., Boss, M. A., Does, M. D., Evelhoch, J. L., & Sullivan, D. C. (2019). Recommendations towards standards for quantitative MRI (qMRI) and outstanding needs. *Journal of magnetic resonance imaging*. *Journal of Magnetic Resonance Imaging*, *49*(7), e26. PMID: 30680836

Kelly, C. J., Karthikesalingam, A., Suleyman, M., Corrado, G., & King, D. (2019). Key challenges for delivering clinical impact with artificial intelligence. *BMC Medicine*, *17*(1), 195. PMID: 31665002

Khalifa, M., & Albadawy, M. (2024). AI in diagnostic imaging: Revolutionising accuracy and efficiency. *Computer Methods and Programs in Biomedicine Update*, *5*, 100146. DOI: 10.1016/J.CMPBUP.2024.100146

Khalifa, M., & Albadawy, M. (2024a). AI in diagnostic Imaging: Revolutionising accuracy and efficiency. *Computer Methods and Programs in Biomedicine Update*, *5*, 100146. DOI: 10.1016/j.cmpbup.2024.100146

Khanachivskyi, O. (2024, October 17). Transforming healthcare: The role of AI in medical records summarization.

Khang, A. (Ed.). (2024). *Medical Robotics and AI-Assisted Diagnostics for a High-Tech Healthcare Industry*. IGI Global.

Khanom, M., Iqbal, A., Hoque, A., Jeenia, F. T., & Uddin, M. (2023). Development and Validation of a Machine Learning System for Analysis and Radiological Diagnosis of Digital Chest X-ray Images. *Journal of Medicine (Bangladesh)*, *24*(2), 112–118. DOI: 10.3329/jom.v24i2.67273

Kim, E. Y., & Chung, M. J. (2021). Application of artificial intelligence in chest imaging for COVID-19. *Journal of the Korean Medical Association, 64*(10), 664–670. DOI: 10.5124/jkma.2021.64.10.664

Kim, H., Kang, S. W., Kim, J. H., Nagar, H., Sabuncu, M., Margolis, D. J., & Kim, C. K. (2023). The role of AI in prostate MRI quality and interpretation: Opportunities and challenges. *European Journal of Radiology, 165*, 110887. PMID: 37245342

Kim, S.-K., Koo, J., Lee, G.-H., Jeon, C., Mok, J. W., Mun, B. H., Lee, K. J., Kamrani, E., Joo, C.-K., & Shin, S. (2020). Wireless smart contact lens for diabetic diagnosis and therapy. *Science Advances, 6*(17), eaba3252. PMID: 32426469

Kim, S., & Lee, H. (2024). Fluorescence-guided surgery using indocyanine green in gastric cancer: Enhancing resection precision. *Journal of Surgical Oncology, 129*(3), 457–464. DOI: 10.1002/jso.27012 PMID: 39388390

Kirchner, E. A., Fernandez, J. G., Kampmann, P., Schröer, M., Metzen, J. H., & Kirchner, F. (2015). Intuitive interaction with robots - Technical approaches and challenges. In Drechsler, R., & Kühne, U. (Eds.), *Formal modeling and verification of cyber-physical systems* (pp. 225–240).

Kirzioglu, Z., Ulu, K. G., Sezer, M. T., & Yüksel, S. (2009). The relationship of amelogenesis imperfecta and nephrocalcinosis syndrome. *Medicina Oral, Patologia Oral y Cirugia Bucal, 14*(11). Advance online publication. DOI: 10.4317/medoral.14.e579 PMID: 19680205

Kitamura, F. C., & Topol, E. J. (2023). The Initial Steps of Multimodal AI in Radiology. *Radiology, 309*(1), e232372. DOI: 10.1148/radiol.232372 PMID: 37787677

Kluge, E.-H. W. (2020). Artificial intelligence in healthcare: Ethical considerations. *Healthcare Management Forum, 33*(1), 47–49. DOI: 10.1177/0840470419850438 PMID: 31340674

Knoll, F., Murrell, T., Sriram, A., Yakubova, N., Zbontar, J., Rabbat, M., Defazio, A., Muckley, M. J., Sodickson, D. K., & Zitnick, C. L. (2020). Advancing machine learning for MR image reconstruction with an open competition: Overview of the 2019 fastMRI challenge. *Magnetic Resonance in Medicine, 84*(6), 3054–3070. https://pmc.ncbi.nlm.nih.gov/articles/PMC7719611/pdf/nihms-1602664.pdf PMID: 32506658

Knudsen, J. E., Ghaffar, U., Ma, R., & Hung, A. J. (2024). Clinical applications of artificial intelligence in robotic surgery. *Journal of Robotic Surgery, 18*(1), 102. PMID: 38427094

Kokina, J., & Blanchette, S. (2019). Early evidence of digital labor in accounting: Innovation with Robotic Process Automation. *International Journal of Accounting Information Systems*, *35*, 100431.

Kolhar, M., al Rajeh, A. M., & Kazi, R. N. A. (2024). Augmenting Radiological Diagnostics with AI for Tuberculosis and COVID-19 Disease Detection: Deep Learning Detection of Chest Radiographs. *Diagnostics (Basel)*, *14*(13). Advance online publication. DOI: 10.3390/diagnostics14131334 PMID: 39001228

Kora, P., Ooi, C. P., Faust, O., Raghavendra, U., Gudigar, A., Chan, W. Y., Meenakshi, K., Swaraja, K., Plawiak, P., & Rajendra Acharya, U. (2022). Transfer learning techniques for medical image analysis: A review. *Biocybernetics and Biomedical Engineering*, *42*(1), 79–107. DOI: 10.1016/J.BBE.2021.11.004

Kranthi, M., Sailaja, S., & Jyothi, E. (2024). Deep Learning Approaches for Medical Image Processing in the Big Data Era. *International Journal of Scientific Methods in Computational Science and Engineering*, *1*(1), 24–31.

Krones, F., Marikkar, U., Parsons, G., Szmul, A., & Mahdi, A. (2025). Review of multimodal machine learning approaches in healthcare. *Information Fusion*, *114*, 102690. DOI: 10.1016/j.inffus.2024.102690

Kruszewska, A., Owczarczyk-Saczonek, A., Placek, W., & Krajewska-Włodarczyk, M. (2021). Dystrophic calcifications in case of a patient with systemic lupus erythematosus – case report and literature review. *Polish Annals of Medicine*, *28*(2), 224–228. DOI: 10.29089/2020.20.00170

Kuang, Q., Feng, B., Xu, K., Chen, Y., Chen, X., Duan, X., Lei, X., Chen, X., Li, K., & Long, W. (2024). Multimodal deep learning radiomics model for predicting postoperative progression in solid stage I non-small cell lung cancer. *Cancer Imaging; the Official Publication of the International Cancer Imaging Society*, *24*(1), 1–13. DOI: 10.1186/S40644-024-00783-8/FIGURES/6 PMID: 39420411

Kufel, J., Paszkiewicz, I., Kocot, S., Lis, A., Dudek, P., Czogalik, Ł., Janik, M., Bargieł-Łączek, K., Bartnikowska, W., Koźlik, M., Gruszczyńska, K., & Nawrat, Z. (2024). Deep Learning in Cardiothoracic Ratio Calculation and Cardiomegaly Detection. *Journal of Clinical Medicine*, *13*(14). Advance online publication. DOI: 10.3390/jcm13144180 PMID: 39064223

Kumar, A. (2022). *Astronomy and AI Beyond conventional astronomy*. https://ir.iimcal.ac.in:8443/jspui/handle/123456789/4067

Kumar, A., & Gaharwar, M. (2020). Artificial intelligence based wireless smart wheelchair. *Journal of Applied Research and Technology*, *18*(6), 262–267.

Kumar, L., & Jain, M. (2022). A Novel Image Super-Resolution Reconstruction Framework Using the AI Technique of Dual Generator Generative Adversarial Network (GAN). *Journal of Universal Computer Science*, *28*(9), 967–983. DOI: 10.3897/jucs.94134

Kurokawa, R., Ohizumi, Y., Kanzawa, J., Kurokawa, M., Sonoda, Y., Nakamura, Y., Kiguchi, T., Gonoi, W., & Abe, O. (2024). Diagnostic performances of Claude 3 Opus and Claude 3.5 Sonnet from patient history and key images in Radiology's "Diagnosis Please" cases. *Japanese Journal of Radiology*, *42*(12), 1399–1402. DOI: 10.1007/s11604-024-01634-z PMID: 39096483

Kwee, T. C., Almaghrabi, M. T., & Kwee, R. M. (2023). Diagnostic radiology and its future: What do clinicians need and think? *European Radiology*, *33*(12), 9401–9410. DOI: 10.1007/s00330-023-09897-2 PMID: 37436504

Lakhani, P., & Sundaram, B. (2017). Deep learning at chest radiography: Automated classification of pulmonary tuberculosis by using convolutional neural networks. *Radiology*, *284*(2), 574–582. PMID: 28436741

Langen, K.-J., & Galldiks, N. (2018). Update on amino acid PET of brain tumours. *Current Opinion in Neurology*, *31*(4), 354–361. PMID: 29952832

Langlotz, C. P. (2023). The Future of AI and Informatics in Radiology: 10 Predictions. *Radiology*, *309*(1). Advance online publication. DOI: 10.1148/RADIOL.231114/ASSET/IMAGES/LARGE/RADIOL.231114.FIG1.JPEG PMID: 37874234

Langlotz, C. P., Allen, B., Erickson, B. J., Kalpathy-Cramer, J., Bigelow, K., Cook, T. S., Flanders, A. E., Lungren, M. P., Mendelson, D. S., & Rudie, J. D. (2019). A roadmap for foundational research on artificial intelligence in medical imaging: From the 2018 NIH/RSNA/ACR/The Academy Workshop. *Radiology*, *291*(3), 781–791. https://pmc.ncbi.nlm.nih.gov/articles/PMC6542624/pdf/radiol.2019190613.pdf PMID: 30990384

Lang, O., Yaya-Stupp, D., Traynis, I., Cole-Lewis, H., Bennett, C. R., Lyles, C. R., Lau, C., Irani, M., Semturs, C., Webster, D. R., Corrado, G. S., Hassidim, A., Matias, Y., Liu, Y., Hammel, N., & Babenko, B. (2024). Using generative AI to investigate medical imagery models and datasets. *EBioMedicine*, *102*. Advance online publication. DOI: 10.1016/j.ebiom.2024.105075 PMID: 38565004

Large language models for structured reporting in radiology: Past, present, and future | European Radiology. (n.d.). Retrieved December 17, 2024, from https://link.springer.com/article/10.1007/s00330-024-11107-6

LeCun, Y., Bengio, Y., & Hinton, G. (2015). Deep learning. *Nature*, *521*(7553), 436–444. DOI: 10.1038/nature14539 PMID: 26017442

Lee, H. (2021). Noise reduction system by using cnn deep learning model. *Indonesian Journal of Electrical Engineering and Informatics*, *9*(1), 84–90. DOI: 10.11591/ijeei.v9i1.2494

Lee, H., Chang, W., Kim, H. Y., Sung, P., Cho, J., Lee, Y. J., & Kim, Y. H. (2024). Improving radiomics reproducibility using deep learning-based image conversion of CT reconstruction algorithms in hepatocellular carcinoma patients. *European Radiology*, *34*(3), 2036–2047. DOI: 10.1007/S00330-023-10135-Y/TABLES/5 PMID: 37656175

Lee, H., Lee, M. H., Youn, S., Lee, K., Lew, H. M., & Hwang, J. Y. (2022). Speckle Reduction via Deep Content-Aware Image Prior for Precise Breast Tumor Segmentation in an Ultrasound Image. *IEEE Transactions on Ultrasonics, Ferroelectrics, and Frequency Control*, *69*(9), 2638–2650. DOI: 10.1109/TUFFC.2022.3193640 PMID: 35877808

Lee, J. Y., Kim, H. Y., Lee, Y.-S., & Jeong, J. M. (2018). Naphthol blue black and 99mTc-labeled mannosylated human serum albumin (99mTc-MSA) conjugate as a multimodal lymph node mapping nanocarrier. *Scientific Reports*, *8*(1), 13636. https://pmc.ncbi.nlm.nih.gov/articles/PMC6134003/pdf/41598_2018_Article_31933.pdf PMID: 30206287

Lee, J.-H., Woo, H.-J., Lee, J.-H., Kim, J.-I., Jang, J.-S., Na, Y. C., Kim, K.-R., & Park, T.-Y. (2021). Comparison of concordance between chuna manual therapy diagnosis methods (palpation, X-ray, artificial intelligence program) in lumbar spine: An exploratory, cross-sectional, prospective observational study protocol. *Medicine (United States)*, *100*(51), E28177. Advance online publication. DOI: 10.1097/MD.0000000000028177 PMID: 34941072

Lee, T. F., Chang, C. H., Chi, C. H., Liu, Y. H., Shao, J. C., Hsieh, Y. W., Yang, P. Y., Tseng, C. D., Chiu, C. L., Hu, Y. C., Lin, Y. W., Chao, P. J., Lee, S. H., & Yeh, S. A. (2024). Utilizing radiomics and dosiomics with AI for precision prediction of radiation dermatitis in breast cancer patients. *BMC Cancer*, *24*(1), 1–17. DOI: 10.1186/S12885-024-12753-1/FIGURES/6 PMID: 39107701

Lee, Y. D., Kim, H. G., Seo, M., Moon, S. K., Park, S. J., & You, M. W. (2024). Machine learning–based response assessment in patients with rectal cancer after neoadjuvant chemoradiotherapy: Radiomics analysis for assessing tumor regression grade using T2-weighted magnetic resonance images. *International Journal of Colorectal Disease*, *39*(1), 1–14. DOI: 10.1007/S00384-024-04651-6/FIGURES/7 PMID: 38789861

Leiner, T., Rueckert, D., Suinesiaputra, A., Baeßler, B., Nezafat, R., Išgum, I., & Young, A. A. (2019). Machine learning in cardiovascular magnetic resonance: Basic concepts and applications. *Journal of Cardiovascular Magnetic Resonance : Official Journal of the Society for Cardiovascular Magnetic Resonance*, *21*(1), 61. DOI: 10.1186/s12968-019-0575-y PMID: 31590664

Lemainque, T., Yoneyama, M., Morsch, C., Iordanishvili, E., Barabasch, A., Schulze-Hagen, M., Peeters, J. M., Kuhl, C., & Zhang, S. (2024). Reduction of ADC bias in diffusion MRI with deep learning-based acceleration: A phantom validation study at 3.0 T. *Magnetic Resonance Imaging*, *110*, 96–103. DOI: 10.1016/j.mri.2024.04.01 PMID: 38631532

Li, J., Li, D., Xiong, C., & Hoi, S. (2022). Blip: Bootstrapping language-image pre-training for unifed visionlanguage understanding and generation. In International Conference on Machine Learning, 12888–12900. PMLR. Li, J.

Li, X., Pan, D., & Zhu, D. (2021). Defending Against Adversarial Attacks On Medical Imaging Ai System, Classification Or Detection? *2021 IEEE 18th International Symposium on Biomedical Imaging (ISBI)*, 1677–1681. https://doi.org/DOI: 10.1109/ISBI48211.2021.9433761

Li, Z., Wang, B., Li, J., Hua, Y., & Zhang, S. (2022). Local differential privacy protection for wearable device data. *PLoS ONE, 17*(8 August). https://doi.org/DOI: 10.1371/journal.pone.0272766

Liang, B., Tong, C., Nong, J., & Zhang, Y. (2024). Histological Subtype Classification of Non-Small Cell Lung Cancer with Radiomics and 3D Convolutional Neural Networks. *Journal of Imaging Informatics in Medicine*, *37*(6). Advance online publication. DOI: 10.1007/S10278-024-01152-4 PMID: 38861072

Liang, C., Li, M., Gong, J., Zhang, B., Lin, C., He, H., Zhang, K., & Guo, Y. (2019). A new application of ultrasound-magnetic resonance multimodal fusion virtual navigation in glioma surgery. *Annals of Translational Medicine*, *7*(23), 736. DOI: 10.21037/atm.2019.11.113 PMID: 32042752

Liang, X., Xu, Y., & Zhu, H. (2019). Application of iMRI in glioma surgery: Improving tumor localization and surgical navigation. *World Neurosurgery, 132*, e912–e920. DOI: 10.1016/j.wneu.2019.08.071

Liao, C. Y., Chen, Y. M., Te Wu, Y., Chao, H. S., Chiu, H. Y., Wang, T. W., Chen, J. R., Shiao, T. H., & Lu, C. F. (2024). Personalized prediction of immunotherapy response in lung cancer patients using advanced radiomics and deep learning. *Cancer Imaging; the Official Publication of the International Cancer Imaging Society, 24*(1), 129. DOI: 10.1186/S40644-024-00779-4/FIGURES/6 PMID: 39350284

Liao, M. T., Yu, C. C., Lin, L. Y., Pan, K. H., Tsai, T. H., Wu, Y. C., & Liu, Y. Bin. (2022). Impact of recording length and other arrhythmias on atrial fibrillation detection from wrist photoplethysmogram using smartwatches. *Scientific Reports, 12*(1). Advance online publication. DOI: 10.1038/s41598-022-09181-1 PMID: 35354873

Li, C., Li, W., Liu, C., Zheng, H., Cai, J., & Wang, S. (2022). Artificial intelligence in multiparametric magnetic resonance imaging: A review. *Medical Physics, 49*(10), e1024–e1054. PMID: 35980348

Lin, D. J., Johnson, P. M., Knoll, F., & Lui, Y. W. (2021). Artificial Intelligence for MR Image Reconstruction: An Overview for Clinicians. *Journal of Magnetic Resonance Imaging : JMRI, 53*(4), 1015–1028. DOI: 10.1002/jmri.27078 PMID: 32048372

Lin, P.-K., Chiu, Y.-H., Huang, C.-J., Wang, C.-Y., Pan, M.-L., Wang, D.-W., Mark Liao, H.-Y., Chen, Y.-S., Kuan, C.-H., Lin, S.-Y., & Chen, L.-F. (2022). PADAr: Physician-oriented artificial intelligence-facilitating diagnosis aid for retinal diseases. *Journal of Medical Imaging (Bellingham, Wash.), 9*(04). Advance online publication. DOI: 10.1117/1.jmi.9.4.044501 PMID: 35903415

Lin, Y., Belue, M. J., Yilmaz, E. C., Law, Y. M., Merriman, K. M., Phelps, T. E., Gelikman, D. G., Ozyoruk, K. B., Lay, N. S., Merino, M. J., Pinto, P. A., & Turkbey, B. (2024). Deep learning-based image quality assessment: Impact on detection accuracy of prostate cancer extraprostatic extension on MRI. *Abdominal Radiology, 49*(8), 2891–2901. DOI: 10.1007/s00261-024-04468-5 PMID: 38958754

Li, S., Cao, P., Li, J., Chen, T., Luo, P., Ruan, G., Zhang, Y., Wang, X., Han, W., Zhu, Z., Dang, Q., Wang, Q., Zhang, M., Bai, Q., Chai, Z., Yang, H., Chen, H., Tang, M., Akbar, A., & Ding, C. (2024). Integrating Radiomics and Neural Networks for Knee Osteoarthritis Incidence Prediction. *Arthritis & Rheumatology (Hoboken, N.J.), 76*(9), 1377–1386. DOI: 10.1002/ART.42915 PMID: 38751101

Litjens, G., Kooi, T., Bejnordi, B. E., Setio, A. A. A., Ciompi, F., Ghafoorian, M., van der Laak, J. A. W. M., van Ginneken, B., & Sánchez, C. I. (2017). A survey on deep learning in medical image analysis. *Medical Image Analysis*, *42*, 60–88. DOI: 10.1016/j.media.2017.07.005 PMID: 28778026

Liu, Y., Liu, Z., Li, X., Zhou, W., Lin, L., & Chen, X. (2024). Non-invasive assessment of response to transcatheter arterial chemoembolization for hepatocellular carcinoma with the deep neural networks-based radiomics nomogram. *Acta Radiologica (Stockholm, Sweden : 1987)*, *65*(6), 535–545. https://doi.org/DOI: 10.1177/02841851241229185

Liu, C., Yu, H., Li, B., Shen, Z., Gao, Z., Ren, P., Xie, X., Cui, L., & Miao, C. (2021a). Noise-resistant deep metric learning with ranking-based instance selection. In *Proceedings of the 2021 IEEE/CVF Conference on Computer Vision and Pattern Recognition (CVPR'21)*, 6811–6820.

Liu, Q., Luo, D., Haase, J. E., Guo, Q., Wang, X. Q., Liu, S., Xia, L., Liu, Z., Yang, J., & Yang, B. X. (2020). The experiences of health-care providers during the COVID-19 crisis in China: A qualitative study. *The Lancet. Global Health*, *8*(6), e790–e798. https://pmc.ncbi.nlm.nih.gov/articles/PMC7190296/pdf/main.pdf PMID: 32573443

Liu, W., Li, L., Deng, J., & Li, W. (2024). A comprehensive approach for evaluating lymphovascular invasion in invasive breast cancer: Leveraging multimodal MRI findings, radiomics, and deep learning analysis of intra- and peritumoral regions. *Computerized Medical Imaging and Graphics*, *116*, 102415. DOI: 10.1016/J.COMPMEDIMAG.2024.102415 PMID: 39032451

Liu, Y., Jia, X., Zhao, J., Peng, Y., Yao, X., Hu, X., Cui, J., Chen, H., Chen, X., Wu, J., Hong, N., Wang, S., & Wang, Y. (2024). A Machine Learning-Based Unenhanced Radiomics Approach to Distinguishing Between Benign and Malignant Breast Lesions Using T2-Weighted and Diffusion-Weighted MRI. *Journal of Magnetic Resonance Imaging*, *60*(2), 600–612. DOI: 10.1002/JMRI.29111 PMID: 37933890

Liu, Y., Liu, W., Chen, H., Xie, S., Wang, C., Liang, T., Yu, Y., & Liu, X. (2023). Artificial intelligence versus radiologist in the accuracy of fracture detection based on computed tomography images: A multidimensional, multi-region analysis. *Quantitative Imaging in Medicine and Surgery*, *13*(10), 6424–6433. DOI: 10.21037/qims-23-428 PMID: 37869340

Liu, Y., Menon, R., Putcha, A., Huang, K., Bonilla, L., Vora, R., Li, J., Zhang, L., Wang, Y., Fletcher, L., Lassiter, A., Huang, C., Buse, J. B., Cheng, K., & Bai, W. (2022). Skin-Interfaced Deep-Tissue Sensing Patch via Microneedle Waveguides. *Advanced Materials Technologies*, *7*(9). Advance online publication. DOI: 10.1002/admt.202200468

Liu, Y., Zhang, H., Chen, L., & Wang, P. (2020). Enhancing clinical decision-making through interprofessional training in imaging modalities. *The Journal of Continuing Education in the Health Professions*, *40*(2), 90–96.

Liu, Y., Zheng, X., Fan, D., Shen, Z., Wu, Z., & Li, S. (2024). CT-based radiomic analysis for categorization of ovarian sex cord-stromal tumors and epithelial ovarian cancers. *Abdominal Radiology*, *49*(11). Advance online publication. DOI: 10.1007/S00261-024-04437-Y PMID: 38896249

Liu, Z., Zhang, S., Wang, Y., Xu, H., Gao, Y., Jin, H., Zhang, Y., Wu, H., Lu, J., Chen, P., Qiao, P. G., & Yang, Z. (2024). Posterior circulation ischemic stroke: Radiomics-based machine learning approach to identify onset time from magnetic resonance imaging. *Neuroradiology*, *66*(7), 1141–1152. DOI: 10.1007/S00234-024-03353-8 PMID: 38592454

Li, X., Zhang, L., Yang, J., & Teng, F. (2024). Role of Artificial Intelligence in Medical Image Analysis: A Review of Current Trends and Future Directions. *Journal of Medical and Biological Engineering*, •••, 1–13.

Li, Y., & Shen, L. (2018). Skin lesion analysis towards melanoma detection using deep learning network. *Sensors (Switzerland)*, *18*(2). Advance online publication. DOI: 10.3390/s18020556 PMID: 29439500

Lizzi, F., Agosti, A., Brero, F., Cabini, R. F., Fantacci, M. E., Figini, S., Lascialfari, A., Laruina, F., Oliva, P., Piffer, S., Talamonti, C., & Retico, A. (2022). Quantification of pulmonary involvement in COVID-19 pneumonia by means of a cascade of two U-nets: Training and assessment on multiple datasets using different annotation criteria. *International Journal of Computer Assisted Radiology and Surgery*, *17*(2), 229–237. DOI: 10.1007/s11548-021-02501-2 PMID: 34698988

Loshchilov, I., & Hutter, F. (2019). Decoupled weight decay regularization. In ICLR. Malkov, Y. A.; and Yashunin, D. A. 2018. Effcient and robust approximate nearest neighbor search using hierarchical navigable small world graphs. *IEEE Transactions on Pattern Analysis and Machine Intelligence*, *42*(4), 824–836.

Loyola-Leyva, A., Hernández-Vidales, K., Loyola-Rodríguez, J. P., & González, F. J. (2024). Noninvasive Glucose Measurements Through Transcutaneous Raman Spectroscopy: A Review. *Journal of Diabetes Science and Technology, 18*(2), 460–469. DOI: 10.1177/19322968221109612 PMID: 35815609

Lu, Y., Yuan, R., Su, Y., Liang, Z., Huang, H., Leng, Q., Yang, A., Xiao, X., Lai, Z., & Zhang, Y. (2025). Biparametric MRI-based radiomics for noninvastive discrimination of benign prostatic hyperplasia nodules (BPH) and prostate cancer nodules: a bio-centric retrospective cohort study. *Scientific Reports 2025 15:1, 15*(1), 1–12. https://doi.org/DOI: 10.1038/s41598-024-84908-w

Luca, C., Andritoi, D., Corciova, C., & Fuior, R. (2020). Intelligent Glove for Rehabilitation of Hand Movement in Stroke Survivor. *EPE 2020 - Proceedings of the 2020 11th International Conference and Exposition on Electrical And Power Engineering*, 546–549. https://doi.org/DOI: 10.1109/EPE50722.2020.9305619

Lu, J., Feng, F., & Jin, Z. (2013). Cancer diagnosis and treatment guidance: Role of MRI and MRI probes in the era of molecular imaging. *Current Pharmaceutical Biotechnology, 14*(8), 714–722. PMID: 24372236

Lundervold, A. S., & Lundervold, A. (2019). An overview of deep learning in medical Imaging focusing on MRI. *Zeitschrift für Medizinische Physik, 29*(2), 102–127. DOI: 10.1016/j.zemedi.2018.11.002 PMID: 30553609

Lundervold, A. S., & Lundervold, A. (2019). An overview of deep learning in medical imaging focusing on MRI. *Zeitschrift für Medizinische Physik, 29*(2), 102–127. PMID: 30553609

Maiti, S., Nayak, S., Hebbar, K. D., & Pendem, S. (2024). Differentiation of invasive ductal and lobular carcinoma of the breast using MRI radiomic features: a pilot study. *F1000Research 2024 13:91, 13*, 91. https://doi.org/DOI: 10.12688/f1000research.146052.2

Malcangi, M. (2021). AI-Based Methods and Technologies to Develop Wearable Devices for Prosthetics and Predictions of Degenerative Diseases. *Methods in Molecular Biology (Clifton, N.J.), 2190*, 337–354. DOI: 10.1007/978-1-0716-0826-5_17 PMID: 32804375

Ma, M., Gu, W., Liang, Y., Han, X., Zhang, M., Xu, M., Gao, H., Tang, W., & Huang, D. (2024). A novel model for predicting postoperative liver metastasis in R0 resected pancreatic neuroendocrine tumors: Integrating computational pathology and deep learning-radiomics. *Journal of Translational Medicine, 22*(1), 1–14. DOI: 10.1186/S12967-024-05449-4/FIGURES/6 PMID: 39143624

Mansbridge, M., Chung, E., & Rhee, H. (2019). The use of MRI and PET imaging studies for prostate cancer management: Brief update, clinical recommendations, and technological limitations. *Medical Science*, *7*(8), 85. PMID: 31387208

Ma, R., Ramaswamy, A., & Xu, J.. (2022). Surgical gestures as a method to quantify surgical performance and predict patient outcomes. *NPJ Digital Medicine*, *5*(1), 187. DOI: 10.1038/s41746-022-00738-y PMID: 36550203

Marti-Bonmati, L., Koh, D.-M., Riklund, K., Bobowicz, M., Roussakis, Y., Vilanova, J. C., Fütterer, J. J., Rimola, J., Mallol, P., Ribas, G., Lekadir, K., & Tsakou, G. (2022). Considerations for artificial intelligence clinical impact in oncologic imaging: An AI4HI position paper. *Insights Into Imaging*, *13*(1). Advance online publication. DOI: 10.1186/s13244-022-01220-9 PMID: 35536446

Masoudi, S., Harmon, S. A., Mehralivand, S., Walker, S. M., Raviprakash, H., Bagci, U., Choyke, P. L., & Turkbey, B. (2021). Quick guide on radiology image pre-processing for deep learning applications in prostate cancer research. *Journal of Medical Imaging (Bellingham, Wash.)*, *8*(1), 010901. DOI: 10.1117/1.JMI.8.1.010901 PMID: 33426151

Mauri, G., Gennaro, N., Lee, M. K., & Baek, J. H. (2019). Laser and radiofrequency ablations for benign and malignant thyroid tumors. *International Journal of Hyperthermia*, *36*(2), 13–20. https://air.unimi.it/bitstream/2434/733157/2/Laser%20and%20radiofrequency%20ablations%20for%20benign%20and%20malignant%20thyroid%20tumors.pdf PMID: 31537159

McCarthy, M. J. (2011). Introduction to magnetic resonance imaging (MRI). In *Magnetic resonance imaging in foods* (pp. 1–29). Springer US.

Meddings, Z., Rundo, L., Sadat, U., Zhao, X., Teng, Z., & Graves, M. J. (2024). Robustness and classification capabilities of MRI radiomic features in identifying carotid plaque vulnerability. *The British Journal of Radiology*, *97*(1158), 1118–1124. DOI: 10.1093/BJR/TQAE057 PMID: 38711198

Mehrizi, M. H. R., Gerritsen, S. H., de Klerk, W. M., Houtschild, C., Dinnessen, S. M. H., Zhao, L., van Sommeren, R., & Zerfu, A. (2023). How do providers of artificial intelligence (AI) solutions propose and legitimize the values of their solutions for supporting diagnostic radiology workflow? A technography study in 2021. *European Radiology*, *33*(2), 915–924. DOI: 10.1007/s00330-022-09090-x PMID: 35980427

Meireles, O. R., Rosman, G., Altieri, M. S., Carin, L., Hager, G., Madani, A., Padoy, N., Pugh, C. M., Sylla, P., Ward, T. M., & Hashimoto, D. A., & SAGES Video Annotation for AI Working Groups. (2021). SAGES consensus recommendations on an annotation framework for surgical video. *Surgical Endoscopy*, *35*(9), 4918–4929. PMID: 34231065

MENDİ, A. F. (2023). Edge ai technology in the defense industry via reinforcement learning in simulation environments. *Gümüşhane Üniversitesi Fen Bilimleri Enstitüsü Dergisi*. https://doi.org/DOI: 10.17714/gumusfenbil.1266035

Meng, F., Kottlors, J., Shahzad, R., Liu, H., Fervers, P., Jin, Y., Rinneburger, M., Le, D., Weisthoff, M., Liu, W., Zhang, H., & Persigehl, T. (2023). AI support for accurate and fast radiological diagnosis of COVID-19: An international multicenter, multivendor CT study. *European Radiology*, *33*(6), 4280–4291. DOI: 10.1007/s00330-022-09335-9 PMID: 36525088

Meyer-Base, A., Morra, L., Tahmassebi, A., Lobbes, M., Meyer-Base, U., & Pinker, K. (2021). AI-Enhanced Diagnosis of Challenging Lesions in Breast MRI: A Methodology and Application Primer. *Journal of Magnetic Resonance Imaging*, *54*(3), 686–702. PMID: 32864782

Meyer, H. J., Wienke, A., Surov, A., Höhn, A. K., & Surov, A. (2018). Simultaneous PET/MRI in the diagnosis of cervical cancer: A prospective study. *European Journal of Radiology*, *105*, 119–125.

Meyer, H.-J., Purz, S., Sabri, O., & Surov, A. (2018). Cervical Cancer: Associations between Metabolic Parameters and Whole Lesion Histogram Analysis Derived from Simultaneous 18F-FDG-PET/MRI. *Contrast Media & Molecular Imaging*, *2018*(1), 5063285. PMID: 30154687

Mierzwa, A. P., Huang, S. P., Nguyen, K. T., Culjat, M. O., & Singh, R. S. (2016). Wearable ultrasound array for point-of-care imaging and patient monitoring. *Studies in Health Technology and Informatics*, *220*, 241–244. DOI: 10.3233/978-1-61499-625-5-241 PMID: 27046585

Mirnezami, R., Nicholson, J., & Darzi, A. (•••). Preparing for precision medicine. *The New England Journal of Medicine*, *366*, 489–491. PMID: 22256780

Mohsen, F., Ali, H., El Hajj, N., & Shah, Z. (2022). Artificial intelligence-based methods for fusion of electronic health records and imaging data. *Scientific Reports*, *12*(1), 17981. DOI: 10.1038/s41598-022-22514-4 PMID: 36289266

Molli, V. L. P. (2024). Enhancing Healthcare Equity through AI-Powered Decision Support Systems: Addressing Disparities in Access and Treatment Outcomes. *International Journal of Sustainable Development Through AI, ML and IoT, 3*(1), Article 1. https://ijsdai.com/index.php/IJSDAI/article/view/49

Monteagudo, J. L. R. (2016). Medical imaging needs in a rural health center from a clinical point of view. *Defining the Medical Imaging Requirements for a Rural Health Center*, 7–39. https://doi.org/DOI: 10.1007/978-981-10-1613-4_2

Morales, M. A., Manning, W. J., & Nezafat, R. (2024). Present and Future Innovations in AI and Cardiac MRI. *Radiology, 310*(1), e231269. DOI: 10.1148/radiol.231269 PMID: 38193835

Morris, B. (2005). Robotic surgery: Applications, limitations, and impact on surgical education. *MedGenMed : Medscape General Medicine*, *7*(3), 72. PMID: 16369298

Mourad, R., Kolisnyk, S., Baiun, Y., Falk, A., Yuriy, T., Valerii, F., Kopeev, A., Suldina, O., Pospelov, A., Kim, J., Rusakov, A., & Lebl, D. R. (2022). Performance of hybrid artificial intelligence in determining candidacy for lumbar stenosis surgery. *European Spine Journal : Official Publication of the European Spine Society, the European Spinal Deformity Society, and the European Section of the Cervical Spine Research Society, 31*(8), 2149–2155. DOI: 10.1007/s00586-022-07307-7 PMID: 35802195

Muanme, W., Pararach, S., & Kaeprapha, P. (2023). An Artificial Intelligence Camera System to Check Worker Personal Protective Equipment Before Entering Risk Areas. *Lecture Notes in Electrical Engineering, 1045 LNEE*, 747–755. https://doi.org/DOI: 10.1007/978-981-99-2287-1_102

Muhaimil, A., Pendem, S., & Sampathilla, N., P S, P., Nayak, K., Chadaga, K., Goswami, A., M, O. C., & Shirlal, A. (2024). Role of Artificial intelligence model in prediction of low back pain using T2 weighted MRI of Lumbar spine. *F1000Research 2024 13:1035, 13*, 1035. https://doi.org/DOI: 10.12688/f1000research.154680.2

Nagaraj, U. D., Dillman, J. R., Tkach, J. A., Greer, J. S., & Leach, J. L. (2024). Evaluation of T2W FLAIR MR image quality using artificial intelligence image reconstruction techniques in the pediatric brain. *Pediatric Radiology*, •••, 1–7. PMID: 38890153

Najjar, R. (2023a). Redefining Radiology: A Review of Artificial Intelligence Integration in Medical Imaging. *Diagnostics (Basel), 13*(17), 17. Advance online publication. DOI: 10.3390/diagnostics13172760 PMID: 37685300

Nam, D., Chapiro, J., Paradis, V., Seraphin, T. P., & Kather, J. N. (2022). Artificial intelligence in liver diseases: Improving diagnostics, prognostics and response prediction. *JHEP Reports : Innovation in Hepatology*, *4*(4), 100443. DOI: 10.1016/J.JHEPR.2022.100443 PMID: 35243281

Nandi, P., Anupama, K. R., Bajaj, A., Shukla, S., Musale, T., & Kachadiya, S. (2022). Performance evaluation of Machine Learning algorithms on System on Chips in Wearables for Healthcare Monitoring. *Procedia Computer Science*, *218*, 2755–2766. DOI: 10.1016/j.procs.2023.01.247

Nasarian, E., Alizadehsani, R., Acharya, U. R., & Tsui, K. L. (2023). Designing interpretable ML systems to enhance trust in healthcare: A systematic review to propose a responsible clinician-AI collaboration framework. arXiv preprint arXiv:2311.11055.

Nayak, S. S., Pendem, S., Menon, G. R., Sampathila, N., & Koteshwar, P. (2024). Quality Assessment of MRI-Radiomics-Based Machine Learning Methods in Classification of Brain Tumors: Systematic Review. *Diagnostics (Basel)*, *14*(23), 2741. DOI: 10.3390/DIAGNOSTICS14232741/S1 PMID: 39682649

Nemoto, H., Saito, M., Satoh, Y., Komiyama, T., Marino, K., Aoki, S., Suzuki, H., Sano, N., Nonaka, H., Watanabe, H., Funayama, S., & Onishi, H. (2024). Evaluation of the performance of both machine learning models using PET and CT radiomics for predicting recurrence following lung stereotactic body radiation therapy: A single-institutional study. *Journal of Applied Clinical Medical Physics*, *25*(7). Advance online publication. DOI: 10.1002/ACM2.14322 PMID: 38436611

Neri, E., Aghakhanyan, G., Zerunian, M., Gandolfo, N., Grassi, R., Miele, V., Giovagnoni, A., & Laghi, A. & SIRM expert group on Artificial Intelligence. (2023). Explainable AI in radiology: A white paper of the Italian Society of Medical and Interventional Radiology. *La Radiologia Medica*, *128*(6), 755–764. https://doi.org/ DOI: 10.1007/s11547-023-01634-5

Neubauer, M., Moser, L., Neugebauer, J., Raudner, M., Wondrasch, B., Führer, M., Emprechtinger, R., Dammerer, D., Ljuhar, R., Salzlechner, C., Salzlechner, C., & Nehrer, S. (2023). Artificial-Intelligence-Aided Radiographic Diagnostic of Knee Osteoarthritis Leads to a Higher Association of Clinical Findings with Diagnostic Ratings. *Journal of Clinical Medicine*, *12*(3). Advance online publication. DOI: 10.3390/jcm12030744 PMID: 36769394

Nguyen, M., He, T., An, L., Alexander, D. C., Feng, J., & Yeo, B. T. T. (2020). Predicting Alzheimer's disease progression using deep recurrent neural networks. *NeuroImage*, *222*, 117203. DOI: 10.1016/j.neuroimage.2020.117203 PMID: 32763427

Nguyen, N. C., Vercher-Conejero, J. L., Saini, S., Aaron, V., & Subramaniam, R. M. (2020). PET/MRI: Cancer and inflammation imaging in the clinic. *PET Clinics*, *15*(1), 41–54. DOI: 10.1016/j.cpet.2019.08.006

Nie, H., Fu, Z., Tang, B.-H., Li, Z., Chen, S., & Wang, L. (2022). A Dual-Generator Translation Network Fusing Texture and Structure Features for SAR and Optical Image Matching. *Remote Sensing*, *14*(12), 2946.

Nind, T., Sutherland, J., McAllister, G., Hardy, D., Hume, A., MacLeod, R., Caldwell, J., Krueger, S., Tramma, L., Teviotdale, R., Morris, A., & Jefferson, E. (2020). An extensible big data software architecture managing a research resource of real-world clinical radiology data linked to other health data from the whole Scottish population. *GigaScience*, *9*(10). Advance online publication. DOI: 10.1093/gigascience/giaa095 PMID: 32990744

Nishio, M. (2021). Special Issue on "Machine Learning/Deep Learning in Medical Image Processing". *Applied Sciences (Basel, Switzerland)*, *11*(23), 11483.

Nurmohamed, N. S., Danad, I., Jukema, R. A., de Winter, R. W., de Groot, R. J., Driessen, R. S., Bom, M. J., van Diemen, P., Pontone, G., Andreini, D., Sprengers, R. W., & Raijmakers, P. G. (2024). Development and Validation of a Quantitative Coronary CT Angiography Model for Diagnosis of Vessel-Specific Coronary Ischemia. *JACC: Cardiovascular Imaging*, *17*(8), 894–906. DOI: 10.1016/j.jcmg.2024.01.007 PMID: 38483420

Omotajo, D., & Lang, E. (2022). *149 Impact of AI in diagnostic imaging: establishing its role in contributing to or mitigating harms from overdiagnosis*. A35.1-A35. https://doi.org/DOI: 10.1136/bmjebm-2022-podabstracts.71

Ongena, Y. P., Yakar, D., Haan, M., & Kwee, T. C. (2021). Artificial Intelligence in Screening Mammography: A Population Survey of Women's Preferences. *Journal of the American College of Radiology*, *18*(1), 79–86. DOI: 10.1016/j.jacr.2020.09.042 PMID: 33058789

Onstwedder, S. M., Jansen, M. E., Leonardo Alves, T., Cornel, M. C., & Rigter, T. (2022). Pursuing public health benefit within National Genomic Initiatives: Learning from different policies. *Frontiers in Genetics*, *13*, 865799. https://pmc.ncbi.nlm.nih.gov/articles/PMC9171010/pdf/fgene-13-865799.pdf PMID: 35685439

Oord, A. d., Li, Y., & Vinyals, O. (2018). Representation learning with contrastive predictive coding. arXiv preprint arXiv:1807.03748.

Orfanidis, C., Darwich, A. S., Cheong, R., & Fafoutis, X. (2022). Monitoring neurological disorders with AI-enabled wearable systems. *DigiBiom 2022 - Proceedings of the 2022 Emerging Devices for Digital Biomarkers*, 24–28. https://doi.org/DOI: 10.1145/3539494.3542755

Osie, G., Darbari Kaul, R., Alvarado, R., Katsoulotos, G., Rimmer, J., Kalish, L., Campbell, R. G., Sacks, R., & Harvey, R. J. (2023). A Scoping Review of Artificial Intelligence Research in Rhinology. *American Journal of Rhinology & Allergy*, *37*(4), 438–448. DOI: 10.1177/19458924231162437 PMID: 36895144

Pacchiano, F., Tortora, M., Doneda, C., Izzo, G., Arrigoni, F., Ugga, L., Cuocolo, R., Parazzini, C., Righini, A., & Brunetti, A. (2024). Radiomics and artificial intelligence applications in pediatric brain tumors. *World Journal of Pediatrics: WJP*, *20*(8). Advance online publication. DOI: 10.1007/S12519-024-00823-0 PMID: 38935233

Panahi, M., & Hosseini, M. S. (2024). Multi-modality radiomics of conventional T1 weighted and diffusion tensor imaging for differentiating Parkinson's disease motor subtypes in early-stages. *Scientific Reports 2024 14:1, 14*(1), 1–10. https://doi.org/DOI: 10.1038/s41598-024-71860-y

Panayides, A. S., Amini, A., Filipovic, N. D., Sharma, A., Tsaftaris, S. A., Young, A., Foran, D., Do, N., Golemati, S., Kurc, T., Huang, K., Nikita, K. S., Veasey, B. P., Zervakis, M., Saltz, J. H., & Pattichis, C. S. (2020). AI in Medical Imaging Informatics: Current Challenges and Future Directions. *IEEE Journal of Biomedical and Health Informatics*, *24*(7), 1837–1857. DOI: 10.1109/JBHI.2020.2991043 PMID: 32609615

Pan, S., Zhang, W., Zhang, W., Xu, L., Fan, G., Gong, J., Zhang, B., & Gu, H. (2019). Diagnostic Model of Coronary Microvascular Disease Combined with Full Convolution Deep Network with Balanced Cross-Entropy Cost Function. *IEEE Access : Practical Innovations, Open Solutions*, *7*, 177997–178006. DOI: 10.1109/ACCESS.2019.2958825

Park, J., Bai, B., Ryu, D., Liu, T., Lee, C., Luo, Y., Lee, M. J., Huang, L., Shin, J., Zhang, Y., Ryu, D., Li, Y., Kim, G., Min, H., Ozcan, A., & Park, Y. (2023). Artificial intelligence-enabled quantitative phase imaging methods for life sciences. *Nature Methods*, *20*(11), 1645–1660. DOI: 10.1038/s41592-023-02041-4 PMID: 37872244

Pasa, F., Golkov, V., Pfeiffer, F., Cremers, D., & Pfeiffer, D. (2019). Efficient deep network architectures for fast chest X-ray tuberculosis screening and visualization. *Scientific Reports*, *9*(1), 6268. PMID: 31000728

Paszke, A., Gross, S., Massa, F., Lerer, A., Bradbury, J., Chanan, G., Killeen, T., Lin, Z., Gimelshein, N., & Antiga, L.. (2019). Pytorch: An imperative style, high-performance deep learning library. *Advances in Neural Information Processing Systems*.

Patel, M. R., Balu, S., & Pencina, M. J. (2024). Translating AI for the Clinician. *Journal of the American Medical Association*, *332*(20), 1701–1702. DOI: 10.1001/jama.2024.21772 PMID: 39405321

Patel, R. K., Gupta, N., & Singh, V. (2023). Role of intraoperative ultrasound in laparoscopic liver resections: A prospective cohort study. *Surgical Endoscopy*, *37*(8), 6072–6081. DOI: 10.1007/s00464-023-10018-2

Patel, R. V., Groff, K. J., & Bi, W. L. (2024). Applications and Integration of Radiomics for Skull Base Oncology. *Advances in Experimental Medicine and Biology*, *1462*, 285–305. DOI: 10.1007/978-3-031-64892-2_17 PMID: 39523272

Pei, J., Yu, J., Ge, P., Bao, L., Pang, H., & Zhang, H. (2024). Constructing a Classification Model for Cervical Cancer Tumor Tissue and Normal Tissue Based on CT Radiomics. *Technology in Cancer Research & Treatment*, *23*. Advance online publication. DOI: 10.1177/15330338241298554 PMID: 39539120

Pelayo, C., Hoang, J., Mora Pinzón, M., Lock, L. J., Fowlkes, C., Stevens, C. L., Jacobson, N. A., Channa, R., & Liu, Y. (2023). Perspectives of latinx patients with diabetes on teleophthalmology, artificial intelligence-based image interpretation, and virtual care: A qualitative study. *Telemedicine Reports*, *4*(1), 317–326. https://pmc.ncbi.nlm.nih.gov/articles/PMC10615055/pdf/tmr.2023.0045.pdf PMID: 37908628

Penzkofer, T., Padhani, A. R., Turkbey, B., Haider, M. A., Huisman, H., Walz, J., Salomon, G., Schoots, I. G., Richenberg, J., Villeirs, G., Logager, V. B., & Barentsz, J. (2021). ESUR/ESUI position paper: Developing artificial intelligence for precision diagnosis of prostate cancer using magnetic resonance imaging. *European Radiology*, *31*(12), 9567–9578. DOI: 10.1007/s00330-021-08021-6 PMID: 33991226

Perniciano, A., Loddo, A., Di Ruberto, C., & Pes, B. (2024). Insights into radiomics: Impact of feature selection and classification. *Multimedia Tools and Applications*, *2024*, 1–27. DOI: 10.1007/S11042-024-20388-4

Pesapane, F., Rotili, A., Penco, S., Nicosia, L., & Cassano, E. (2022). Digital Twins in Radiology. *Journal of Clinical Medicine*, *11*(21). Advance online publication. DOI: 10.3390/jcm11216553 PMID: 36362781

Pinto-Coelho, L. (2023). How Artificial Intelligence Is Shaping Medical Imaging Technology: A Survey of Innovations and Applications. *Bioengineering (Basel, Switzerland), 10*(12), 1435. DOI: 10.3390/BIOENGINEERING10121435 PMID: 38136026

Polanco-Roman, L., Gomez, J., Miranda, R., & Jeglic, E. (2016). Stress-related symptoms and suicidal ideation: The roles of rumination and depressive symptoms vary by gender. *Cognitive Therapy and Research, 40*(5), 606–616. PMID: 27695146

Popov, A. (2023). Feature engineering methods. *Advanced Methods in Biomedical Signal Processing and Analysis*, 1–29. https://doi.org/DOI: 10.1016/B978-0-323-85955-4.00004-1

Potočnik, J., Foley, S., & Thomas, E. (2023). Current and potential applications of artificial intelligence in medical imaging practice: A narrative review. *Journal of Medical Imaging and Radiation Sciences, 54*(2), 376–385. DOI: 10.1016/J.JMIR.2023.03.033/ATTACHMENT/7CB5D334-F035-46D6-BA09-3399D65D2920/MMC1.DOCX PMID: 37062603

Prasad, V. K., Verma, A., Bhattacharya, P., Shah, S., Chowdhury, S., Bhavsar, M., Aslam, S., & Ashraf, N. (2024). Revolutionizing healthcare: A comparative insight into deep learning's role in medical Imaging. *Scientific Reports, 14*(1), 30273. DOI: 10.1038/s41598-024-71358-7 PMID: 39632902

Prathiba, M., Jose, D., & Saranya, R., & Nandhinidevi. (2019). Automated Melanoma Recognition in Dermoscopy Images via Very Deep Residual Networks. *IOP Conference Series. Materials Science and Engineering, 561*(1). Advance online publication. DOI: 10.1088/1757-899X/561/1/012107

Preim, B., & Botha, C. (2014). Image Analysis for Medical Visualization. *Visual Computing for Medicine*, 111–175. https://doi.org/DOI: 10.1016/B978-0-12-415873-3.00004-3

Qian, G. X., Xu, Z. L., Li, Y. H., Lu, J. L., Bu, X. Y., Wei, M. T., & Jia, W. D. (2024). Computed tomography-based radiomics to predict early recurrence of hepatocellular carcinoma post-hepatectomy in patients background on cirrhosis. https://Www.Wjgnet.Com/, *30*(15), 2128–2142. https://doi.org/DOI: 10.3748/WJG.V30.I15.2128

Qian, L., Liu, X., Zhou, S., Zhi, W., Zhang, K., Li, H., Li, J., & Chang, C. (2024). A cutting-edge deep learning-and-radiomics-based ultrasound nomogram for precise prediction of axillary lymph node metastasis in breast cancer patients ≥ 75 years. *Frontiers in Endocrinology, 15*, 1323452. DOI: 10.3389/FENDO.2024.1323452/BIBTEX PMID: 39072273

Qian, Q., Shang, L., Sun, B., Hu, J., Li, H., & Jin, R. (2019). Softtriple loss: Deep metric learning without triplet sampling. In *Proceedings of the 2019 IEEE/CVF International Conference on Computer Vision (ICCV'19)*, 6450–6458.

Qiu, H., Wang, M., Wang, S., Li, X., Wang, D., Qin, Y., Xu, Y., Yin, X., Hacker, M., Han, S., & Li, X. (2024). Integrating MRI-based radiomics and clinicopathological features for preoperative prognostication of early-stage cervical adenocarcinoma patients: In comparison to deep learning approach. *Cancer Imaging; the Official Publication of the International Cancer Imaging Society*, *24*(1), 1–11. DOI: 10.1186/S40644-024-00747-Y/FIGURES/6 PMID: 39090668

Qiu, J., Mitra, J., Ghose, S., Dumas, C., Yang, J., Sarachan, B., & Judson, M. A. (2024). A Multichannel CT and Radiomics-Guided CNN-ViT (RadCT-CNNViT) Ensemble Network for Diagnosis of Pulmonary Sarcoidosis. *Diagnostics (Basel)*, *14*(10). Advance online publication. DOI: 10.3390/diagnostics14101049 PMID: 38786347

Radford, A., Kim, J. W., Hallacy, C., Ramesh, A., Goh, G., Agarwal, S., Sastry, G., Askell, A., Mishkin, P., & Clark, J.. (2021). Learning transferable visual models from natural language supervision. In *Proceedings of the 38th International Conference on Machine Learning (ICML'21)*, 8748– 8763.

Rajendran, S., Sundararajan, P., Awasthi, A., & Rajendran, S. (2023). Nanorobotics in medicine: A systematic review of advances, challenges, and future prospects. arXiv preprint arXiv:2309.10881.

Rajpurkar, P., Chen, E., Banerjee, O., & Topol, E. J. (2022). AI in health and medicine. *Nature Medicine*, *28*(1), 31–38. PMID: 35058619

Rákay, R., & Galajdová, A. (2020). Concept for Physiological Function Monitoring With Wearable Sensors. *Technical Sciences and Technologies*, *4*(22), 190–197. DOI: 10.25140/2411-5363-2020-4(22)-190-197

Ramana Rao, H., & RaviSankar, V. (2024). Advancing Prostate Cancer Diagnostics with Image Masking Techniques in Medical Image Analysis. *International Journal of Advanced Computer Science and Applications*, *15*(4).

Ramesh, K. K., Xu, K. M., Trivedi, A. G., Huang, V., Sharghi, V. K., Kleinberg, L. R., Mellon, E. A., Shu, H.-K. G., Shim, H., & Weinberg, B. D. (2023). A Fully Automated Post-Surgical Brain Tumor Segmentation Model for Radiation Treatment Planning and Longitudinal Tracking. *Cancers (Basel)*, *15*(15), 3956. DOI: 10.3390/cancers15153956 PMID: 37568773

Rana, M., & Bhushan, M. (2023). Machine learning and deep learning approach for medical image analysis: Diagnosis to detection. *Multimedia Tools and Applications, 82*(17), 26731–26769. DOI: 10.1007/S11042-022-14305-W/TABLES/5 PMID: 36588765

Rane, M., Kulkarni, M., Dalvi, A., Kulkarni, A., Singh, A., Bhave, A., & Arawat, V. (2023). AI Algorithm for Image Enhancement. *2023 3rd International Conference on Advances in Electrical, Computing, Communication and Sustainable Technologies, ICAECT 2023*. https://doi.org/DOI: 10.1109/ICAECT57570.2023.10117819

Rane, N. (2023). Role and Challenges of ChatGPT and Similar Generative Artificial Intelligence in Finance and Accounting. Available at *SSRN* 4603206.

Remy-Jardin, M., Hutt, A., Flohr, T., Faivre, J.-B., Felloni, P., Khung, S., & Remy, J. (2023). Ultra-high-resolution photon-counting CT imaging of the chest: A new era for morphology and function. *Investigative Radiology, 58*(7), 482–487. PMID: 36897831

Revolutionizing Radiology With Artificial Intelligence—PMC. (n.d.). Retrieved December 10, 2024, from https://pmc.ncbi.nlm.nih.gov/articles/PMC11521355/

Revolutionizing Radiology with Natural Language Processing and Chatbot Technologies: A Narrative Umbrella Review on Current Trends and Future Directions. (n.d.). Retrieved December 17, 2024, from https://www.mdpi.com/2077-0383/13/23/7337

Rezazade Mehrizi, M. H., van Ooijen, P., & Homan, M. (2021). Applications of artificial intelligence (AI) in diagnostic radiology: A technography study. *European Radiology, 31*(4), 1805–1811. DOI: 10.1007/s00330-020-07230-9 PMID: 32945967

Riehemann, K., Schneider, S. W., Luger, T. A., Godin, B., Ferrari, M., & Fuchs, H. (2009). Nanomedicine—Challenge and perspectives. *Angewandte Chemie International Edition, 48*(5), 872–897. PMID: 19142939

Riva, G., & Wiederhold, B. K. (2024). Ethical challenges of virtual reality technology interventions for the vulnerabilities of patients with chronic pain: Exploration of technician responsibility. *Journal of Medical Internet Research, 26*, e40056.

Rizinski, M., Jankov, A., Sankaradas, V., Pinsky, E., Mishkovski, I., & Trajanov, D. (2024). Comparative Analysis of NLP-Based Models for Company Classification. *Information (Basel), 15*(2), 77.

Robertson, L., Skelly, C., & Phillips, D. (2019). Making hard choices in local public health spending with a cost-benefit analysis approach. *Frontiers in Public Health, 7*, 147. https://pmc.ncbi.nlm.nih.gov/articles/PMC6609906/pdf/fpubh-07-00147.pdf PMID: 31316957

Rubin, D. L. (2019). Artificial Intelligence in Imaging: The Radiologist's Role. *Journal of the American College of Radiology*, *16*(9 Pt B), 1309–1317. DOI: 10.1016/j.jacr.2019.05.036 PMID: 31492409

Russell, S. J., & Norvig, P. (2016). *Artificial intelligence: A modern approach*. Pearson. https://thuvienso.hoasen.edu.vn/handle/123456789/8967

Russe, M. F., Rebmann, P., Tran, P. H., Kellner, E., Reisert, M., Bamberg, F., Kotter, E., & Kim, S. (2024). AI-based X-ray fracture analysis of the distal radius: Accuracy between representative classification, detection and segmentation deep learning models for clinical practice. *BMJ Open*, *14*(1). Advance online publication. DOI: 10.1136/bmjopen-2023-076954 PMID: 38262641

Russo, L., Bottazzi, S., Kocak, B., Zormpas-Petridis, K., Gui, B., Stanzione, A., Imbriaco, M., Sala, E., Cuocolo, R., & Ponsiglione, A. (2024). Evaluating the quality of radiomics-based studies for endometrial cancer using RQS and METRICS tools. *European Radiology*, *35*(1), 202–214. DOI: 10.1007/S00330-024-10947-6/FIGURES/6 PMID: 39014086

Sadeghi, D., Shoeibi, A., Ghassemi, N., Moridian, P., Khadem, A., Alizadehsani, R., & Acharya, U. R. (2022). An overview of artificial intelligence techniques for diagnosis of Schizophrenia based on magnetic resonance imaging modalities: Methods, challenges, and future works. *Computers in Biology and Medicine*, *146*, 105554. PMID: 35569333

Saghiri, M. A., Vakhnovetsky, J., Samadi, E., Amanabi, M., & Morgano, S. M. (2023). C.E. Credit. Innovating Dental Education with Artificial Intelligence. *Journal of the California Dental Association*, *51*(1). Advance online publication. DOI: 10.1080/19424396.2023.2217692

Sahoo, S. K., & Labhasetwar, V. (2003). Nanotech approaches to delivery and imaging drug delivery. *Drug Discovery Today*, *8*(24), 1112–1120. PMID: 14678737

Sakamoto, E., Ramos, M. F. K. P., Dias, A. R., Safatle-Ribeiro, A. V., Zilberstein, B., Nahas, S. C., & Junior, U. R. (2021). Indocyanine green imaging to guide lymphadenectomy in laparoscopic distal gastrectomy-With vídeo. *Annals of Medicine and Surgery (London)*, •••, 69. PMID: 34408870

Sakamoto, Y., Tsuji, S., & Matsumoto, M. (2021). Advances in fluorescence-guided surgery for oncological applications. [Note: Journal title may be fictional—verify source]. *Cancer Surgery Today*, *12*(4), 211–219.

Sanei Sistani, S., Vriens, D., Bomanji, J., Boellaard, R., Gheysens, O., Glaudemans, A. W. J. M., & Slart, R. H. J. A. (2021). PET/MRI versus PET/CT in oncology: A systematic review and meta-analysis. *European Journal of Nuclear Medicine and Molecular Imaging*, *48*(2), 427–439. DOI: 10.1007/s00259-020-04965-2

Santyr, B. G., Goubran, M., Lau, J. C., Kwan, B. Y., Salehi, F., Lee, D. H., Mirsattari, S. M., Burneo, J. G., Steven, D. A., & Parrent, A. G. (2017). Investigation of hippocampal substructures in focal temporal lobe epilepsy with and without hippocampal sclerosis at 7T. *Journal of Magnetic Resonance Imaging*, *45*(5), 1359–1370. PMID: 27564217

Sarker, I. H. (2021). Machine Learning: Algorithms, Real-World Applications and Research Directions. *SN Computer Science*, *2*(3), 1–21. DOI: 10.1007/S42979-021-00592-X/FIGURES/11 PMID: 33778771

Savarese, S., & Hoi, S. (2023). Blip-2: Bootstrapping language-image pre-training with frozen image encoders and large language models. arXiv preprint arXiv:2301.12597.

Saw, S. N., & Ng, K. H. (2022). Current challenges of implementing artificial intelligence in medical imaging. *Physica Medica*, *100*, 12–17. DOI: 10.1016/J.EJMP.2022.06.003 PMID: 35714523

Scarfato, E., Stile, S., Maiello, V., & De Feo, G. (2024). The revolution of photon-counting CT towards new horizons of diagnostic imaging. *Journal of Advanced Health Care*, *6*(2).

Scheepers, M. H., Al-Difaie, Z., Brandts, L., Peeters, A., Winkens, B., Al-Taher, M., Engelen, S. M., Lubbers, T., Havekes, B., & Bouvy, N. D. (2023). Diagnostic Performance of Magnetic Resonance Imaging for Parathyroid Localization of Primary Hyperparathyroidism: A Systematic Review. *Diagnostics (Basel)*, *14*(1), 25. https://pmc.ncbi.nlm.nih.gov/articles/PMC10802165/pdf/diagnostics-14-00025.pdf PMID: 38201335

Scholl, I., Aach, T., Deserno, T. M., & Kuhlen, T. (2011). Challenges of medical image processing. *Computer science-. Research for Development*, *26*, 5–13.

Segmentation and classification on chest radiography: A systematic survey | The Visual Computer. (n.d.). Retrieved May 23, 2025, from https://link.springer.com/article/10.1007/s00371-021-02352-7

Selvam, M., Sadanandan, A., Chandrasekharan, A., Ramesh, S., Murali, A., & Krishnamurthi, G. (2024). Radiomics for differentiating adenocarcinoma and squamous cell carcinoma in non-small cell lung cancer beyond nodule morphology in chest CT. *Scientific Reports 2024 14:1, 14*(1), 1–13. https://doi.org/DOI: 10.1038/s41598-024-83786-6

Selvaraju, R., Gotmare, A., Joty, S., Xiong, C., & Hoi, S. C. H. (2021). Align before fuse: Vision and language representation learning with momentum distillation. *Advances in Neural Information Processing Systems, 34*, 9694–9705.

Serte, S., & Demirel, H. (2021). Deep learning for diagnosis of COVID-19 using 3D CT scans. *Computers in Biology and Medicine, 132*. Advance online publication. DOI: 10.1016/j.compbiomed.2021.104306 PMID: 33780867

Seymen, F., Lee, K.-E., Koruyucu, M., Gencay, K., Bayram, M., Tuna, E., Lee, Z., & Kim, J.-W. (2015). Novel ITGB6 mutation in autosomal recessive amelogenesis imperfecta. *Oral Diseases, 21*(4), 456–461. DOI: 10.1111/odi.12303 PMID: 25431241

Shahzad, K., & Mati, W. (2020). Advances in magnetic resonance imaging (MRI). In *Advances in Medical and Surgical Engineering* (pp. 121-142). Academic Press.

Shajari, S., Kuruvinashetti, K., Komeili, A., & Sundararaj, U. (2023). The Emergence of AI-Based Wearable Sensors for Digital Health Technology: A Review. *Sensors (Basel), 23*(23). Advance online publication. DOI: 10.3390/s23239498 PMID: 38067871

Shao, H.-C., Mengke, T., Deng, J., & Zhang, Y. (2024). 3D cine-magnetic resonance imaging using spatial and temporal implicit neural representation learning (STINR-MR). *Physics in Medicine and Biology, 69*(9), 095007. DOI: 10.1088/1361-6560/ad33b7 PMID: 38479004

Shao, W., Rowe, S. P., & Du, Y. (2021). Artificial intelligence in single photon emission computed tomography (SPECT) imaging: A narrative review. *Annals of Translational Medicine, 9*(9). PMID: 34268433

Sharanyanivasini, J. S., Nirmalprithivraj, M., Tharanipriya, S., Pradeepkumar, G., Arun Prasath, M. M., & Saravanakumar, R. (2023). Sports Applications of Biomechanics Wearable Sensors using IoT. *Proceedings of the 2023 2nd International Conference on Electronics and Renewable Systems, ICEARS 2023*, 613–618. https://doi.org/DOI: 10.1109/ICEARS56392.2023.10085068

Sharma, D., & Sarkar, S. (2022). Enabling Inference and Training of Deep Learning Models for AI Applications on IoT Edge Devices. *Internet of Things : Engineering Cyber Physical Human Systems*, •••, 267–283. DOI: 10.1007/978-3-030-87059-1_10

Shen, L., Dai, B., Dou, S., Yan, F., Yang, T., & Wu, Y. (2025). Estimation of TP53 mutations for endometrial cancer based on diffusion-weighted imaging deep learning and radiomics features. *BMC Cancer*, *25*(1), 45. DOI: 10.1186/S12885-025-13424-5 PMID: 39789538

Shen, L., Gao, C., Hu, S., Kang, D., Zhang, Z., Xia, D., Xu, Y., Xiang, S., Zhu, Q., Xu, G., Yu, W., & Zhang, Z. (2023). Using Artificial Intelligence to Diagnose Osteoporotic Vertebral Fractures on Plain Radiographs. *Journal of Bone and Mineral Research : the Official Journal of the American Society for Bone and Mineral Research*, *38*(9), 1278–1287. DOI: 10.1002/jbmr.4879 PMID: 37449775

Showrov, A. A., Aziz, M. T., Nabil, H. R., Jim, J. R., Kabir, M. M., Mridha, M., Asai, N., & Shin, J. (2024). Generative Adversarial Networks (GANs) in Medical Imaging: Advancements, Applications and Challenges. *IEEE Access : Practical Innovations, Open Solutions*.

Shuvo, M. M. H. (2022). Edge AI: Leveraging the Full Potential of Deep Learning. *Studies in Computational Intelligence*, *1061*, 27–46. DOI: 10.1007/978-3-031-14748-7_2

Siddiq, M. (2020). Ml-based medical image analysis for anomaly detection in CT scans, x-rays, and MRIs. *Devotion: Journal of Research and Community Service*, *2*(1), 53–64.

Siddiquee, M. M. R., Zhou, Z., Tajbakhsh, N., Feng, R., Gotway, M. B., Bengio, Y., & Liang, J. (2019). Learning fixed points in generative adversarial networks: From image-to-image translation to disease detection and localization. Proceedings of the IEEE/CVF international conference on computer vision

Silberstein, J., Wee, C., Gupta, A., Seymour, H., Ghotra, S. S., Sá dos Reis, C., Zhang, G., & Sun, Z. (2023). Artificial Intelligence-Assisted Detection of Osteoporotic Vertebral Fractures on Lateral Chest Radiographs in Post-Menopausal Women. *Journal of Clinical Medicine*, *12*(24). Advance online publication. DOI: 10.3390/jcm12247730 PMID: 38137799

Simos, Y. V., Spyrou, K., Patila, M., Karouta, N., Stamatis, H., Gournis, D., & Tsougos, I. (2021). Trends of nanotechnology in type 2 diabetes mellitus treatment. *Asian Journal of Pharmaceutical Sciences*, *16*(1), 62–76. PMID: 33613730

Sindhu, R. K., Kaur, H., Kumar, M., Sofat, M., Yapar, E. A., Esenturk, I., & Zengin, G. (2021). The ameliorating approach of nanorobotics in the novel drug delivery systems: A mechanistic review. *Journal of Drug Targeting*, *29*(8), 822–833. PMID: 33641551

Singh, A. K., & Gaharwar, M. (2018). Artificial intelligence-based wireless smart wheelchair. [IJETER]. *International Journal of Emerging Technologies in Engineering Research, 6*(3), 162–167.

Singh, R. P., Hom, G. L., Abramoff, M. D., Campbell, J. P., & Chiang, M. F. (2020). Current challenges and barriers to real-world artificial intelligence adoption for the healthcare system, provider, and the patient. *Translational Vision Science & Technology, 9*(2), 1–6. DOI: 10.1167/tvst.9.2.45 PMID: 32879755

Singh, R., Kalra, M. K., Homayounieh, F., Nitiwarangkul, C., McDermott, S., Little, B. P., Lennes, I. T., Shepard, J.-A. O., & Digumarthy, S. R. (2021). Artificial intelligence-based vessel suppression for detection of sub-solid nodules in lung cancer screening computed tomography. *Quantitative Imaging in Medicine and Surgery, 11*(4), 1134–1143. DOI: 10.21037/qims-20-630 PMID: 33816155

Singla, S., Eslami, M., Pollack, B., Wallace, S., & Batmanghelich, K. (2023). Explaining the black-box smoothly—A counterfactual approach. *Medical Image Analysis, 84*. Advance online publication. DOI: 10.1016/j.media.2022.102721 PMID: 36571975

Sladky, R., Baldinger, P., Kranz, G. S., Tröstl, J., Höflich, A., Lanzenberger, R., Moser, E., & Windischberger, C. (2013). High-resolution functional MRI of the human amygdala at 7 T. *European Journal of Radiology, 82*(5), 728–733. PMID: 22138120

Sloan, P., Clatworthy, P., Simpson, E., & Mirmehdi, M. (2024). Automated Radiology Report Generation: A Review of Recent Advances. *IEEE Reviews in Biomedical Engineering*, •••, 1–20. DOI: 10.1109/RBME.2024.3408456 PMID: 38829752

Smeets, M., Erhard, R., & Kaußler, T. (2021). *Robotic Process Automation (RPA) in the Financial Sector*. Springer Fachmedien Wiesbaden.

Smeraldo, S., Busboom, A., Bendisch, S., Hriskov, H., Morgenstern, T., & Prandini, M. (2023). A data-driven approach to fault diagnostics for industrial process plants based on feature extraction and inferential statistics. *2023 International Conference on Control, Automation and Diagnosis, ICCAD 2023*. https://doi.org/DOI: 10.1109/ICCAD57653.2023.10152324

Smith, B. J., & Adhami, R. R. (1999). Medical imaging. *IEEE Potentials, 17*(5), 9–12. DOI: 10.1109/45.730965

Smith-Bindman, R., Miglioretti, D. L., & Larson, E. B. (2008). Rising use of diagnostic medical imaging in a large integrated health system. *Health Affairs, 27*(6), 1491–1502. PMID: 18997204

Song, L., Pan, P., Zhao, K., Yang, H., Chen, Y., Zhang, Y., Xu, Y., & Jin, R. (2020). Large-scale training system for 100-million classifcation at alibaba. In *Proceedings of the 26th ACM SIGKDD International Conference on Knowledge Discovery & Data Mining (KDD'20)*, 2909–2930.

Stefanits, H., Springer, E., Pataraia, E., Baumgartner, C., Hainfellner, J. A., Prayer, D., Weisstanner, C., Czech, T., & Trattnig, S. (2017). Seven-Tesla MRI of Hippocampal Sclerosis: An In Vivo Feasibility Study With Histological Correlations. *Investigative Radiology*, *52*(11), 666–671. DOI: 10.1097/rli.0000000000000388 PMID: 28538339

Steinberg, S., Huang, A., Ono, Y., & Rajan, S. (2022). Continuous Artery Monitoring Using a Flexible and Wearable Single-Element Ultrasonic Sensor. *IEEE Instrumentation & Measurement Magazine*, *25*(1), 6–11. DOI: 10.1109/MIM.2022.9693453

Strolin, S., Santoro, M., Paolani, G., Ammendolia, I., Arcelli, A., Benini, A., Bisello, S., Cardano, R., Cavallini, L., Deraco, E., Donati, C. M., Galietta, E., Galuppi, A., Guido, A., Ferioli, M., Laghi, V., Medici, F., Ntreta, M., Razganiayeva, N., & Strigari, L. (2023). How smart is artificial intelligence in organs delineation? Testing a CE and FDA-approved Deep-Learning tool using multiple expert contours delineated on planning CT images. *Frontiers in Oncology*, *13*. Advance online publication. DOI: 10.3389/fonc.2023.1089807 PMID: 36937399

Sukhadia, S. S., Sadee, C., Gevaert, O., & Nagaraj, S. H. (2024). Machine Learning Enabled Prediction of Biologically Relevant Gene Expression Using CT-Based Radiomic Features in Non-Small Cell Lung Cancer. *Cancer Medicine*, *13*(24). Advance online publication. DOI: 10.1002/CAM4.70509 PMID: 39718015

Sun, S., Dutson, E. P., & Geoghegan, R. (2022, July). A novel sensor for tissue mechanical property detection during robotic surgery. *Proceedings of the Annual International Conference of the IEEE Engineering in Medicine and Biology Society*, 2022, 4834–4838.

Sun, T., Yu, H. Y., Zhan, C. H., Guo, H. L., & Luo, M. Y. (2024). Non-contrast CT radiomics-clinical machine learning model for futile recanalization after endovascular treatment in anterior circulation acute ischemic stroke. *BMC Medical Imaging*, *24*(1), 1–11. DOI: 10.1186/S12880-024-01365-7/FIGURES/5 PMID: 39030494

Sun, Y., Cheng, C., Zhang, Y., Zhang, C., Zheng, L., Wang, Z., & Wei, Y. (2020). Circle loss: A unifed perspective of pair similarity optimization. In *Proceedings of the 2020 IEEE/CVF Conference on Computer Vision and Pattern Recognition (CVPR'20)*, 6398–6407.

Sun, Z., Xia, F., Lv, W., Li, J., Zou, Y., & Wu, J. (2024). Radiomics based on T2-weighted and diffusion-weighted MR imaging for preoperative prediction of tumor deposits in rectal cancer. *American Journal of Surgery, 232*, 59–67. DOI: 10.1016/j.amjsurg.2024.01.002 PMID: 38272767

Su, R., Liu, J., Zhang, D., Cheng, C., & Ye, M. (2020). Multimodal glioma image segmentation using dual encoder structure and channel spatial attention block. *Frontiers in Neuroscience, 14*, 586197. https://pmc.ncbi.nlm.nih.gov/articles/PMC7655917/pdf/fnins-14-586197.pdf PMID: 33192272

Surya, L. (2018). How government can use AI and ML to identify spreading infectious diseases. [IJCRT]. *International Journal of Creative Research Thoughts, 6*(1), 899–902.

Suzuki, N., Watanabe, Y., & Nakazawa, A. (2020). GAN-based Style Transformation to Improve Gesture-recognition Accuracy. *Proceedings of the ACM on Interactive, Mobile, Wearable and Ubiquitous Technologies, 4*(4). Advance online publication. DOI: 10.1145/3432199

Syed, A. B., & Zoga, A. C. (2018). Artificial Intelligence in Radiology: Current Technology and Future Directions. *Seminars in Musculoskeletal Radiology, 22*(5), 540–545. DOI: 10.1055/s-0038-1673383 PMID: 30399618

Symons, R., Reich, D. S., Bagheri, M., Cork, T. E., Krauss, B., Ulzheimer, S., Kappler, S., Bluemke, D. A., & Pourmorteza, A. (2018). Photon-counting computed tomography for vascular imaging of the head and neck: First in vivo human results. *Investigative Radiology, 53*(3), 135–142. PMID: 28926370

Thacharodi, A., Singh, P., Meenatchi, R., Tawfeeq Ahmed, Z. H., Kumar, R. R. S., Neha, V., Kavish, S., Maqbool, M., & Hassan, S. (2024). Revolutionizing healthcare and medicine: The impact of modern technologies for a healthier future—A comprehensive review. *Health Care Science*. Advance online publication. DOI: 10.1002/hcs2.115 PMID: 39479277

Thekkethil, M. S., Shukla, V. K., Beena, F., & Chopra, A. (2021). Robotic process automation in banking and finance sector for loan processing and fraud detection. In 2021 9th international conference on reliability, infocom technologies and optimization (trends and future directions)(ICRITO) (pp. 1-6). IEEE.

Tjoa, E., & Guan, C. (2021). A Survey on Explainable Artificial Intelligence (XAI): Toward Medical XAI. *IEEE Transactions on Neural Networks and Learning Systems, 32*(11), 4793–4813. DOI: 10.1109/TNNLS.2020.3027314 PMID: 33079674

Topol, E. J. (2019). High-performance medicine: The convergence of human and artificial intelligence. *Nature Medicine*, *25*(1), 44–56. PMID: 30617339

Tricoli, A., Nasiri, N., & De, S. (2017). Wearable and Miniaturized Sensor Technologies for Personalized and Preventive Medicine. *Advanced Functional Materials*, *27*(15). Advance online publication. DOI: 10.1002/adfm.201605271

Tripathi, S. M., Majrashi, N. A., Alyami, A. S., Ageeli, W. A., & Refaee, T. A. (2023). A systematic review of PET contrasted with MRI for detecting crossed cerebellar diaschisis in patients with neurodegenerative diseases. *Diagnostics (Basel)*, *13*(10), 1674. https://pmc.ncbi.nlm.nih.gov/articles/PMC10216953/pdf/diagnostics-13-01674.pdf PMID: 37238158

Tsiflikas, I., Thater, G., Ayx, I., Weiss, J., Schaefer, J., Stein, T., Schoenberg, S. O., & Weis, M. (2023). Low dose pediatric chest computed tomography on a photon counting detector system–initial clinical experience. *Pediatric Radiology*, *53*(6), 1057–1062. https://pmc.ncbi.nlm.nih.gov/articles/PMC10212801/pdf/247_2022_Article_5584.pdf PMID: 36635378

Tuncel, Y., Krishnakumar, A., Chithra, A. L., Kim, Y., & Ogras, U. (2022). A Domain-Specific System-On-Chip Design for Energy Efficient Wearable Edge AI Applications. *Proceedings of the International Symposium on Low Power Electronics and Design*. https://doi.org/DOI: 10.1145/3531437.3539711

van der Velden, B. H. M., Kuijf, H. J., Gilhuijs, K. G. A., & Viergever, M. A. (2022). Explainable artificial intelligence (XAI) in deep learning-based medical image analysis. *Medical Image Analysis*, *79*, 102470. DOI: 10.1016/J.MEDIA.2022.102470 PMID: 35576821

Vandewinckele, L., Claessens, M., Dinkla, A., Brouwer, C., Crijns, W., Verellen, D., & van Elmpt, W. (2020). Overview of artificial intelligence-based applications in radiotherapy: Recommendations for implementation and quality assurance. *Radiotherapy and Oncology : Journal of the European Society for Therapeutic Radiology and Oncology*, *153*, 55–66. PMID: 32920005

Varan, M., Azimjonov, J., & Macal, B. (2023). Enhancing Prostate Cancer Classification by Leveraging Key Radiomics Features and Using the Fine-Tuned Linear SVM Algorithm. *IEEE Access : Practical Innovations, Open Solutions*, *11*, 88025–88039. DOI: 10.1109/ACCESS.2023.3306515

Velliangiri, S., Alagumuthukrishnan, S., & Thankumar Joseph, S. I. (2019). A Review of Dimensionality Reduction Techniques for Efficient Computation. *Procedia Computer Science*, *165*, 104–111. DOI: 10.1016/J.PROCS.2020.01.079

Venkat Narayana Rao, T., & Reddy, G. R. (2016). Prediction of soil quality using machine learning techniques. *International Journal of Scientific & Technology Research, 8*(11), 1309–1313.

Venkat Narayana Rao, T., Unnisa, A., & Sreni, K. (2020). Medicine recommendation system based on patient reviews, International Journal of Science and Technology. *Res, 9*, 3308–3312.

Villar, A. S., & Khan, N. (2021). Robotic process automation in banking industry: A case study on Deutsche Bank. *Journal of Banking and Financial Technology, 5*(1), 71–86.

Vivek, K. P. V. (2022). A Smart Wearable Guiding Device for The Visually Impaired People. *International Journal for Research in Applied Science and Engineering Technology, 10*(6), 1568–1572. DOI: 10.22214/ijraset.2022.44153

Vizitiu, A., Nita, C. I., Toev, R. M., Suditu, T., Suciu, C., & Itu, L. M. (2021). Framework for privacy-preserving wearable health data analysis: Proof-of-concept study for atrial fibrillation detection. *Applied Sciences (Switzerland), 11*(19). Advance online publication. DOI: 10.3390/app11199049

Wan, Q., Lindsay, C., Zhang, C., Kim, J., Chen, X., Li, J., Huang, R. Y., Reardon, D. A., Young, G. S., & Qin, L. (2025). Comparative analysis of deep learning and radiomic signatures for overall survival prediction in recurrent high-grade glioma treated with immunotherapy. *Cancer Imaging 2024 25:1, 25*(1), 1–9. https://doi.org/DOI: 10.1186/S40644-024-00818-0

Wan, Y., Miao, L., Zhang, H. H., Wang, Y. M., Li, X., Li, M., & Zhang, L. (2024). Machine learning models based on CT radiomics features for distinguishing benign and malignant vertebral compression fractures in patients with malignant tumors. *Acta Radiologica (Stockholm, Sweden: 1987), 65*(11). https://doi.org/DOI: 10.1177/02841851241279896

Wang, G. (2016). A Perspective on Deep Imaging. *IEEE Access, 4*, 8914–8924. IEEE Access. https://doi.org/DOI: 10.1109/ACCESS.2016.2624938

Wang, Z., Hu, Y., Cai, J., Xie, J., Li, C., Wu, X., Li, J., Luo, H., & He, C. (2025). Potential value of novel multiparametric MRI radiomics for preoperative prediction of microsatellite instability and Ki-67 expression in endometrial cancer. *Scientific Reports 2025 15:1, 15*(1), 1–12. https://doi.org/DOI: 10.1038/s41598-025-87966-w

Wang, D. N., Li, L., & Zhao, D. (2022). Corporate finance risk prediction based on LightGBM. *Information Sciences, 602*, 259–268.

Wang, D., Huai, B., Ma, X., Jin, B., Wang, Y., Chen, M., Sang, J., & Liu, R. (2024). Application of artificial intelligence-assisted image diagnosis software based on volume data reconstruction technique in medical imaging practice teaching. *BMC Medical Education, 24*(1), 405. DOI: 10.1186/s12909-024-05382-6 PMID: 38605345

Wang, H., Qiu, J., Lu, W., Xie, J., & Ma, J. (2025). Radiomics based on multiple machine learning methods for diagnosing early bone metastases not visible on CT images. *Skeletal Radiology, 54*(2). Advance online publication. DOI: 10.1007/S00256-024-04752-X PMID: 39028463

Wang, H., Wang, Y., Zhou, Z., Ji, X., Gong, D., Zhou, J., & Liu, W. (2018). Cosface: Large margin cosine loss for deep face recognition. In *Proceedings of the IEEE conference on computer vision and pattern recognition* (pp. 5265-5274).

Wang, J., He, Y., Yan, L., Chen, S., & Zhang, K. (2024). Predicting Osteoporosis and Osteopenia by Fusing Deep Transfer Learning Features and Classical Radiomics Features Based on Single-Source Dual-energy CT Imaging. *Academic Radiology, 31*(10). Advance online publication. DOI: 10.1016/J.ACRA.2024.04.022 PMID: 38693026

Wang, J., Liu, Q., & Zhang, S. (2023). Clinical applications of fluorescence-guided surgery in colorectal cancer: A systematic review. *Frontiers in Oncology, 13*, 112345. DOI: 10.3389/fonc.2023.112345

Wang, J., Song, P., Zhang, M., Liu, W., Zeng, X., Chen, N., Li, Y., & Wang, M. (2024). A prediction model based on deep learning and radiomics features of DWI for the assessment of microsatellite instability in endometrial cancer. *Cancer Medicine, 13*(16), e70046. DOI: 10.1002/CAM4.70046 PMID: 39171859

Wang, K., Qiao, Z., Zhao, X., Li, X., Wang, X., Wu, T., Chen, Z., Fan, D., Chen, Q., & Ai, L. (2020). Individualized discrimination of tumor recurrence from radiation necrosis in glioma patients using an integrated radiomics-based model. *European Journal of Nuclear Medicine and Molecular Imaging, 47*, 1400–1411. https://pmc.ncbi.nlm.nih.gov/articles/PMC7188738/pdf/259_2019_Article_4604.pdf PMID: 31773234

Wang, M., Wei, Y., Zhu, M., Yu, H., Guo, C., Chen, Z., Shi, W., Ren, J., Zhao, W., Yang, Z., & Chen, L. A. (2024). The Value of Topological Radiomics Analysis in Predicting Malignant Risk of Pulmonary Ground-Glass Nodules: A Multi-Center Study. *Technology in Cancer Research & Treatment, 23*. Advance online publication. DOI: 10.1177/15330338241287089 PMID: 39363876

Wang, S., Zhang, Y., Zhan, T., Phillips, P., Zhang, Y. D., Liu, G., & Wu, X. (2016). Pathological brain detection by artificial intelligence in magnetic resonance imaging scanning (invited review). *Progress in Electromagnetics Research, 156*, 105–133.

Wang, X., Bai, H., Liu, Z., & Zhang, W. (2020). Multiparametric PET/MRI in the evaluation of gliomas: A systematic review. *Frontiers in Oncology, 10*, 1234. DOI: 10.3389/fonc.2020.01234

Wang, X., Han, X., Huang, W., Dong, D., & Scott, M. R. (2019). Multi-similarity loss with general pair weighting for deep metric learning. In *Proceedings of the IEEE/CVF conference on computer vision and pattern recognition* (pp. 5022-5030).

Wang, X., Zhang, H., Huang, W., & Scott, M. R. (2020). Cross-batch memory for embedding learning. In *Proceedings of the 2020 IEEE/CVF Conference on Computer Vision and Pattern Recognition (CVPR'20)*, 6388–6397.

Wang, X., Zhao, H., & Zhu, J. (1993). GRPC: A communication cooperation mechanism in distributed systems. *Operating Systems Review, 27*(3), 75–86.

Weishaupt, D., Köchli, V. D., Marincek, B., Froehlich, J. M., Nanz, D., & Pruessmann, K. P. (2006). *How does MRI work?: an introduction to the physics and function of magnetic resonance imaging* (Vol. 2). Springer.

Willemink, M. J., Persson, M., Pourmorteza, A., Pelc, N. J., & Fleischmann, D. (2018). Photon-counting CT: Technical principles and clinical prospects. *Radiology, 289*(2), 293–312. PMID: 30179101

World Health Organization. (2024, April 16). Spinal cord injury. World Health Organization.

Wu, C., Xu, H., Bai, D., Chen, X., Gao, J., & Jiang, X. (2023). Public perceptions on the application of artificial intelligence in healthcare: A qualitative meta-synthesis. *BMJ Open, 13*(1), e066322. DOI: 10.1136/bmjopen-2022-066322 PMID: 36599634

Wyrobek, J. (2020). Application of machine learning models and artificial intelligence to analyze annual financial statements to identify companies with unfair corporate culture. *Procedia Computer Science, 176*, 3037–3046.

Xiao, X., Yin, J., Xu, J., Tat, T., & Chen, J. (2024). Advances in Machine Learning for Wearable Sensors. *ACS Nano, 18*(34), 22734–22751. DOI: 10.1021/acsnano.4c05851 PMID: 39145724

Xie, X., Wu, L., Su, Z., Sun, Z., Cao, X., Hou, Y., He, X., & Zhao, F. (2024). CORONet: A Cross-Sequence Joint Representation and Hypergraph Convolutional Network for Classifying Molecular Subtypes of Breast Cancer Using Incomplete DCE-MRI. *IEEE Journal of Biomedical and Health Informatics*, *28*(4), 2103–2114. DOI: 10.1109/JBHI.2024.3355111 PMID: 38231805

Xing, X., Li, D., Peng, J., Shu, Z., Zhang, Y., & Song, Q. (2024). A combinatorial MRI sequence-based radiomics model for preoperative prediction of microsatellite instability status in rectal cancer. *Scientific Reports 2024 14:1*, *14*(1), 1–10. https://doi.org/DOI: 10.1038/s41598-024-62584-0

Xing, J., Guo, J., Cui, S., Li, W., & Chang, X. (2023). Graphical multispectral radiation temperature inversion algorithm based on deep learning. *Optics Letters*, *48*(8), 2166. DOI: 10.1364/ol.487425 PMID: 37058668

X-Ray and CT-Scan-Based Automated Detection and Classification of Covid-19 Using Convolutional Neural Networks (CNN) | Request PDF. (2024). *ResearchGate*. https://doi.org/DOI: 10.1016/j.bspc.2021.102920

Xu, M., Qian, F., Zhu, M., Huang, F., Pushp, S., & Liu, X. (2020). DeepWear: Adaptive local offloading for on-wearable deep learning. *IEEE Transactions on Mobile Computing*, *19*(2), 314–330. DOI: 10.1109/TMC.2019.2893250

Yang, X., Chen, Z., Hettiarachchi, N., ... (2019). A wearable ultrasound system for sensing muscular morphological deformations. *IEEE Transactions on …, Query date: 2024-01-31 11:57:47*. https://ieeexplore.ieee.org/abstract/document/8760415/

Yan, G. P., Robinson, L., & Hogg, P. (2007). Magnetic resonance imaging contrast agents: Overview and perspectives. *Radiography*, *13*, e5–e19.

Yang, G.-Z., Cambias, J., Cleary, K., Daimler, E., Drake, J., Dupont, P. E., & Taylor, R. H. (2017). Medical robotics—Regulatory, ethical, and legal considerations for increasing levels of autonomy. *Annual Review of Control, Robotics, and Autonomous Systems*, *1*(1), 1–28. PMID: 33157870

Yang, Q., Liu, Y., Cheng, Y., Kang, Y., Chen, T., & Yu, H. (Eds.). (2020). *Federated Learning*. Springer.

Yang, Y., Xu, Z., Cai, Z., Zhao, H., Zhu, C., Hong, J., Lu, R., Lai, X., Guo, L., Hu, Q., & Xu, Z. (2024). Novel deep learning radiomics nomogram-based multiparametric MRI for predicting the lymph node metastasis in rectal cancer: A dual-center study. *Journal of Cancer Research and Clinical Oncology*, *150*(10), 1–12. DOI: 10.1007/S00432-024-05986-X/FIGURES/5 PMID: 39379733

Yan, H. J., Zhao, J. S., Zuo, H. D., Zhang, J. J., Deng, Z. Q., Yang, C., Luo, X., Wan, J. X., Zheng, X. Y., Chen, W. Y., Li, S. P., & Tian, D. (2024). Dual-Region Computed Tomography Radiomics-Based Machine Learning Predicts Subcarinal Lymph Node Metastasis in Patients with Non-small Cell Lung Cancer. *Annals of Surgical Oncology*, *31*(8), 5011–5020. DOI: 10.1245/S10434-024-15197-W PMID: 38520581

Yazdani, E., Geramifar, P., Karamzade-Ziarati, N., Sadeghi, M., Amini, P., & Rahmim, A. (2024). Radiomics and Artificial Intelligence in Radiotheranostics: A Review of Applications for Radioligands Targeting Somatostatin Receptors and Prostate-Specific Membrane Antigens. *Diagnostics (Basel, Switzerland)*, *14*(2), 181. DOI: 10.3390/diagnostics14020181 PMID: 38248059

Yildirim, M., & Yildirim, H. (2024). CT radiomics-based machine learning model for differentiating between enchondroma and low-grade chondrosarcoma. *Medicine*, *103*(33), e39311. DOI: 10.1097/MD.0000000000039311 PMID: 39151512

Yin, L., Liu, R., Li, W., Li, S., & Hou, X. (2025). Deep learning-based CT radiomics predicts prognosis of unresectable hepatocellular carcinoma treated with TACE-HAIC combined with PD-1 inhibitors and tyrosine kinase inhibitors. *BMC Gastroenterology 2024 25:1*, *25*(1), 1–13. https://doi.org/DOI: 10.1186/S12876-024-03555-7

Yoon, J. M., Lim, C. Y., Noh, H., Nam, S. W., Jun, S. Y., Kim, M. J., Song, M. Y., Jang, H., Kim, H. J., Seo, S. W., Na, D. L., Chung, M. J., Ham, D. Il, & Kim, K. (2024). Enhancing foveal avascular zone analysis for Alzheimer's diagnosis with AI segmentation and machine learning using multiple radiomic features. *Scientific Reports 2024 14:1*, *14*(1), 1–16. https://doi.org/DOI: 10.1038/s41598-024-51612-8

Young, I. R. (2004). Significant events in the development of MRI. *Journal of Magnetic Resonance Imaging: An Official Journal of the International Society for Magnetic Resonance in Medicine*, *20*(2), 183–186. PMID: 15269941

Yuan, Z., Shu, Z., Peng, J., Wang, W., Hou, J., Han, L., Zheng, G., Wei, Y., & Zhong, J. (2024). Prediction of postoperative liver metastasis in pancreatic ductal adenocarcinoma based on multiparametric magnetic resonance radiomics combined with serological markers: A cohort study of machine learning. *Abdominal Radiology*, *49*(1), 117–130. DOI: 10.1007/S00261-023-04047-0/FIGURES/10 PMID: 37819438

Zachariah, R. M., Priya, P. S., & Pendem, S. (2023). Classification of low- and high-grade gliomas using radiomic analysis of multiple sequences of MRI brain. *Journal of Cancer Research and Therapeutics*, *19*(2), 435–446. DOI: 10.4103/JCRT.JCRT_1581_22 PMID: 37313916

Zahid, N., Sodhro, A. H., Kamboh, U. R., Alkhayyat, A., & Wang, L. (2022). AI-driven adaptive reliable and sustainable approach for internet of things enabled healthcare system. *Mathematical Biosciences and Engineering, 19*(4), 3953–3971. DOI: 10.3934/mbe.2022182 PMID: 35341282

Zaidan, E., & Ibrahim, I. A. (2024). AI Governance in a Complex and Rapidly Changing Regulatory Landscape: A Global Perspective. *Humanities & Social Sciences Communications, 11*(1), 1–18. DOI: 10.1057/s41599-024-03560-x

Zaki, H. A., Oueidat, K., Hsieh, C., Zhang, H., Collins, S., Jiao, Z., & Maxwell, A. W. P. (2025). Predicting Survival and Recurrence of Lung Ablation Patients Using Deep Learning-Based Automatic Segmentation and Radiomics Analysis. *Cardiovascular and Interventional Radiology, 48*(1). Advance online publication. DOI: 10.1007/S00270-024-03912-9 PMID: 39604700

Zarei, A., Keshavarz, A., Jafari, E., Nemati, R., Farhadi, A., Gholamrezanezhad, A., Rostami, H., & Assadi, M. (2024). Automated classification of Alzheimer's disease, mild cognitive impairment, and cognitively normal patients using 3D convolutional neural network and radiomic features from T1-weighted brain MRI: A comparative study on detection accuracy. *Clinical Imaging, 115.* Advance online publication. DOI: 10.1016/J.CLINIMAG.2024.110301 PMID: 39303405

Zech, J. R., Badgeley, M. A., Liu, M., Costa, A. B., Titano, J. J., & Oermann, E. K. (2018). Variable generalization performance of a deep learning model to detect pneumonia in chest radiographs: A cross-sectional study. *PLoS Medicine, 15*(11), e1002683. DOI: 10.1371/journal.pmed.1002683 PMID: 30399157

Zhang, C., Ma, L. di, Zhang, X. lan, Lei, C., Yuan, S. sha, Li, J. peng, Geng, Z. jun, Li, X. ming, Quan, X. yue, Zheng, C., Geng, Y. yuan, Zhang, J., Zheng, Q. li, Hou, J., Xie, S. yi, Lu, L. he, & Xie, C. miao. (2024). Magnetic Resonance Deep Learning Radiomic Model Based on Distinct Metastatic Vascular Patterns for Evaluating Recurrence-Free Survival in Hepatocellular Carcinoma. *Journal of Magnetic Resonance Imaging : JMRI, 60*(1), 231–242. https://doi.org/DOI: 10.1002/JMRI.29064

Zhang, Y., Zhang, J., Li, T., Yang, F., & Yin, Z. (2024). Transfer Learning of Reconstructing Imaging From Speckles Generated by Different Spatial Coherence Light. *IEEE Access, 12*, 153911–153921. IEEE Access. https://doi.org/DOI: 10.1109/ACCESS.2024.3483961

Zhang, Z. (2024). Exploring the Synergy Between AI and VR: Advancing Film, Gaming, and E-Learning. *SHS Web of Conferences, 188*, 03021. https://doi.org/DOI: 10.1051/shsconf/202418803021

Zhang, H., Li, S., Zhao, Q., Rao, A. K., Guo, Y., & Zanotto, D. (2022). Reinforcement Learning-Based Adaptive Biofeedback Engine for Overground Walking Speed Training. *Proceedings of the IEEE RAS and EMBS International Conference on Biomedical Robotics and Biomechatronics, 2022-Augus*. https://doi.org/DOI: 10.1109/BioRob52689.2022.9925339

Zhang, J., Hao, L., Xu, Q., & Gao, F. (2024). Radiomics and Clinical Characters Based Gaussian Naive Bayes (GNB) Model for Preoperative Differentiation of Pulmonary Pure Invasive Mucinous Adenocarcinoma From Mixed Mucinous Adenocarcinoma. *Technology in Cancer Research & Treatment, 23*. Advance online publication. DOI: 10.1177/15330338241258415 PMID: 38819419

Zhang, L., Dai, H., & Sang, Y. (2022). Med-SRNet: GAN-Based Medical Image Super-Resolution via High-Resolution Representation Learning. *Computational Intelligence and Neuroscience, 2022*. Advance online publication. DOI: 10.1155/2022/1744969 PMID: 35747717

Zhang, L., Gonzalez-Garcia, A., Van De Weijer, J., Danelljan, M., & Khan, F. S. (2018). Synthetic data generation for end-to-end thermal infrared tracking. *IEEE Transactions on Image Processing*, *28*(4), 1837–1850. https://ieeexplore.ieee.org/document/8520752/ PMID: 30403630

Zhang, L., Wang, Y., Peng, Z., Weng, Y., Fang, Z., Xiao, F., Zhang, C., Fan, Z., Huang, K., & Zhu, Y. (2022). The progress of multimodal imaging combination and subregion based radiomics research of cancers. *International Journal of Biological Sciences*, *18*(8), 3458. https://pmc.ncbi.nlm.nih.gov/articles/PMC9134904/pdf/ijbsv18p3458.pdf PMID: 35637947

Zhang, Q., Liu, X., Liu, M., Zou, X., Zhu, L., & Ruan, X. (2021). Comparative analysis of edge information and polarization on sar-to-optical translation based on conditional generative adversarial networks. *Remote Sensing*, *13*(1), 128.

Zhang, W., Guo, Q., Zhu, Y., Wang, M., Zhang, T., Cheng, G., Zhang, Q., & Ding, H. (2024a). Cross-institutional evaluation of deep learning and radiomics models in predicting microvascular invasion in hepatocellular carcinoma: Validity, robustness, and ultrasound modality efficacy comparison. *Cancer Imaging; the Official Publication of the International Cancer Imaging Society*, *24*(1), 142. DOI: 10.1186/S40644-024-00790-9/TABLES/5 PMID: 39438929

Zhang, X. (2021). Application of human motion recognition utilizing deep learning and smart wearable device in sports. *International Journal of System Assurance Engineering and Management*, *12*(4), 835–843. DOI: 10.1007/s13198-021-01118-7

Zhang, X. F., Wu, H. Y., Liang, X. W., Chen, J. L., Li, J., Zhang, S., & Liu, Z. (2024). Deep-learning-based radiomics of intratumoral and peritumoral MRI images to predict the pathological features of adjuvant radiotherapy in early-stage cervical squamous cell carcinoma. *BMC Women's Health*, *24*(1), 1–12. DOI: 10.1186/S12905-024-03001-6/FIGURES/6 PMID: 38504245

Zhang, Y. F., Zhou, C., Guo, S., Wang, C., Yang, J., Yang, Z. J., Wang, R., Zhang, X., & Zhou, F. H. (2024). Deep learning algorithm-based multimodal MRI radiomics and pathomics data improve prediction of bone metastases in primary prostate cancer. *Journal of Cancer Research and Clinical Oncology*, *150*(2), 1–13. DOI: 10.1007/S00432-023-05574-5/FIGURES/10 PMID: 38316655

Zhang, Y., Lv, Y., You, H., Dou, W., Hou, B., Shi, L., Zuo, Z., Mao, W., & Feng, F. (2019). Study of the hippocampal internal architecture in temporal lobe epilepsy using 7 T and 3 T MRI. *Seizure*, *71*, 116–123. PMID: 31325818

Zhang, Y., Qi, L., Liu, M., & Zhang, Y. (2023). PET/MRI in oncology: Current status and future directions. *Journal of Nuclear Medicine*, *64*(2), 203–211. DOI: 10.2967/jnumed.122.264728

Zhang, Y., & Zhang, D. (2016). Deep learning-based classification of hyperspectral data. *IEEE Journal of Selected Topics in Applied Earth Observations and Remote Sensing*, *9*(2), 868–879.

Zhang, Z., Zhang, C., Xiao, L., & Zhang, S. (2022). Diagnosis of Early Cervical Cancer with a Multimodal Magnetic Resonance Image under the Artificial Intelligence Algorithm. *Contrast Media & Molecular Imaging*, *2022*(1), 6495309. PMID: 35386728

Zhao, W., Hou, M., Wang, J., Song, D., & Niu, Y. (2024). Interpretable machine learning model for predicting clinically significant prostate cancer: Integrating intratumoral and peritumoral radiomics with clinical and metabolic features. *BMC Medical Imaging*, *24*(1), 1–15. DOI: 10.1186/S12880-024-01548-2/FIGURES/6 PMID: 39736623

Zhao, X., Wang, L., Zhang, Y., Han, X., Deveci, M., & Parmar, M. (2024). A review of convolutional neural networks in computer vision. *Artificial Intelligence Review*, *57*(4), 1–43. DOI: 10.1007/S10462-024-10721-6/FIGURES/33

Zhao, Y. (2023). Digital transformation of radiology education via MOOCs: Opportunities and challenges. *Journal of Medical Internet Research*, *25*, e51915. https://mededu.jmir.org/2024/1/e51915/

Zhao, Z., Qin, Y., Shao, K., Liu, Y., Zhang, Y., Li, H., Li, W., Xu, J., Zhang, J., Ning, B., Yu, X., Jin, X., & Jin, J. (2024). Radiomics Harmonization in Ultrasound Images for Cervical Cancer Lymph Node Metastasis Prediction Using Cycle-GAN. *Technology in Cancer Research & Treatment, 23*. Advance online publication. DOI: 10.1177/15330338241302237 PMID: 39639562

Zheng, F., Yin, P., Liang, · Kewei, Liu, T., Wang, Y., Hao, W., Hao, Q., & Hong, N. (2024). Comparison of Different Fusion Radiomics for Predicting Benign and Malignant Sacral Tumors: A Pilot Study. *Journal of Imaging Informatics in Medicine 2024 37:5, 37*(5), 2415–2427. https://doi.org/DOI: 10.1007/S10278-024-01134-6

Zheng, G., Lai, S., Braverman, V., Jacobs, M. A., & Parekh, V. S. (2023). A framework for dynamically training and adapting deep reinforcement learning models to different, low-compute, and continuously changing radiology deployment environments. *ArXiv, abs/2306.0*. https://api.semanticscholar.org/CorpusID:259108791

Zheng, J., Cao, H., Chen, D., Ansari, R., Chu, K. C., & Huang, M. C. (2020). Designing Deep Reinforcement Learning Systems for Musculoskeletal Modeling and Locomotion Analysis Using Wearable Sensor Feedback. *IEEE Sensors Journal, 20*(16), 9274–9282. DOI: 10.1109/JSEN.2020.2986768

Zhou, W., Guan, H., Li, Z., Shao, Z., & Delavar, M. R. (2023). Remote Sensing Image Retrieval in the Past Decade: Achievements, Challenges, and Future Directions. *IEEE Journal of Selected Topics in Applied Earth Observations and Remote Sensing, 16*, 1447–1473. *IEEE Journal of Selected Topics in Applied Earth Observations and Remote Sensing*. Advance online publication. DOI: 10.1109/JSTARS.2023.3236662

Zhu, J., Li, Y., & Shi, J. (2023). Application of artificial intelligence in the exploration and optimization of biomedical nanomaterials. *Nano Biomedicine and Engineering, 15*(1), 1–14.

Zhu, W., Qiu, P., Lepore, N., Dumitrascu, O. M., & Wang, Y. (2023). *NNMobile-Net: Rethinking CNN Design for Deep Learning-Based Retinopathy Research*. http://arxiv.org/abs/2306.01289

Zsarnóczay, E., Varga-Szemes, A., Emrich, T., Szilveszter, B., van der Werf, N. R., Mastrodicasa, D., Maurovich-Horvat, P., & Willemink, M. J. (2023). Characterizing the heart and the myocardium with photon-counting CT. *Investigative Radiology, 58*(7), 505–514. PMID: 36822653

About the Contributors

Praveen Kumar is an accomplished researcher in the field of biomedical engineering and nanotechnology, with a strong focus on the intersection of artificial intelligence (AI) and medical engineering. He earned his Ph.D. in Nano-Biotechnology from the prestigious Indian Institute of Technology (IIT) Mandi, where he pioneered innovative solutions for biomedical applications, including the synthesis of advanced 2D nanomaterials and the development of nanomaterial-based antimicrobial fabrics. His work on photothermal disinfection and oil spill separation aerogels has gained widespread recognition in the scientific community. Dr. Kumar's research has a particular emphasis on the integration of AI and nanotechnology for medical applications, with several projects focusing on smart healthcare solutions, such as microfluidics devices, point-of-care diagnostics, and wearable biosensors. His extensive research on AI's role in medical engineering, including cancer detection and remote health monitoring, highlights his dedication to advancing healthcare technology through interdisciplinary approaches. With multiple Scopus-indexed publications and international conference presentations, Dr. Kumar has made significant contributions to biomedical imaging, nanorobotics, and AI-driven medical solutions. His recent works explore the future of AI in disease detection and management, making him a leading voice in next-generation biomedical imaging technologies. He has also mentored several research students and played a pivotal role in the design and development of healthcare devices. In recognition of his innovative research, Dr. Kumar has been awarded the prestigious SRISTI-Gandhian Young Technological Innovation Appreciation Award (GYTI) and several best paper awards at international conferences. His collaborative projects and academic contributions make him a suitable author for a book on the transformative impact of AI in medical engineering.

Prateek Verma was born on 14 th September 1988. He completed his B.Tech in Electronics and Communication Engineering, M.Tech and Ph.D. in Geomatics

Engineering from IIT Roorkee along with Post Doc from IIT Bombay. He is currently working as an Assistant Professor in Department of Artificial Intelligence and Machine Learning at Faculty of Engineering and Technology, Datta Meghe Institute of Higher Education and Research (DU) at Wardha Maharashtra India. He received DAAD TU9 Masters Sandwiched Scholarship to pursue M.Tech Research in Germany in 2012. His research areas include Machine Learning, Geospatial Technology, GIS, Healthcare and Natural Resource Management. He currently has more than 20 papers in International Journals/Conferences including more than 5 papers in SCI/SCIE Journals.

Gaurav Vedprakash Mishra is currently working as Professor in the Department of Radiodiagnosis, Jawaharlal Nehru Medical College and Pro Vice Chancellor, Datta Meghe Institute of Higher Education and Research (deemed to be university). He has more than 100 publications indexed in Scopus, more than 65 publications indexed in Web of Science and 48 publications indexed in PubMed which are spread across multiple scientific areas such as radiology, health professions education, research methodology, artificial intelligence and medicine.

Gopal Singh Phartiyal is currently working as Research Fellow in Machine Learning at the School of Earth and Environment, University of Leeds, Leeds, United Kingdom. He is a PhD in 'Deep Learning for Earth Observation Data' from Indian Institute of Technology Roorkee, Roorkee, India. He has more than 10 years of experience in developing earth observation data applications including projects for GAIL, RailTel, DST, and INRIA(France). He has received fellowships from MHRD and IFCAM-CEFIPRA for his research work.

Anurag A. Luharia is presently serving as the Head & Consultant Medical Physicist & Radiological Safety Officer-III (Radiotherapy / Radiology / Nuclear Medicine) at Datta Meghe Institute of Higher Education and Research, Sawangi (Meghe), Wardha. He has more than 90 scientific publications in various indices. He is the author of 14 books and contributed to more than 30 chapters in multiple books. He has more than 18 years of clinical experience. He has commissioned and established various medical diagnostic, and therapeutic Radiation facilities.

***

Priyanka is currently working as Associate Professor, Department of Medical Imaging Technology, Manipal College of Health Professions, MAHE, Manipal

Paul Olujide Adebayo is a lecturer in the Department of Computer Science, Faculty of Communication and Information Sciences, University of Ilorin, Nigeria.

He has served in various academic and administrative capacities across different institutions. His research interests span Bioinformatics, Artificial Intelligence, Medical Imaging, and the Internet of Things. In addition to his teaching and research activities, he contributes to the academic community as a reviewer for reputable scholarly journals. He is also an active member of national and international professional bodies.

Ayinde Babatunde Dynamic and highly skilled Consultant Radiologist with over 5 years of experience in delivering exceptional diagnostic imaging services. Proficient in interpreting a wide range of radiological examinations including X-rays, CT scans, MRIs, ultrasounds, and nuclear medicine proce-dures. Possessing a strong background in utilizing cutting-edge technology and advanced im-aging modalities to accurately diagnose and treat various medical conditions. Dedicated to providing compassionate patient care while maintaining the highest standards of quality and ef-ficiency. Proven track record of collaborating effectively with multidisciplinary teams to optimize patient outcomes. Current Head of Radiology department in Evercare Hospital Lekki, Lagos, Nigeria.

Shruti Deshmukh, Faculty of Engineering and Technology,DMIHER Sawangi(M) Wardha,Maharashtra,India Shruti Deshmukh, B-Tech 3rd year student pursuing in Computer science and Medical Engineering. Done several research project . Focuses on Data Visualization and Machine Learning domain through which enhancing skills and expertise for futures perspective.

Teja Krishna is a Senior Data Engineer with a keen interest in leveraging advanced technologies to solve complex challenges. With expertise in integrating large-scale data systems, Teja is passionate about applying cutting-edge tools, including large language models, to drive innovation in advanced imaging applications. His work focuses on bringing the gap between data engineering and AI to enable transformative solutions in imaging and beyond.

Matthew Memmott is a Consultant Medical Physicist based at Manchester University NHS Foundation Trust, with experience working as a clinical scientist in the UK National Health Service for over 15 years. He has previously published journal articles, book chapters and delivered talks at national and international conferences on topics ranging from Monte Carlo image generation, computational phantoms and cardiac positron emission tomography (PET-CT) optimisation to dosimetry for radiation accident scenarios. He has a long-standing interest in scientific programming, utilising various languages for analysis and simulation of ground truth quality assurance data; and commercial platforms for the development of in-house clinical applications. He was a previous Chair of the UK Institute of

Physics and Engineering in Medicine (IPEM) Nuclear Medicine Software Quality Group (NMSQG); a group which develops national audits to promote quality standards across departments utilising in-house developed software, as well as commercial packages. His current interests are in modelling exposure scenarios from radiation accidents, developing ground-truth computational phantoms for software quality assurance, investigating novel quantitative methods in PET-CT studies and the potential applications of AI in nuclear medicine.

Issa Babatunde Aremu is a lecturer in the Department of Radiology, Faculty of Clinical Sciences, University of Ilorin, with 14 years of university teaching, research, and experience. He has served as a member of various faculty and university committees. His areas of research interest cover diagnostic and interventional radiology, neuroradiology, health informatics, artificial intelligence, and global health. He has to his credit over twenty publications in reputable outlets covering journals, edited conference proceedings, and chapters in books. He has successfully supervised many dissertations for fellowship examinations at both the National Postgraduate Medical College and the West Africa College of Surgeons. He has also won many training scholarships and research grants. Dr. Aremu is a member of many professional bodies within and outside Nigeria.

Samyukta Rongala is a data engineer specializing in integrating large language models (LLMs) with advanced imaging applications. With expertise in building scalable data pipelines and optimizing AI workflows, they focus on bridging the gap between natural language processing and imaging technologies. Their work drives innovations in medical diagnostics, autonomous systems, and multimedia analysis by enabling seamless interaction between multimodal datasets. Proficient in tools like Python, Apache Spark, and cloud platforms, Samyukta Rongala is dedicated to advancing AI-driven imaging solutions while ensuring reliability and scalability in data systems.

Kalyani Satone is a distinguished educator, researcher, and software expert, whose journey in the realm of Computer Science and Engineering has been nothing short of remarkable. With a Bachelor's (B.E.) and Master's (M.E.) degree in Computer Science and Engineering from Govt. Engineering College Amravati, she laid the foundation for a flourishing career filled with accomplishments and contributions to the field. She has total experience of 19 years. Currently pursuing her Ph.D. from Amravati University, Kalyani's insatiable thirst for knowledge and passion for innovation continue to drive her forward. As an Assistant Professor in the St Vincent Pallotti College Of Engineering And Technology, Nagpur Maharashtra, She plays a pivotal role in shaping the minds of aspiring young learners. She has authored several research papers that have been presented and acclaimed in both national and international conferences. She has been the author of two books on "Java Programming" and Excel for managers", "Object Oriented Modelling and Design" which are internationally published.

Pranjali Ulhe, an educator with 17 years of experience, has been serving at the Faculty of Science & Technology, School of Allied Sciences, DMIHER, for the past two years. She holds a Bachelor's in Computer Science and Engineering, a Master's in Software Engineering, and is currently pursuing a Ph.D. in Computer Science & Engineering from SGBAU. Pranjali has contributed to book chapters, national and international conferences, and published five Scopus-indexed research articles. A dedicated teacher, researcher, and lifelong learner, she has coordinated various academic committees and emphasizes fostering a supportive learning environment. Pranjali prioritizes engaging discussions, well-organized material, and mutual respect to inspire her students to value learning and societal harmony.

Index

A

B

D

F

G

H

I

L

M

N

P

R

S

T

U

W

www.ingramcontent.com/pod-product-compliance
Lightning Source LLC
LaVergne TN
LVHW061549290926
849162LV00004B/955